Quantitative Methods for Health Research

A Practical Interactive Guide to Epidemiology and Statistics

Nigel Bruce, Daniel Pope and Debbi Stanistreet

Division of Public Health, University of Liverpool, UK

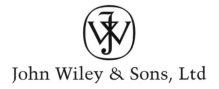

John Wiley & Sons, Ltd

Other Wiley Editorial Offices

John Wiley & Sons Inc., 111 River Street, Hoboken, NJ 07030, USA

Jossey-Bass, 989 Market Street, San Francisco, CA 94103-1741, USA

Wiley-VCH Verlag GmbH, Boschstr. 12, D-69469 Weinheim, Germany

John Wiley & Sons Australia Ltd, 33 Park Road, Milton, Queensland 4064, Australia

John Wiley & Sons (Asia) Pte Ltd, 2 Clementi Loop #02-01, Jin Xing Distripark, Singapore 129809

John Wiley & Sons Canada Ltd, 6045 Freemont Blvd, Mississauga, Ontario, L5R 4J3

Wiley also publishes its books in a variety of electronic formats. Some content that appears in print may not be available
in electronic books.

Library of Congress Cataloging in Publication Data

Bruce, Nigel, 1955–
    Quantitative methods for health research : a practical interactive guide / Nigel Bruce, Daniel Pope,
    and Debbi Stanistreet.
        p.   ;   cm.
    Includes bibliographical references and index.
    ISBN 978-0-470-02274-0 (cloth : alk. paper) — ISBN 978-0-470-02275-7 (pbk. : alk. paper)
    1. Medicine—Research—Methodology.   2. Health—Research—Methodology.
    3. Epidemiology—Research—Methodology.   4. Epidemiology.
    I. Pope, Daniel, 1969–   II. Stanistreet, Debbi, 1963–   III. Title.
    [DNLM: 1. Epidemiologic Methods.   2. Biomedical Research—methods.
    3. Biometry—methods. WA 950 B918q 2008]
    RA852.B78 2008
    362.1072′4—dc22

                                                                                            2008002734

British Library Cataloguing in Publication Data

A catalogue record for this book is available from the British Library

ISBN 978-0-470-02274-0 (H/B)   978-0-470-02275-7 (P/B)

Typeset in 10/12pt Times by Integra Software Services Pvt. Ltd, Pondicherry, India
Printed and bound in Great Britain by CPI Antony Rowe, Chippenham, Wiltshire

Quantitative Methods for Health Research

Contents

Preface

Introduction

Welcome to *Quantitative Methods for Health Research*, a study programme designed to introduce you to the knowledge and skills required to make sense of published health research, and to begin designing and carrying out studies of your own.

The book is based closely on materials developed and tested over almost ten years with the Master of Public Health (MPH) programme at the University of Liverpool, UK. A key theme of our approach to teaching and learning is to ensure a reasonable level of theoretical knowledge (as this helps to provide a solid basis to knowledge), while placing at least as much emphasis on the application of theory to practice (to demonstrate what actually happens when theoretical 'ideals' come up against reality). For these reasons, the learning materials have been designed around a number of published research studies and information sources that address a variety of topics from the UK, Europe and developing countries. The many aspects of study design and analysis illustrated by these studies provide examples which are used to help you understand the fundamental principles of good research, and to practise these techniques yourself.

The MPH programme on which this book is based, consists of two postgraduate taught modules, one **Introductory**, the other **Advanced**, each of which requires 150 hours of study (including assessments), and provides 15 postgraduate credits (1 unit). As students and tutors using the book may find it convenient to follow a similar module-based approach, the content of chapters has been organised to make this as simple as possible. The table summarising the content of each chapter on pages xi to xiii indicates which sections (together with page numbers) relate to the introductory programme, and which to the advanced programme.

The use of computer software for data analysis is a fundamental area of knowledge and skills for the application of epidemiological and statistical methods. A complementary study programme in data analysis using SPSS (Statistical Package for the Social Sciences) has been prepared; this relates closely to the structure and content of the book. Full details of this study programme, including the data sets used for data analysis exercises, are available on the companion web site for this book www.wileyeurope.com/college/bruce.

The book also has a number of other features designed to enhance learning effectiveness, summarised in the following sections.

Learning objectives

Specific, detailed learning objectives are provided at the start of each chapter. These set out the nature and level of knowledge, understanding and skills required to achieve a good standard at Masters level, and can be used as one point of reference for assessing progress.

Resource papers and information sources

All sections of published studies that are absolutely required, in order to follow the text and answer self-assessment exercises, (see below) are reproduced as excerpts in the book. However, we strongly recommend that all resource papers be obtained and read fully, as indicated in the text. This will greatly enhance understanding of how the methods and ideas discussed in the book are applied in practice, and how research papers are prepared. All papers are fully referenced, and the majority are recent and in journals that are easily available through higher education establishments.

Key terms

In order to help identify which concepts and terms are most important, those regarded as core knowledge appear in **bold italic** font, thus. These can be used as another form of self-assessment, as a good grasp of the material covered in this book will only have been achieved if all these key terms are familiar and understood.

Self assessment exercises

Each chapter includes self-assessment exercises, which are an integral part of the study programme. These have been designed to assess and consolidate understanding of theoretical concepts and competency in practical techniques. The exercises have also been designed to be worked through as they are encountered, as many of the answers expand on issues that are introduced in the main text. The answers and discussion for these exercises are provided at the end of each chapter.

Mathematical aspects of statistics

Many people find the mathematical aspects of statistical methods, such as formulae and mathematical notation, quite challenging. It is useful however, to gain a basic mathematical understanding of the most commonly used statistical concepts and methods. We recognise that creating the expectation of much more in-depth knowledge for all readers would be very demanding, and arguably unnecessary.

On the other hand, readers with more affinity for and knowledge of mathematics may be interested to know more, and such understanding is important for more advanced research work and data analysis. In order to meet these objectives, all basic concepts, simple mathematical formulae, etc., the understanding of which can be seen as core knowledge are included in the main text. More detailed explanations, including some more complex formulae and examples, are included in statistical reference sections [RS], marked with a start and finish as indicated below.

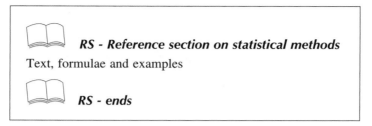

RS - Reference section on statistical methods

Text, formulae and examples

RS - ends

This book does not set out to provide detailed mathematical explanations of statistical methods as there are plenty of other books that do so and can be referred to if required.

We hope that you will enjoy this study programme, and find that it meets your expectations and needs.

Organisation of subject matter by chapter

The following table summarises the subject content for each chapter, indicating which sections are introductory and which advanced.

Chapter content and level

| | Introductory | | | Advanced |

Chapter	Level	Pages	Topics covered
1. Philosophy of science and introduction to epidemiology	Introductory	1–28	• Approaches to scientific research • What is epidemiology? • What is Statistics? • Formulating a research question • Rates, incidence and prevalence • Concepts of prevention
2. Routine data sources and descriptive epidemiology	Introductory	29–110	• Routine collection of health information • Descriptive epidemiology • Information on the environment • Displaying, describing and presenting data • Association and correlation • Summary of routinely available data relevant to health • Descriptive epidemiology in action, ecological studies and the ecological fallacy • Overview of epidemiological study designs
3. Standardisation	Introductory	111–128	• Rationale for standardisation • Indirect standardisation • Direct standardisation

Chapter	Level	Pages	Topics covered
4. Surveys	Introductory	129–192	• Rationale for survey methods • Sampling methods • The sampling frame • Sampling error, sample size and confidence intervals • Response rates • Measurement, questionnaire design, validity • Data types and presentation: categorical and continuous
5. Cohort studies	Introductory	193–256	• Rationale for cohort study methods • Obtaining a sample • Measurement and measurement error • Follow-up for mortality and morbidity • Basic analysis – relative risk, hypothesis testing: the t-test and the chi-squared test • Introduction to the problem of confounding
	Advanced		• Sample size for cohort studies • Simple linear regression • Multiple linear regression: dealing with confounding factors
6. Case-control studies	Introductory	257–306	• Rationale for case-control study methods • Selecting cases and controls • Matching – to match or not? • The problem of bias • Basic analysis – the odds ratio for unmatched and matched designs
	Advanced		• Sample size for case control studies • Matching with more than one control • Multiple logistic regression
7. Intervention studies	Introductory	307–362	• Rationale for intervention study methods • The randomised controlled trial (RCT) • Randomisation • Blinding, controls and ethical considerations • Basic analysis of trial outcomes: analysis by intention to treat
	Advanced		• Adjustment when confounding factors are not balanced by randomisation • Sample size for intervention studies • Testing more complex health interventions • Factorial design • Cluster randomisation, community randomised trials, quasi-experimental designs, cross-over trials
8. Life tables, survival analysis and Cox regression	Advanced	363–392	• Nature of survival data • Kaplan – Meier survival curves • Cox proportional hazards regression • Introduction to life tables

Chapter	Level	Pages	Topics covered
9. Systematic reviews and meta-analysis	Advanced	393–432	• Purpose of systematic reviews • Method of systematic review • Method of meta-analysis • Special considerations in systematic reviews and meta-analysis of observational studies • The Cochrane Collaboration
10. Prevention strategies and evaluation of screening	Advanced	433–470	• Relative and attributable risk, population attributable risk and attributable fraction • High-risk and population approaches to prevention • Measures and techniques used in the evaluation of screening programmes, including sensitivity, specificity, predictive value and receiver operator characteristic (ROC) curves • Methodological issues and bias in studies of screening programme effectiveness • Cohort and period effects
11. Probability distributions, hypothesis testing and Bayesian methods	Advanced	471–526	• Theoretical probability distributions • Steps in hypothesis testing • Transformation of data • Paired t-test • One-way analysis of variance • Non-parametric tests for paired data, two or more independent groups, and for more than two groups • Spearman's rank correlation • Fisher's exact test • Guide to choosing an appropriate test • Multiple significance testing • Introduction to Bayesian methods

Acknowledgements

The preparation of this book has involved the efforts of a number of people whose support we wish to acknowledge. Francine Watkins for preparing the first section of Chapter 1 'Approaches to Scientific Research'. Jo Reeve for preparing Section 5 of Chapter 2. 'A Summary of Routinely Available Data'. Paul Blackburn for assistance with graphics and obtaining permission for reproduction of the resource papers, and input into the data management and analysis course. Chris West for his advice on statistical methods, and input into the data management and analysis course. Nancy Cleave and Gill Lancaster for their invaluable contributions to early versions of the statistical components of the materials. Our students and programme tutors who have provided much valued, constructive feedback that has helped to guide the development of the materials upon which this book is based. The staff at Wiley for their encouragement and support. Chris and Ian at Ty Cam for providing a tranquil, e-mail free refuge in a beautiful part of Denbighshire.

1

Philosophy of science and introduction to epidemiology

Introduction and learning objectives

In this chapter, we will begin by looking at different approaches to *scientific research*, how these have arisen, and the importance of recognising that there is no single, 'right way' to carry out investigations in the health field. We will then go on to explore the *research task*, discuss what is meant by *epidemiology* and *statistics*, and look at how these two disciplines are introduced and developed in the book. The next section introduces the concept of *rates* for measuring the frequency of disease or characteristics we are interested in, and in particular the terms *incidence* and *prevalence*. These definitions and uses of rates are fundamental ideas with which you should be familiar before we look in more detail at research methods and study design. In the final section, we will look at key concepts in disease prevention, including the commonly used terms *primary, secondary* and *tertiary* prevention.

The reason for starting with a brief exploration of the nature of scientific methods is to see how historical and social factors have influenced the biomedical and social research traditions that we take for granted today. This will help you understand your own perceptions of, and assumptions about, health research, based on the knowledge and experience you have gained to date. It will also help you understand the scientific approach being taken in this book, and how this both complements, and differs from, that developed in books and courses on qualitative research methods – as and when you may choose to study these. Being able to draw on a range of research traditions and their associated methods is especially important for the discipline of public health, but also for many other aspects of health and health care.

Learning objectives

By the end of Chapter 1, you should be able to do the following:

Quantitative Methods for Health Research   Nigel Bruce, Daniel Pope and Debbi Stanistreet
© 2008 John Wiley & Sons, Ltd

- Briefly describe the philosophical differences between the main approaches to research that are used in the health field.

- Describe what is meant by epidemiology, and list the main uses to which epidemiological methods and thought can be put.

- Describe what is meant by statistics, and list the main uses to which statistical methods and thought can be put.

- Define and calculate rates, prevalence and incidence, and give examples of their use.

- Define primary, secondary and tertiary prevention and give examples of each.

1.1 Approaches to scientific research

1.1.1 History and nature of scientific research

Scientific research in health has a long history going back to the classical period. There are threads of continuity, as well as new developments in thinking and techniques, which can be traced from the ancient Greeks, through the fall of the Roman Empire, the Dark Ages and the Renaissance, to the present time. At each stage, science has influenced, and been influenced by, the culture and philosophy of the time. Modern scientific methods reflect these varied historical and social influences. So it is useful to begin this brief exploration of scientific health research by reflecting on our own perceptions of science, and how our own views of the world fit with the various ways in which research can be approached. As you read this chapter you might like to think about the following questions:

- What do you understand by the terms *science*, and *scientific research*, especially in relation to health?

- How has your understanding of research developed?

- What type of research philosophy best fits your view of the world, and the problems you are most interested in?

Thinking about the answers to these questions will help you understand what we are trying to achieve in this section, and how this can best support the research interests that you have and are likely to develop in the years to come. The history and philosophy of science is of course a whole subject in its own right, and this is of necessity a very brief introduction.

Scientific reasoning and epidemiology

Health research involves many different scientific disciplines, many of which you will be familiar with from previous training and experience. Here we are focusing principally on epidemiology, which is concerned with the study of the distribution and determinants of disease within and between populations. In epidemiology, as we shall see subsequently, there is an emphasis on *empiricism*, that is, the study of observable phenomena by scientific methods, detailed observation and accurate measurement. The scientific approach to epidemiological investigation has been described as:

- **Systematic** – there is an agreed system for performing observations and measurement.

- **Rigorous** – the agreed system is followed exactly as prescribed.

- **Reproducible** – all the techniques, apparatus and materials used in making the observations and measurements are written down in enough detail to allow another scientist to reproduce the same process.

- **Repeatable** – scientists often repeat their own observations and measurements several times in order to increase the reliability of the data. If similar results are obtained each time, the researcher can be confident the phenomena have been accurately recorded.

These are characteristics of most epidemiological study designs and will be an important part of the planning and implementation of the research. However, this approach is often taken for granted by many investigators in the health field (including epidemiologists) as the only way to conduct research. Later we will look at some of the criticisms of this approach to scientific research but first we need to look in more detail at the reasoning behind this perspective.

Positivism

The assumptions of contemporary epidemiological investigations are associated with a view of science and knowledge known as *positivism*. Positivism is a philosophy that developed in the eighteenth century in a period known as the Enlightenment, a time when scientists stopped relying on religion, conjecture and faith to explain phenomena, and instead began to use reason and rational thought. This period saw the emergence of the view that it is only by using scientific thinking and practices that we can reveal the truth about the world (Bilton *et al.*, 2002).

Positivism assumes a stable observable reality that can be measured and observed. So, for positivists, scientific knowledge is proven knowledge, and theories are therefore derived in a systematic, rigorous way from observation and experiment. This approach to studying human life is the same approach that scientists take to study the natural world. Human beings are believed by positivists to exist in causal relationships that can be empirically observed, tested and measured (Bilton *et al.*, 2002), and to behave in accordance with various laws. As this reality exists whether we look for it or not, it is the role of scientists to reveal its existence, but not to attempt to understand the inner meanings of these laws or express personal opinions about these laws. One of the primary characteristics of a positivist approach is that the researcher takes an objective distance from the phenomena so that the description of the investigation can be detached and undistorted by emotion or personal bias (Davey, 1994). This means that within epidemiology, various study designs and techniques have been developed to increase objectivity, and you will learn more about these in later chapters.

Induction and deduction

There are two main forms of scientific reasoning – *induction* and *deduction*. Both have been important in the development of scientific knowledge, and it is useful to appreciate the difference between the two in order to understand the approach taken in epidemiology.

Induction

With inductive reasoning, researchers make repeated observations and use this evidence to generate theories to explain what they have observed. For example, if a researcher made a number of observations in different settings of women cooking dinner for their husbands, they might then inductively derive a general theory:

> All women cook dinner for their husbands.

Deduction

Deduction works in the opposite way to induction, starting with a theory (known as an *hypothesis*) and then testing it by observation. Thus, a very important part of deductive reasoning is the formulation of the hypothesis – that is, the provisional assumption researchers make about the population or phenomena they wish to study before starting with observations. A good hypothesis must enable the researcher to test it through a series of *empirical observations*. So, in deductive reasoning, the hypothesis would be:

> All women will cook dinner for their husbands.

Observations would then be made in order to test the validity of this statement. This would allow researchers to check the consistency of the hypothesis against their observations, and if necessary the hypothesis can be discarded or refined to accommodate the observed data. So, if they found even one woman not cooking for her husband, the hypothesis would have to be re-examined and modified. This characterises the approach taken in epidemiology and by positivists generally.

One of the most influential science philosophers of recent times was Karl Popper (1902–1994), who argued that hypotheses can never be proved true for all time and scientists should aim to refute their own hypothesis even if this goes against what they believe (Popper, 1959). He called this the *hypothetico-deductive method*, and in practice this means that an hypothesis should be capable of being falsified and then modified. Thus, to be able to claim the hypothesis is true would mean that all routes of investigation had been carried out. In practice, this is impossible, so research following this method does not set out with the intention of proving that an hypothesis is true. In due course we will see how important this approach is for epidemiology and in the statistical methods used for testing hypotheses.

Alternative approaches to research

It is important to be aware that positivism is only one approach to scientific research. Positivism has been criticised by some researchers, in particular social scientists, who think it is an inappropriate approach to studies of human behaviour. From this perspective, they believe that human beings can behave irrationally and do not always act in accordance with any observable rules or laws. This makes them different from phenomena in the natural world, and so they need to be studied in a different way. Positivism has also been criticised because it does not allow for the view that human beings act in response to others around them; that is, that they interpret their own behaviour in response to others. As Green and Thorogood (2004, p. 12) argue:

> Unlike atoms (or plants or planets), human beings make sense of their place in the world, have views on researchers who are studying them, and behave in ways that are not determined in law-like ways. They are complex, unpredictable, and reflect on their behaviour. Therefore, the methods and aims of the natural sciences are unlikely to be useful for studying people and social behaviour: instead of explaining people and society, research should aim to understand human behaviour.

Social scientists therefore tend to have a different belief about how we should research human beings. Consequently, they are more likely to take an *inductive* approach to research because they would argue that they do not want to make assumptions about the social world until they have observed it in and for itself. They, therefore, do not want to formulate hypotheses because they believe these are inappropriate for making sense of human action. Rather, they believe that human action cannot be explained but must be understood.

While positivists are concerned mainly with observing patterns of behaviour, other researchers principally wish to understand human behaviour. This latter group requires a different starting point that will encompass their view of the world, or different *theoretical positions* to make sense of the world. It turns out that there are many different positions that can be adopted, and while we cannot go into them all here, we will use one example to illustrate this perspective.

Interpretative approaches

An interpretative approach assumes an interest in the meanings underpinning human action, and the role of the researcher is therefore to unearth that meaning. The researcher would not look to measure the reality of the world but would seek to understand how people interpret the world around them (Green and Thorogood, 2004).

Let's look at an example of this in respect of asthma. A *positivist* approach to researching this condition may be to obtain a series of objective measurements of symptoms and lung function by a standard procedure on a particular sample of people over a specified period of time. An *interpretative* approach might involve talking in-depth to fewer participants to try to understand how their symptoms affect their lives. Obviously, in order to do this, these two 'types' of researchers would need to use very different approaches. Those planning the interpretative research would be more likely to use *qualitative methods* (interviews, focus groups, participatory methods, etc.), while positivists (for example, epidemiologists) would choose *quantitative methods* (surveys, cohort studies, etc., involving lung-function measurements and highly structured questionnaires). These two different approaches are called *research paradigms* and would therefore produce different types of information.

Interpretative researchers would also criticise positivists for their belief that researchers can have an objective, unimpaired and unprejudiced stance in the research that allows them to make value-free statements. Interpretative researchers accept that researchers are human beings and therefore cannot stand objectively apart from the research. In a sense they are part of the research, as their presence can influence the nature and outcome of the research. Whether or not you agree with the criticism of positivism, you need to be aware that there are alternative approaches to conducting research that neither prioritise objectivity nor set out to measure 'reality'.

One of the most influential writers on the scientific method was Thomas Kuhn (1922–1996) (Davey, 1994). He argued that one scientific paradigm – one 'conceptual worldview' – may be the dominant one at a particular period in history. Over time, this is challenged, and eventually replaced by another view (paradigm), which then becomes accepted as the most important and influential. These revolutions in science were termed 'paradigm shifts'. Although challenged by other writers, this perspective suggests that scientific methods we may take for granted as being the only or best way to investigate health and disease, are to an extent the product of historical and social factors, and can be expected to evolve – and maybe change substantively – over time.

Exercise for reflection

1. Make brief notes on the type of scientific knowledge and research with which you are most familiar.

2. Is this predominantly positivistic (hypothetico-deductive) or interpretative in nature, or is it more of a mixture?

There are no 'answers' provided for this exercise, as it is intended for personal reflection.

1.1.2   What is epidemiology?

The term *epidemiology* is derived from the following three Greek words:

Epi – among
Demos – the people
Logos – discourse

We can translate this in more modern terms into *'The study of the distribution and determinants of disease frequency in human populations'*. The following exercise will help you to think about the uses to which the discipline of epidemiology is put.

Self-Assessment Exercise 1.1.1

Make a list of some of the *applications* of epidemiological methods and thought that you can think of. In answering this, avoid listing types of epidemiological study that you may already know of. Try instead to think in general terms about the practical outcomes and applications of these methods.

Answers in Section 1.5

This exercise shows the very wide application of epidemiological methods and thought. It is useful to distinguish between two broad functions of epidemiology, one very practical, the other more philosophical:

- The range of epidemiological research methods provides a toolbox for obtaining the best scientific information in a given situation (assuming, that is, you have established that a positivist approach is most appropriate for the topic under study!).

- Epidemiology helps us use knowledge about the population determinants of health and disease to inform the full range of investigative work, from the choice of research methods, through analysis and interpretation, to the application of findings in policy. With experience, this becomes a way of thinking about health issues, over and above the mere application of good methodology.

You will find that your understanding of this second point grows as you learn about epidemiological methods and their application. This is so because epidemiology provides the means of describing the characteristics of populations, comparing them, and analysing and interpreting the differences, as well as the many social, economic, environmental, behavioural, ecological and genetic factors that determine those differences.

1.1.3 What are statistics?

A statistic is a numerical fact. Your height and weight and the average daily rainfall in Liverpool are examples of statistics. The academic discipline of statistics is concerned with the collection, presentation, analysis and interpretation of numerical information (also called *quantitative* information).

Statistics are everywhere!

We are surrounded by, and constantly bombarded with, information from many sources - from the cereal box, to unemployment figures, the football results and opinion polls, to articles in scientific journals. The science of statistics allows us to make sense of this information and is thus a fundamental tool for investigation in many disciplines, including health, education, economics, agriculture and politics, to name but a few. The next exercise encourages you to explore how statistics are used in everyday life.

Self-Assessment Exercise 1.1.2

Look at a recent newspaper (hard copy or website for a newspaper, or, for example, the BBC news website (http://news.bbc.co.uk)) and find up to five items in which statistics are used. List the ways in which numerical information is presented.

Examples in Section 1.5

The scientific term for pieces of information is **data**. The singular is **datum**, meaning a single piece of information, such as, for example, one person's weight. A set of data may consist of many items, such as the heights, weights, blood pressures, smoking habits and exercise level of several hundred people. In its raw state, this mass of figures tells us little. There are two ways in which we use statistics to help us interpret data:

- To **describe** the group about which the data have been collected. This may be a group of people, or a group of hospitals, or a group of laboratory cultures. We describe the group by summarising the information into a few meaningful numbers and pictures.

- To **infer** something about the population of which the group studied is a part. We often want to know something about a population, such as everyone aged over 65 in Liverpool, but, practically, can collect information about only a subset of that population. This 'subset' is called a sample, and is explored in Chapter 3 on surveys. With inference, we want to know what generalisations to the population can be made from the sample, and with what degree of certainty.

 Self-Assessment Exercise 1.1.3

Can you find one example of **description**, and one example of **inference** in your newspaper or Web search? If you have found an example of making an inference, to which population does it apply?

Examples in Section 1.5

1.1.4 Approach to learning

We will explore the use and interpretation of statistical techniques through a number of published studies. Whether or not you go on to carry out research and use statistical methods yourself, you are certain to be a consumer of statistics through published research. We shall emphasise both the use of appropriate techniques and the critical interpretation of published results. You will also be learning about epidemiology and statistics in an integrated way. This approach recognises that the two disciplines embody many closely related concepts and techniques. There are also certain very distinct qualities, which you will find are emphasised through the more theoretical discussion relating to one or other discipline. Your learning of these research methods is based primarily on practical examples of data and published studies in order to help you to see how epidemiology and statistics are used in practice, and not just in theoretical or ideal circumstances.

Summary

- There is no single, 'right' philosophy of research. The approach taken is determined by many factors, including historical and social influences, and the nature of the problem being investigated.

- As an individual, your education, training and experience will strongly influence the scientific 'paradigm' that you are familiar, and comfortable with.

- A variety of approaches to, and methods for, research is both appropriate and necessary in the health field.

- Epidemiology provides us with a range of research tools, which can be used to obtain the information required for prevention, service provision, and the evaluation of health care. One of the most important contributions of epidemiology is the insight gained about the factors which determine the health of populations.

- Statistics is concerned with the collection, presentation, analysis and interpretation of numerical information. We may use statistical techniques to describe a group (of people, hospitals, etc.) and to make inferences about the population to which the group belongs.

1.2 Formulating a research question

1.2.1 Importance of a well-defined research question

This is arguably the most important section of the whole book. The reason for our saying this is that the methods we use, and ultimately the results that we obtain, must be determined by the question we are seeking to answer.

So, how do we go about formulating that question? This does not (usually) happen instantly, and there is a good deal of debate about how the question ought to be formulated, and how it is formulated in practice. Karl Popper argued that research ideas can come from all kinds of sources. But the idea is not enough on its own, and will usually need working on before it is a clearly formulated *research question*. Here are some of the factors we will have to take into account in fashioning a clear research question:

- What does all the other work on the topic tell us about the state of knowledge, and what aspects need to be addressed next? Our idea might actually arise from a review such as this, and therefore be already fairly well defined, but more often than not, the idea or need arises before we have had a chance to fully evaluate the existing body of knowledge. This will also depend on how far we are into researching a particular subject.

- Different types of problem and topic areas demand, and/or have been traditionally associated with, different research traditions. Does our idea require a positivist approach, with an hypothesis that can be falsified? If so, the research question will need to be phrased in a way that allows this. Alternatively, we might be trying to understand how a certain group of people view a disease and the services provided for them. This question must also be precisely defined, but not in the same way: there is nothing here to be falsified; rather, we wish to gain as full an understanding as possible of people's experience and opinions to guide the development of services.

- If our idea is overambitious, the necessary research may be too demanding, expensive or complex to answer the question(s) in one go. Perhaps it needs to be done in separate studies, or in stages.

In practice, defining the research question does not usually happen cleanly and quickly, but is a process that gradually results in a more and more sharply defined question as the existing knowledge, research options, and other practical considerations are explored and debated. There may appear to be exceptions to this – for instance, a trial of a new drug. On the face of it, the question seems simple enough: the drug is now available, so is it better than existing alternatives or not? However, as we will discover later, the context in which the drug would be used can raise a lot of issues that will play a part in defining the research question.

Although knowledge of appropriate research methods is important in helping you to formulate a clear research question, it is nevertheless useful to start the *process* of developing your awareness of, and skills in, this all-important aspect of research. The following exercise provides an opportunity for you to try this.

 Self-Assessment Exercise 1.2.1

A research idea . . .

> Your work in an urban area involves aspects of the care and management of people with asthma. You are well aware of the contemporary concern about the effect of air pollution on asthma, and the view that while pollution (e.g. ozone, nitrogen oxides) almost certainly exacerbates asthma, this may not be the cause of the underlying asthmatic tendency.
>
> In recent years, you have noticed that asthmatics (especially children) living in the poorest parts of the city seem to suffer more severe and frequent asthma episodes than those living in better-off parts.
>
> Although you recognise that pollution from traffic and industry might be worse in the poorer areas, you have been wondering whether other factors, such as diet (e.g. highly processed foods) or housing conditions such as dampness and associated moulds might be the real cause of the difference.
>
> You have reviewed the literature on this topic and found a few studies which are somewhat conflicting, and do not seem to have distinguished very well between the pollution, diet and housing factors you are interested in.

Have a go at converting the idea described above into a well-formulated research question appropriate for epidemiological enquiry. Note that there is no single, right, research question here. You do not need to describe the study methods you might go on to use.

Specimen answer in Section 1.5

1.2.2   Development of research ideas

We have seen that research is a process which evolves over a period of time. It is influenced by many factors, including other work in the field, the prevalent scientific view, political factors, finance, etc. Research is not a socially isolated activity with a discrete (inspirational) beginning, (perfect) middle and (always happy) ending, Figure 1.2.1.

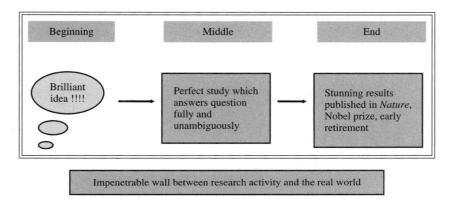

Figure 1.2.1   Research fantasy time

A more realistic way to describe the process of research development is cyclical, as illustrated in Figure 1.2.2. A well-defined and realistic question, which is (as we have seen) influenced by many factors, leads to a study which, it is hoped, provides much of the information required.

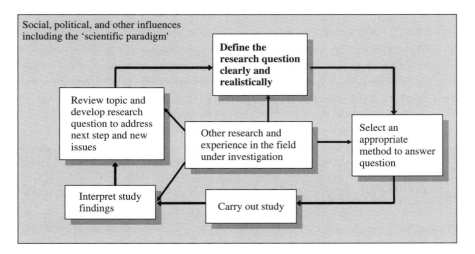

Figure 1.2.2   Research is a process that can usefully be thought of as being cyclical in nature, and subject to many influences from both inside and outside the scientific community

These findings, together with developments in the scientific field as well as social, political or other significant influences, will lead to further development of the research question.

Summary

- Defining a clear research question is a fundamental step in research.

- Well-defined research questions do not (usually) appear instantly!

- Research is a process, which can usefully be thought of as cyclical, albeit subject to many external influences along the way.

1.3 Rates: incidence and prevalence

1.3.1 Why do we need rates?

A useful way to approach this question is by considering the problem that arises when we try to interpret a change in the number of events (which could be deaths, hospital admissions, etc.) occurring during, say, a period of one year in a given setting. Exercise 1.3.1 is an example of this type of problem, and is concerned with an increase in numbers of hospital admissions.

 Self-Assessment Exercise 1.3.1

Over a period of 12 months, the accident and emergency department of a city hospital noted the number of acute medical admissions for people over 65 had increased by 30 per cent. In the previous 5 years, there had been a steady increase of only about 5 per cent per year.

---

1. List the possible reasons for the 30 per cent increase in hospital accident and emergency admissions.

2. What other information could help us interpret the reasons for this sudden increase in admissions?

Answers in Section 1.5

In this exercise we have seen the importance of interpreting changes in numbers of events in the light of knowledge about the ***population*** from which those events arose. This is why we need ***rates***. A rate has a ***numerator*** and a ***denominator***, and must be determined over a specified ***period of time***. It can be defined as follows:

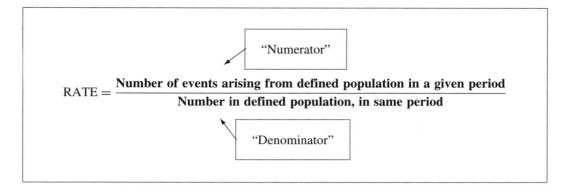

1.3.2 Measures of disease frequency

We will encounter rates on many occasions, as these are a fundamental means of expressing information gathered and analysed in epidemiological research. We can view these as measures of the *frequency* of disease, or of characteristics in the population. Two important general ways of viewing disease frequency are provided by *prevalence* and *incidence*.

1.3.3 Prevalence

The prevalence tells us how many cases of a disease (or people with a characteristic, such as smoking) there are in a given population, at a specified time. The *numerator* is the number of cases, and the *denominator* the population we are interested in.

$$\textit{Prevalence} = \frac{\text{Number of cases at a given time}}{\text{Number in population at that time}}$$

This can be expressed as a percentage, or per 1000 population, or per 10 000, etc., as convenient. The following are therefore examples of prevalence:

- In a primary care trust (PCT), with a population of 400 000, there are 100 000 smokers. The prevalence is therefore 25 per cent, or 250 per 1000.

- In the same PCT, there are known to be 5000 people diagnosed with schizophrenia. The prevalence is therefore 1.25 per cent, or 12.5 per 1000.

Note that these two examples represent 'snapshots' of the situation at a given time. We do not have to ask about people starting or giving up smoking, nor people becoming ill with (or recovering from) schizophrenia. It is a matter of asking, 'in this population, how many are there now?' This snapshot approach to measuring prevalence is known as *point prevalence*, since it refers to one point in time, and is the usual way in which the term prevalence is used. If, on the other hand, we assess prevalence over a period of time, it is necessary to think about cases that exist at the start of the period, and new cases which develop during the period. This measure is known as *period prevalence*, and this, together with point prevalence, is illustrated in Figure 1.2.3 and Exercise 1.3.2.

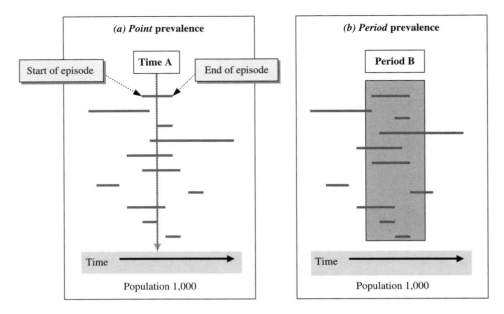

Figure 1.2.3 Period and point prevalence

Point prevalence (Figure 1.2.3a) is assessed at one point in time (time A), whereas period prevalence (Figure 1.2.3b) is assessed over a period (period B). The horizontal bars represent patients becoming ill and recovering after varying periods of time – the start and end of one episode is marked in Figure 1.2.3a. Period prevalence includes everyone who has experienced the disease at some time during this period.

 Self-Assessment Exercise 1.3.2

1. In the above examples (Figure 1.2.3a and b), calculate the point prevalence and period prevalence.

2. Why do the point prevalence and period prevalence differ?

Answers in Section 1.5

1.3.4 Incidence

Whereas *prevalence* gives us a measure of how many cases there are in the population at a given time, *incidence* tells us the rate at which *new* cases are appearing in the population. This is a vital distinction. In order to determine the incidence, we need to know the number of new cases appearing over a specified period of time, and the number of people in the population who could become cases over that same period of time (the 'at-risk' population). This is called *cumulative incidence* (or *incidence rate*) and is calculated as follows:

Incidence rate (also termed 'cumulative incidence')

$$Incidence = \frac{\text{Number of new cases arising from defined population in specified time period}}{\text{Number in defined at risk population over same period of time}}$$

The incidence can be expressed per 1000 per year (or other convenient time period), or per 10 000 per year, etc., as appropriate. Note that incidence is expressed over a specified time period, often taken as one year. Thus, if there were 20 new cases of a disease in a population of 2500 over a period of one year, the incidence, expressed per 1000 per year is as follows:

$$\text{Incidence} = \frac{20}{2,500} \times 1,000$$

This gives a rate of 8 cases per 1000 per year. The denominator, the 'defined population', must be exclusively that population which could become cases (termed *at risk*). For example, if we are considering the rate of hysterectomy (removal of the uterus) among UK women aged 50 years and above, the denominator population must be women over 50, excluding those who have previously had a hysterectomy.

Quite often, however, when a large group of the population is being studied, for example, all men in a city such as Liverpool, the number at risk in this defined population will not be readily available, and an estimate has to be made. In this case the corresponding midyear population estimate is often used as the denominator population, since it is usually available from published official statistics. This means that existing cases who are not 'at risk' of becoming new cases of the disease (because they are already affected) will be included in the denominator of the equation. In this case, the resulting incidence measure will not be much affected so long as the number of existing cases is relatively small in comparison to the total population, but you should be aware that the true incidence of the disease will be slightly underestimated. The following exercise will help you consolidate your understanding of *cumulative incidence*.

Self-Assessment Exercise 1.3.3

1. In the period prevalence diagram in Figure 1.2.3b, how many new cases arose during period B?

2. Surveillance data for episodes of food poisoning in a given population showed that among children aged 0–14 years there had been 78 new cases among boys, and 76 new cases among girls, over a period of 1 year. The population breakdown for the district is as shown in the following table.

Age group	Female	Male
0–14	37 100	41 000
15–24	59 610	60 100
25–44	62 050	57 300
45–64	42 450	39 610
65+	28 790	21 990
Total	**230 000**	**220 000**

Calculate the annual incidence rates per 10 000 for boys aged 0–14 years, and for girls aged 0–14 years. Comment on what you find.

Answers in Section 1.5

1.3.4.1 Person-time

Cumulative incidence assumes that the entire population at risk at the beginning of the study has been followed up for the same amount of time. It therefore measures the proportion of unaffected individuals who, on average, will contract the disease over the specified time period. However, in some study designs, such as cohort studies (described in Chapter 5), people may be entered into the study at different times and then be followed up to a specific end of study date. In addition, some may withdraw from the study, or die, before the end of the study. Study participants will therefore have differing lengths of follow-up.

To account for these varying times of follow-up, a denominator measure known as ***person-time*** is used. This is defined as the sum of each individual's time at risk while remaining free of disease. When person-time is used, incidence is calculated slightly differently, and is known as the ***incidence density***. This is calculated as follows:

Incidence density

$$Incidence = \frac{\text{Number of new cases arising from defined population in specified time period}}{\text{Total at risk person-time of observation}}$$

Since person-time can be counted in various units such as days, months or years, it is important to specify the time units used. For example, if 6 new cases of a disease are observed over a period of 30 person-years, then the incidence would be $6/30 = 0.2$ per person-year or equivalently, 20 per 100 person-years, or 200 per 1000 person-years. If people are lost to follow-up or withdraw from the study prematurely, their time at risk is taken to be the time they were under observation in the study. This next exercise will help with understanding incidence density.

Self-Assessment Exercise 1.3.4

Time of follow-up in study, or until disease develops, for 30 subjects

Subject	Years	Disease	Subject	Years	Disease
1	19.6	N	16	0.6	Y
2	10.8	Y	17	2.1	Y
3	14.1	Y	18	0.8	Y
4	3.5	Y	19	8.9	N
5	4.8	N	20	11.6	Y
6	4.6	Y	21	1.3	Y
7	12.2	N	22	3.4	N
8	14.0	Y	23	15.3	N
9	3.8	Y	24	8.5	Y
10	12.6	N	25	21.5	Y
11	12.8	Y	26	8.3	N
12	12.1	Y	27	0.4	Y
13	4.7	Y	28	36.5	N
14	3.2	N	29	1.1	Y
15	7.3	Y	30	1.5	Y

1. Assuming that all subjects in the table enter the study at the same time and are followed up until they leave the study (end of follow-up) or develop the disease, find the total observation time for the 30 subjects and estimate the incidence density. Give your answer per 1000 (10^3) person-years.

2. It is more usual for follow-up studies to be of limited duration where not all the subjects will develop the disease during the study period. Calculate the incidence density for the same 30 subjects if they were observed for only the first 5 years, and compare this with the rate obtained in question 1.

Answers in Section 1.5

1.3.5   Relationship between incidence, duration and prevalence

There is an important relationship between incidence, illness duration, and prevalence. Consider the following two examples:

- Urinary tract infections among women are seen very commonly in general practice, reflecting the fact that the incidence rate is high. The duration of these infections (with treatment) is usually quite short (a few days), so at any one time there are not as many women with an infection as one might imagine given the high incidence. Thus, the (point) prevalence is not particularly high.

- Schizophrenia is a chronic psychiatric illness from which the majority of sufferers do not recover. Although the incidence is quite low, it is such a long-lasting condition that at any one time the prevalence is relatively high, between 0.5 per cent and 1 per cent, or 5–10 per 1000 in the UK.

Thus, for any given incidence, a condition with a longer duration will have a higher prevalence. Mathematically, we can say that the prevalence is proportional to the product of incidence and average duration. In particular, when the prevalence is low (less than about 10 per cent), the relationship between prevalence, incidence and duration can be expressed as follows:

$$\text{Prevalence} = \text{incidence} \times \text{duration}$$

This formula holds so long as the units concerned are consistent, the prevalence is low, and the duration is constant (or an average can be taken). Thus, if the incidence is 15 per 1000 per year, and the duration is, on average, 26 weeks (0.5 years), then the prevalence will be (15×0.5) per $1000 = 7.5$ per 1000.

Summary

- Rates are a vitally important concept in epidemiology, and allow comparison of information on health and disease from different populations.

- A rate requires a numerator (cases) and a denominator (population), each relating to the same specified time period.

- The prevalence rate is the number of cases in a defined population at a particular point in time (point prevalence), or during a specified period (period prevalence).

- The incidence rate is the number of new cases which occur during a specified time period in a defined at risk population (cumulative incidence).

- Incidence density is a more precise measure of incidence and uses person-time of observation as the denominator.

- Without using rates, comparison of numbers of cases in different populations may be very misleading.

- The relationship between incidence and prevalence is determined by the duration of the condition under consideration.

1.4 Concepts of prevention

1.4.1 Introduction

In this section, we will look at the ways in which we can conceptualise **approaches to prevention**. This is a well-established framework that provides important background to many of the studies we will examine in learning about research methods, as well as for services such as screening. The following examples illustrate three different approaches to prevention. Please read through these, and complete exercise 1.4.1. We will then look at the formal definition of these approaches.

Example 1: Road accidents among children

Accidents are the most common cause of death among children in the UK, and the majority of these accidents occur on the roads. Traffic calming offers one way of reducing the number of childhood deaths arising from road accidents.

Example 2: Breast cancer

Breast cancer is one of the most common cancers among women. Despite this, we know little for certain about the causes beyond genetic, hormonal and possibly some dietary factors. In recent years, mammography, a radiographic examination of the breast, has been routinely offered to women 50–64 years of age. Abnormalities suggestive of cancer are investigated by biopsy (removal of a small piece of tissue for microscopic examination), and if the biopsy is positive, treatment for cancer is carried out.

Example 3: Diabetes and the prevention of foot problems

Diabetes, a disorder of glucose (blood sugar) metabolism, is generally a progressive condition. The actual underlying problem does not usually get better, and control of blood glucose has to be achieved through attention to diet, and usually also with medication, which may be in tablet form or as injected insulin. Associated with this disordered glucose metabolism are a range of chronic degenerative problems, including atherosclerosis (which leads to heart attacks, and poor blood supply to the lower legs and feet), loss of sensation in the feet due to nerve damage, and eye problems. Many of these degenerative processes can be slowed down, and associated problems prevented, by careful management of the diabetes. One important example is care of the foot when blood supply and nerves are affected. This involves education of the diabetic about the problem, and how to care for the foot, and provision of the necessary treatment and support.

 Self-Assessment Exercise 1.4.1

For each of the above examples, describe in everyday language (that is, avoiding technical terms and jargon) how prevention is being achieved. In answering this question, think about the way in which the prevention measure acts on the development and progression of the disease or health problem concerned.

Answers in Section 1.5

1.4.2   Primary, secondary and tertiary prevention

The three examples of prevention that we have just discussed are (respectively) illustrations of *primary, secondary* and *tertiary* prevention. These terms can be defined as follows:

Term	Definition	Example studied
Primary	Prevention of an infection, injury or other disease process from the beginning.	Traffic calming reduces the likelihood of a child's being involved in a collision with a vehicle, and therefore reduces the chance of injury or death from this cause.
Secondary	Early detection of a disease process at a stage where the course of the disease can be stopped or reversed.	Offering mammography to the population of women aged 50–64 allows early detection of breast cancer, and a better chance of successful treatment.
Tertiary	Management of a condition which is already established in such a way as to minimise consequences such as disability and other complications.	The diabetic generally requires lifelong treatment, and the underlying condition cannot be 'cured'. The complications and disability arising from foot problems, for example, can be avoided or ameliorated by an active approach to prevention.

 Self-Assessment Exercise 1.4.2

For each of the following activities, state whether this is primary, secondary or tertiary prevention, giving brief reasons for your answer:

1. Measles immunisation.

2. Five-yearly smear tests for cervical cancer.

3. A well-managed programme of terminal care for a patient with cancer.

4. Use of bed nets impregnated with insecticide in malaria-endemic areas.

5. Smoking-cessation programme in middle-aged men recovering from a heart attack.

Answers in Section 1.5

1.5 Answers to self-assessment exercises

Section 1.1

Exercise 1.1.1

The uses of epidemiological methods and thought: this list is not necessarily exhaustive, but covers the most important applications:

- By studying populations rather than those already in the health-care system, one can gain a more ***representative and complete picture*** of the distribution of disease, and maybe identify the factors which determine who does, and does not, take up health care.

- Describing the frequency of a disease, health problem or risk factor; who is affected, where and when. This may be used for ***planning***, as in epidemic control, service provision, etc.

- Understanding the ***natural history*** of health problems; that is, what happens if there is no treatment or other intervention.

- Understanding the ***causes*** of disease, thus laying the basis for prevention.

- Determining the ***effectiveness*** of health interventions, whether drugs, surgical operations, or health promotion.

- Through an understanding of the determinants of the health of populations, epidemiology contributes to the development of ***prevention policy***.

Thus, while basic research may add to our biologic understanding of why an exposure causes or prevents disease, only epidemiology allows the quantification of the magnitude of the exposure – disease relationship in humans and offers the possibility of altering the risk through intervention. Indeed, epidemiologic research has often provided information that has formed the basis for public health decisions long before the basic mechanism of a particular disease was understood.

(Hennekens and Buring, 1987, p. 13)

Study of groups that are particularly healthy or vulnerable is often the beginning of the search for causes and so of prevention.

(Morris, 1957, p. 263)

Exercise 1.1.2

These are just a few examples of the use of statistics found in newspapers over two days in August 2005. Note the different ways that the information is presented.

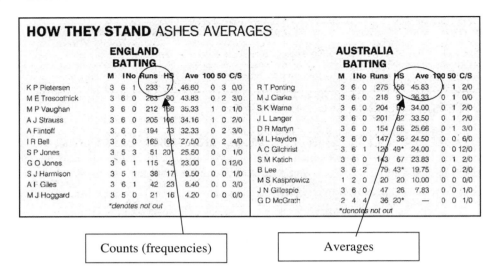

Counts (frequencies)

Averages

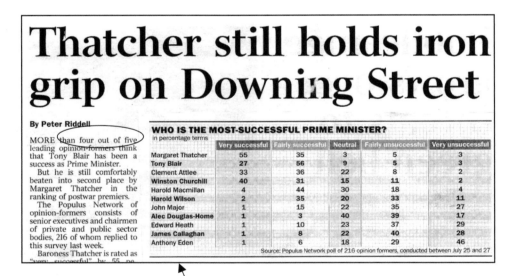

This panel shows results of a poll about the success of UK Prime Ministers. On the first line of the article, results are reported as a ***proportion*** (four out of five), while in the tables ***percentages*** are used.

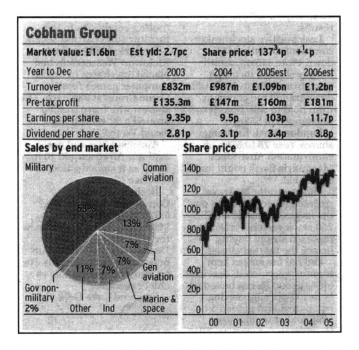

Cobham Group

Market value: £1.6bn   Est yld: 2.7pc   Share price: 137³⁄₄p   +¹⁄₄p

Year to Dec	2003	2004	2005est	2006est
Turnover	£832m	£987m	£1.09bn	£1.2bn
Pre-tax profit	£135.3m	£147m	£160m	£181m
Earnings per share	9.35p	9.5p	103p	11.7p
Dividend per share	2.81p	3.1p	3.4p	3.8p

This panel shows a *pie chart* (bottom left) and a *line graph* (bottom right). Data in the pie chart are presented as *percentages*.

The *table* in the upper section shows total **counts** (turnover, profit) and *averages* of earnings and dividends per share.

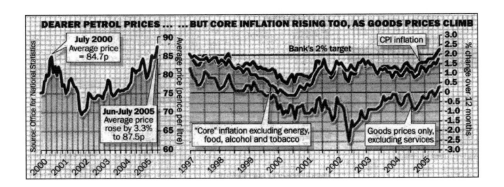

This panel shows quite a range of statistical information, presented as *line graphs* over time (by year).

Included are *average* petrol prices per litre, and the *percentage change* over 12 months in three indices of inflation (which are themselves calculated from the average prices of a range of commodities).

Exercise 1.1.3

Here is one example of *description* of groups (world drinkers), and one example of *inference* (German election poll).

Example 1

This is a *bar chart* presenting average alcohol consumption per adult, calculated from national data (on consumption and adult population). As these are data for the whole country, this represents *description* of groups (countries), not *inference*.

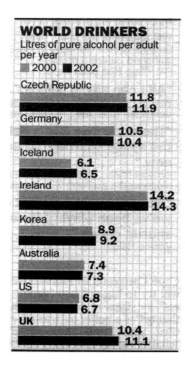

World Drinkers

Example 2

This panel shows results from German opinion polls. The results are in the form of *percentages*, displayed in *line graphs* to show the trends over time. As this is a poll, it is an example of a *sample* being used for *inference* about the opinions of those eligible to vote in the whole German *population*.

You will recognise that the example of the 'most successful prime minister' in Exercise 1.1.2 was also an example of *inference*. These statistics were obtained from a poll of 216 'opinion formers', so the intention is *inference* from this *sample* about the wider *population* of opinion formers.

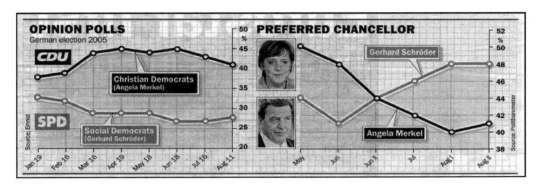

German election poll

Section 1.2

Exercise 1.2.1

This is a complex problem, so don't worry if you have found it challenging. There are many different research questions that could arise from this, depending on the type of research your experience and interests relate to. For example, at one end of the spectrum, a laboratory-based scientist may wish to carry out some physiologically based animal experiments involving chemicals from traffic pollution, food additives and fungal spores (from damp housing). Any kind of laboratory experiment with humans is out of the question, so we will concentrate on epidemiological investigation. The following two research questions represent different levels of investigation. The first aims to start the research process off by describing the situation (from which associations between asthma and other factors can be investigated), while the second takes a more analytical approach. Which one is appropriate would depend on exactly what has already been studied, resources available, etc. You will note that both define the population as children aged 5–15 years, in order to help focus the study.

Research question 1

How are asthma, levels of air pollution, damp housing, consumption of (specified) processed foods, and socio-economic circumstances distributed among children aged 5–15 living in (named city)?

Research question 2

Among children aged 5–15 living in (named city), are the presence and/or frequency of asthma associated with (specified) processed foods or damp housing, after taking account of levels of air pollution?

Section 1.3

Exercise 1.3.1

The reasons for this very large increase could be as follows:

- A *chance* (random) variation (although this is unlikely given the large numbers involved). The role of chance variation is a very important concept in epidemiology and statistical methods, and we will begin to examine this in Chapter 2.

- An *artefact* of the system, such as a change, or error, in the system for recording admissions. This is also unlikely to cause such a dramatic increase, but needs to be considered. The quality of information and how it is defined and handled are also very important issues in research, which we will begin to look at in Chapter 2.

- A *real* increase, which could result from changes in referral procedures by GPs (although this is again unlikely to cause such a large increase in one year, especially given the more gradual increase seen in previous years). A more likely explanation is a sudden increase in the population that the accident and emergency department is serving. Natural increase in population is unlikely, unless there had been an event such as a rapid influx of refugees. Closure of another (smaller) accident and emergency department in the city is the most likely reason for the large increase in the population being served.

The key point here is that, in order to make some judgement about this increase, we need to know the size of the population from which the admissions are coming. If this population has increased by 30 per cent, then, all other things being equal, we would expect the number of admissions to increase by 30 per cent. Changes in numbers of events (whether deaths, cases, admissions, etc.) cannot be interpreted usefully without information on changes in the population from which these events arose.

Exercise 1.3.2

1. Calculation of point and period prevalence. *Point prevalence*: in this diagram, 7 cases were 'active' at time A. With a population of 1000, the point prevalence is $7 \div 1000 = 0.007$. This is a rather untidy way of expressing the prevalence, so we can state it as 0.7 per cent or 7 per 1000. *Period prevalence*: here we have a longer period to consider, during which some cases resolve, and new ones occur. We include the cases that got better, since they were cases at some time during period B. We must also include the new cases that start during period B. A total of 10 cases were 'active' during period B, so the period prevalence is $10 \div 1000 = 0.01$. This can be presented as 1 per cent or 10 per 1000.

2. The point and period prevalence rates differ because, for period prevalence, we included some cases that had not yet recovered and some new cases that appeared during period B.

Exercise 1.3.3

1. During period B, a total of seven new cases arose.

2. The incidence rate for boys aged 0–14 is $(78 \div 41\,000) \times 10000$ per year, $= 19.0$ per 10 000 per year. The incidence rate for girls aged 0–14 is $(76 \div 37\,100) \times 10\,000$ per year, $= 20.5$ per 10 000 per year. So despite the fact that there were more cases among boys, the incidence rate was actually higher among girls. The reason for this is that the population of girls was smaller. This again emphasises why rates are so important.

Exercise 1.3.4

1. The total observation time for the 30 subjects is 261.9 person-years, during which time $n = 20$ subjects developed the disease. The incidence rate is $20/261.9 = 0.0764$ per person-year or 76.4 per 1,000 (10^3) person years.

2. In this case the total observation time is:

$$5 + 5 + 5 + 3.5 + 4.8 + 4.6 + 5 + \ldots + 1.5 = 115.8 \text{ person-years}$$

The total number of cases is now 11 (as we only include cases occurring within the first 5 years), so the incidence rate is $11/115.8 = 0.095$ per person-year or 95.0 per 10^3 person-years. This rate is somewhat higher than that for the longer follow-up.

Section 1.4

Exercise 1.4.1

Road accident prevention

Traffic calming slows vehicles to a speed which markedly reduces the chance of a collision. In addition, traffic calming makes drivers more aware of the likely presence of pedestrians, including children, and this further reduces the chance of an accident occurring. The slower speed also reduces the chance of serious injury or death if a collision between a child and a vehicle does occur. The prevention process here is principally through preventing the accident (injury/death) happening in the first place, but if it does happen, the severity and likelihood of death are reduced.

Breast cancer prevention

From the information we have, it is apparent that we do not yet know enough to prevent most cases of breast cancer from occurring in the first place. What we can do is detect the disease at a stage where, if treated promptly, it is possible to cure the disease in a substantial proportion of affected women. Thus, in contrast to the road accident example, the prevention begins after the disease process has started, but it is at a stage where it is still possible to cure the disease.

Prevention of foot problems in the diabetic

In this last example, the disease process is well established, and cannot be removed or 'cured'. That does not mean that the concept of prevention has to be abandoned, however. In this situation, preventative action (education, support, treatment, etc.) is being used to prevent damage to the skin of the feet, with the infection and ulceration that can follow. Prevention is carried out, despite the fact that the underlying disease remains present.

Exercise 1.4.2

Example	Prevention approach	Reasons/explanation
Measles immunisation	Primary	Immunisation raises immunity of the recipient, and prevents infection.
Smear tests	Secondary	The smear test is a screening procedure, designed to detect the disease process at an early stage. Note that the test on its own is not prevention, as it does not alter the course of the disease: it must be followed up (if positive) by biopsy and treatment as necessary.

(Continued)

Example	Prevention approach	Reasons/explanation
Terminal care	Tertiary	The patient is dying (e.g. from cancer), and nothing can be done to alter that. That does not mean the preventative approach is abandoned. Good terminal care can prevent a lot of pain and emotional distress in both the patient and family/friends. This can have lasting benefits.
Bed nets	Primary	Impregnated bed nets prevent contact between the feeding mosquito and humans, especially at night when most biting occurs. This prevents introduction of the malaria parasite into the body, thus preventing the occurrence of the disease.
Smoking cessation	Tertiary?	This one does not fit definitions easily. Smoking cessation in a healthy younger person could properly be regarded as primary prevention of heart disease. In our example, the men had already had a heart attack. This is not secondary prevention (detection at early stage, etc.). It is probably best seen as tertiary, especially bearing in mind that this smoking cessation should generally be part of a broader rehabilitation package helping the man to get mentally and physically better, reduce his risk of further heart attack, and get back to work or other activity.

2

Routine data sources and descriptive epidemiology

Introduction and learning objectives

In this chapter, we will examine a range of information sources of value to health research, and learn how to present, analyse and interpret this information. Exercises will help you understand how the information is collected, its strengths and weaknesses, and introduce you to methods for presenting and comparing the data. We will finish by looking at how these descriptive epidemiological research methods fit into an overview of study designs, and consider the nature of the research evidence that we have obtained from the methods studied.

Learning objectives

By the end of this chapter, you should be able to do the following:

- Describe the key sources of routinely available data relevant to research in public health and health care, including the census, and examples of registrations (deaths, cancer, etc.), notifiable diseases, service utilisation, surveys and environmental monitoring.

- Examine the uses, strengths and weaknesses of selected examples of routine data.

- Describe the usefulness of studying variations in health, and health determinants, by time, place and person, with examples.

- Calculate and present a frequency distribution for a set of continuous data.

- Display continuous data in a histogram.

- Describe the shape of a distribution of continuous data.

(Continued)

Quantitative Methods for Health Research   Nigel Bruce, Daniel Pope and Debbi Stanistreet
© 2008 John Wiley & Sons, Ltd

- Summarise distributions of continuous data: calculate mean, median and mode, standard deviation and interquartile range, and use appropriately.

- Interpret a scatterplot, describe the relationship between two continuous variables, and interpret a (Pearson) correlation coefficient.

- Describe what is meant by an ecological study, and how the ecological fallacy arises.

- Present an overview of the different types of epidemiological study design, and the nature of descriptive studies in relation to other study designs.

2.1 Routine collection of health information

2.1.1 Deaths (mortality)

We will begin by describing the collection and recording of death data (termed ***mortality data***), drawing on the system used in England and Wales. This includes how the cause of death is decided upon and recorded, and how other information about the person who had died (such as their occupation) is added. The following two stories are about deaths occurring in very different circumstances. Read through these, and as you do so, note down the pathways by which information about the person dying, and the mode of death, is obtained and recorded. Note the roles of relatives, medical staff and other officials, and other significant people such as witnesses.

Story A – an expected death

On a cold January afternoon, tired and laden with shopping, Joan Williams walked slowly up to her front door. Hearing the phone, she put down the bags, and fumbled with the key in her anxiety about the call. Perhaps it was the hospital with news about her mother.

'Hello, Joan Williams,' she said quietly.

'Oh Hello, Mrs Williams, it's Sister Johnson here. I'm afraid your mother has had a relapse. She is conscious, but I think you should come over to the hospital as soon as you can.'

'Yes, of course. . . I'll be there,' she replied.

Joan had been expecting this call for a week or more, but that did not prevent the fear she now felt about what lay ahead. Mechanically, she put away the shopping, as her thoughts drifted back to the summer holidays. Her 79-year-old mother had joined the family for their holiday in Cornwall, and, despite her age she was active and helpful with the children, who were very fond of her. Just before they were due to go home, her mother developed a cough and fever, and was diagnosed as having pneumonia. She improved on antibiotics, but then fell ill again with a recurrence, this time with blood-stained phlegm. She was found to have lung cancer, and for much of the next 6 months was in and out of hospital for palliative radiotherapy, and treatment of chest infections. She had deteriorated a lot in the last few weeks, and Joan knew that her mother was close to death.

When Joan arrived at the infirmary, her mother was unconscious. A few minutes before, she had suffered a heart attack, and apart from monitoring her condition, no other active treatment was to be given. For a while after her mother died, Joan sat beside the bed thinking of all that had happened in the last 6 months, and how she would tell the children. She had not had the responsibility of dealing with the death of a family member before, since her father had been killed on active military service when she was very young. Now she would have to get the death certificate, make all the arrangements for the funeral, and tell the rest of the family. She just wanted to be left alone with her memories of her mother.

The staff at the hospital were very kind though, and helped as much as they could. 'If you come back tomorrow morning, the death certificate will be ready,' Sister Johnson told her. The doctor who filled in the death certificate had to decide on the cause of death, which she put down as myocardial infarction, with the underlying cause as carcinoma of the bronchus. Since a clear diagnosis of the cancer had already been established, and Mrs Williams' mother had been seen both by her GP and at the hospital regularly over the previous 6 months, all the information the doctor needed was in the medical records. The next day, Joan collected the death certificate, and took it to the local registry office, where she had to register the death. The clerk asked her a few more questions about her mother, thanked her as he handed her the disposal order for the undertaker, and said that she could now go ahead with the funeral arrangements.

Walking out into the bright January sunshine, she was grateful that at least this bit of the proceedings had been quite straightforward, though painful nonetheless. She thought of her sister Mary, whose husband had died suddenly at home last year: Mary had suffered terribly with all the delay while the coroner's office spoke to the doctors, and a post-mortem examination was carried out, all the time wondering whether they would order an inquest. At least her mother's death had been expected, and the officials could fill in the forms without all kinds of delays and investigations.

  ### Self-Assessment Exercise 2.1.1

1. Who completed the death certificate for Joan Williams' mother?

   - Sister Johnson
   - the coroner
   - the hospital doctor
   - Joan Williams
   - the registrar of births and deaths.

2. We are interested in how accurately mortality statistics report the true cause of death.

   a) How accurate do you think the information on the certificate was for Mrs Williams' mother?

   b) Do you think a post-mortem examination (autopsy) would have improved the quality of the information?

Answers in Section 2.8

Story B – a sudden, unexpected death

John Evans had been driving trains for over 20 years. Late one Sunday afternoon he experienced the nightmare that all drivers fear more than anything else.

After leaving York on the way south to London, he brought his Intercity train up to full speed as he ran down the beautiful coastal track of East Yorkshire. Rounding a gentle bend at over 120 miles per hour, he noted someone on a bridge about half a mile ahead. That was a common enough sight on this stretch of track, but something about the person's movements held his attention. His heart missed a beat as he realised a man was climbing the parapet, and he instantly applied the brakes, knowing only too well that stopping the train was impossible. Unable to look away, he caught sight of the blank face of a young man as he fell past the windscreen. He barely heard the thud as the man's body went under the train, and there was little left for the forensic scientists. Dental records were enough though, and he was eventually identified as a 24-year-old, homeless man who had been living in a hostel in Hull. He had no record of psychiatric illness, had left no suicide note, and had not told anyone of his intentions.

At the coroner's inquest, only his mother was available to give evidence, as his father had left home when he was very young and died some 5 years before from heart disease. She had not seen her son for 6 months before he died, and on the occasion of their last meeting he had not appeared unduly upset. The train driver also gave his evidence, and he felt certain this was a deliberate act of suicide. However, without evidence of definite suicidal intent such as a note or a record of several previous attempts, the coroner was obliged to return a verdict of 'death uncertain as to whether deliberately or accidentally caused', known as an open verdict.

 Self-Assessment Exercise 2.1.2

1. Why did the coroner not return a verdict of suicide on the homeless man, who seemingly deliberately threw himself under a high-speed train?

2. What proportion of true suicides do you think receive a verdict of suicide, and hence appear in the mortality statistics as such?

Answers in Section 2.8

2.1.2   Compiling mortality statistics: the example of England and Wales

These examples have given you part of the picture of how information about deaths in the UK is obtained and compiled into mortality statistics. Figure 2.1.1 summarises all of the stages for a death (like that of Joan Williams' mother) not requiring notification to the coroner.

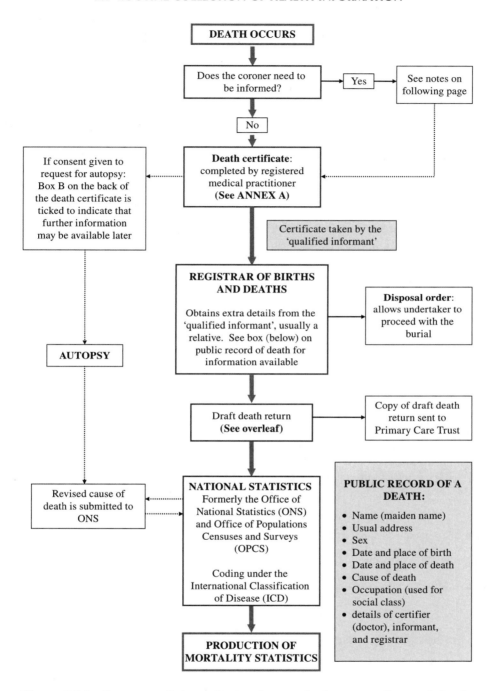

Figure 2.1.1 Summary of the pathways from a death to mortality statistics in England and Wales

The circumstances in which the coroner needs to be involved are summarised in the box below. It is important for you to be aware of these for three reasons:

1. The coroner's inquest will result in more complete information than would otherwise be available.

2. There is usually a delay of several months, and sometimes more than a year, before the inquest is completed, and the information about the cause of death may not enter the mortality statistics until the inquest is closed.

3. The coroner's records are a potentially useful source of information for local research (subject to permission).

Circumstances in which the coroner must be informed of a death

The coroner is an independent judicial officer of the Crown who has a statutory duty to investigate the circumstances of certain categories of death for the protection of the public. These are where the deceased person has:

- died a violent or unnatural death (which includes accidents, suicides, homicides, industrial disease or industrial poisoning)

- died a sudden death of which the cause is unknown

- died in prison (or in such a place or in such circumstances as to require an inquest under any other Act)

- died within 24 hours of admission to hospital, or during a surgical procedure.

Coroners hold inquests for about 12 per cent of deaths, and often use their discretion to decide whether a post-mortem (autopsy) alone provides sufficient evidence of the cause of a sudden death (diseases of the circulation, such as heart attack, account for around 75 per cent of these deaths). In addition, the registrar of deaths is legally obliged to refer a death to the coroner, if it appears from the doctor's death certificate, that (in addition to the categories above):

- the dead person was not attended by a doctor during his/her last illness

- the registrar has been unable to obtain a duly completed death certificate.

Source: Modified from Mathews and Foreman (1993).

2.1.3 Suicide among men

Having looked at how information about deaths is collected, we will now examine some actual data on deaths (known as *mortality data*) to find out what we can learn from simply presenting the information in a graph, and making some comparisons between different years. In this example we will look at mortality rates for suicide among men in England and Wales for the years 1980–2003, Table 2.1.1.

The tenth revision of the *International Statistical Classification of Diseases and Related Health Problems* (ICD-10) was introduced on 1 January 2001. ICD-10 replaced ICD-9, which had been

Table 2.1.1 Death rates per million population per year for 'suicide and self-inflicted injury' for all men, and selected age groups for men and women, England and Wales 1980–2003 (ICD codes E950-E959 for mortality statistics based on ICD-9, 1980–2000 and X60-X84 for mortality statistics based on ICD-10, 2001–2003)

Year	All men	Men 25–34	Men 65–74	Women 25–34
1980	110	130	182	42
1981	114	145	165	47
1982	115	145	173	46
1983	116	140	175	34
1984	118	140	170	38
1985	121	153	169	44
1986	116	146	176	39
1987	113	146	158	38
1988	121	155	162	38
1989	108	147	133	35
1990	117	160	136	38
1991	116	172	108	32
1992	118	159	129	37
1993	108	145	106	32
1994	113	181	109	33
1995	109	168	110	27
1996	103	163	98	37
1997	103	157	91	32
1998	109	186	90	34
1999	108	162	92	35
2000	100	150	99	33
2001	100	157	95	28
2002	98	148	82	35
2003	97	138	85	33

Source: Reproduced with permission from office for National Statistics: cause (Series DH2) available from http://www.statistics.gov.uk

used between 1979 and 2000. As a result, ICD-10 mortality data are not directly comparable with ICD-9. However, overall suicide data are not affected by the change (although codes do vary at the third- and fourth-digit level). If you wish to read about the effect of the introduction of ICD-10 in more detail, see Griffiths and Rooney (1999).

 Self-Assessment Exercise 2.1.3

1. Plot the data in Table 2.1.1 for all men and for each of the two male age groups separately for each year (we will examine the data for women shortly). Use graph paper if you are not yet familiar with computer software for drawing graphs (e.g. MS Excel).

2. Describe what you see for the three groups (all men, 25–34, and 65–74), over the years 1980 to 2003.

Answers in Section 2.8

This exercise illustrates variation in an important measure of health over time, and starts to raise questions about the changes that have occurred since 1980, especially since these are so different for young and older men. Do not spend any more time at this stage on why there are differences between the two age groups, as we will return to the interpretation of these changes shortly.

2.1.4 Suicide among young women

We will now look at the same information on suicide rates for young women.

 Self-Assessment Exercise 2.1.4

1. Using data for women aged 25–34 (Table 2.1.1), add the rates to your male mortality graph.

2. What do you observe about the trends for women aged 25–34 and men in the same age group.

Answers in Section 2.8

2.1.5 Variations in deaths of very young children

Here is another striking example of how an important health indicator, in this case the ***infant mortality rate*** (IMR), varies between different groups in society. The IMR for a given area (e.g. country, region or district) is defined as:

$$IMR = \frac{\text{The number of deaths per year occurring within the first year of life}}{\text{Total number of } \textit{live} \text{ births in the year}} \times 1000$$

The IMR is one of the best indicators we have of the health status of a population, and generally relates quite closely to the level of socio-economic development. This is true for both developed and developing countries, and for this reason it is widely used as an indicator of health and development, either on its own or combined with other information.

Table 2.1.2 is taken from the annual review of the Registrar General on childhood, infant and perinatal deaths, in England and Wales for the year 2002 and shows IMRs for children in a number of groupings as defined by the National Statistics Socio-Economic Classification (NS SEC) based on occupation of the child's father. This information is recorded by the registrar of births and deaths when the parents go to register the death (Figure 2.1.1).

Since 2001, this classification has replaced social class based on occupation and socio-economic group in official statistics. There are three versions of the classification, the eight-class version, the five-class version and the three-class version. The data used in this example are classified into the eight-class version ranging from 'large employers and higher managerial' to 'never worked

Table 2.1.2 Mortality rates for live-born children less than 1 year of age (infant mortality rate – IMR), expressed per 1000 live births; England and Wales 2002

NS SEC (See table footnotes)	Infant (IMR)
1.1	2.95
1.2	3.26
2	3.64
3	5.57
4	4.87
5	4.01
6	7.20
7	6.58
8	(see text)
Not classified	10.83

Classification of NS SEC categories is as follows: 1.1 – large employers and higher managerial, 1.2 – higher professional, 2 – lower managerial and professional, 3 – intermediate, 4 – small employers and account workers, 5 – lower supervisory and technical, 6 – semi-routine, 7 – routine, 8 – never worked and long-term unemployed.
Source: Reproduced with permission from Office for National Statistics (2002).

and long-term unemployed'. Data for group 8, 'never worked and long-term unemployed', are not shown in the table, as the number of births in this group was extremely small ($n = 15$).

 Self-Assessment Exercise 2.1.5

1. What is the ratio of the IMR for children in group 7 compared to group 1.1?

2. Briefly list the reasons that you think could explain the striking variations in IMR across these SEC groups in England and Wales.

Answers in Section 2.8

Summary

- The accuracy of mortality statistics (including the cause of death and information about the deceased person) depends on the accuracy of death certificate completion.

- Autopsies and coroner's inquests provide additional information for those deaths on which they are performed.

- Variations in levels of mortality, e.g. by time, or between groups defined by socio-economic circumstances, can provide valuable insight into possible causes of disease and death.

2.2 Descriptive epidemiology

2.2.1 What is 'descriptive epidemiology'?

In the last section we looked at some dramatic differences between gender and social groups in trends in suicide rates over time, and in infant mortality. These two examples show how a relatively simple study of data over time, and between the sexes (suicide) or socio-economic groups (IMR), which we can term differences between groups of persons, can begin to throw light on very important issues that might determine health. This is the essence of *descriptive epidemiology*, in which we can begin to learn about the determinants of population health by exploring the patterns of variation in measures of health (in this case the suicide and infant mortality rates), and factors which tell us something about what is causing these variations. So far, we have looked at variations by time and person, and we will shortly add a third dimension to this which is variation by place.

Descriptive epidemiology is the study of variations in measures of population health by *time, person and place*.

So, what seems at first sight to be a very simple investigative technique nevertheless sets us thinking about fundamental social, economic and environmental issues that are among the most important influences on health and the incidence of disease.

2.2.2 International variations in rates of lung cancer

In this final part of our discussion of routine mortality statistics, we will look at variations in death rates for lung cancer in two European countries. Table 2.2.1 shows the numbers of deaths, and death rates per 100 000 population, from lung cancer among women aged 65–74 for Austria (2000) and Ireland (1999).

Table 2.2.1 Numbers of deaths and death rates per 100 000 per year from lung cancer

Country (year)	number of deaths	rate per 100 000/year
Austria (2000)	247	65.2
Ireland (1999)	171	134.6

Source: Reproduced with permission from World Health Organisation (2007).

 Self-Assessment Exercise 2.2.1

1. Describe the differences between the data for the two countries.

2. What reasons can you think of that might explain these differences (in answering this question, it is useful to think about whether observed differences relate to chance, are an artefact, or are real).

Answers in Section 2.8

In the two examples of suicide data we have been considering, the data were collected by the system outlined in Figure 2.1.1, and were for England and Wales. The systems used in different countries vary in a number of respects, and this should be borne in mind when comparing data across countries. The following table summarises key information on mortality statistics preparation in Ireland and Austria, taken from the 1996 WHO Mortality Statistics Annual.

Country	% deaths medically certified	% deaths occurring in hospital, etc.	% deaths for which autopsy performed	Follow-up enquiries where doubt about cause	Coding procedure	Remarks on coverage of mortality statistics
Ireland	100	62	65+: 4% All: 7%	Yes	Centrally coded	All deaths in country; nationals dying abroad excluded
Austria	100	59	65+: 31% All: 34%	Yes: 3–4% of deaths	Centrally coded	Resident foreigners included; nationals resident abroad excluded

 Self-Assessment Exercise 2.2.2

1. What differences are there between the two systems for collecting mortality data?

2. Do you think this could have influenced the reported lung cancer data? If so, in what way?

3. In the light of this new information, would you alter your views about the likely cause(s) of the large difference in lung cancer death rates for women aged 65–74 in the two countries?

Answers in Section 2.8

2.2.3 Illness (morbidity)

So far in this chapter, we have looked at data on deaths, which are termed *mortality* statistics. Although death is an important and useful measure of disease, especially where accurate information is available on the cause, we also want to know about episodes of disease not resulting in death. The term used for episodes of illness is *morbidity*.

Good information on mortality is more easily available than for morbidity. This is because, in most countries, it is a legal requirement that all deaths be certified by a doctor, and officially registered. Thus, in a country such as the UK, although there are some inconsistencies and inaccuracies in the way certificates are completed, virtually all deaths are recorded, and the information in the mortality statistics is of a reasonably high standard of accuracy (although this does vary by age and cause of death). By contrast, not all episodes of illness are recorded with anything like the level of attention that attends the certification of a death, and the recording that is done is determined primarily by the contact that the ill person has with the health system:

- Many illness episodes are not brought to the attention of the health-care system, and so are not recorded. This is a very important perspective to bear in mind, and one of the reasons why studies of the *prevalence* of illness often require population surveys (Chapter 4).

- Episodes of illness brought to the attention of primary care are often recorded inconsistently, although, increasingly, GPs record episodes of certain conditions in disease registers (e.g. asthma, diabetes), and some information about all consultations on computer. Although some of this information may be made available with permission, there are nevertheless inconsistencies in methods of recording, and between different systems.

- More serious conditions requiring investigation and treatment in hospital have more detailed records (attendances at accident and emergency, as outpatients and as inpatients), but it is only the data transferred onto *patient information systems* that are potentially available for analysis.

2.2.4   Sources of information on morbidity

For these reasons, information on the majority of illness episodes in the population is not available for routine analysis in the way that all deaths are. Having said that, there are some sources that do provide this type of information, such as, for instance, on illness episodes seen in general practice. Until recently, the *National Morbidity Studies* have been the main source of GP morbidity data for England and Wales. These surveys commenced in the 1950s and obtained information approximately every 10 years in selected practices until 1991–2. This has now been superseded by the General Practice Research Database, and you can read more about this in Section 2.5.4. There are also systems for the routine recording of some key disease types, two of the most important examples being the *notification of infectious diseases*, and the *registration of cancers*. We will now examine some examples of infectious disease notification.

2.2.5   Notification of infectious disease

Despite the decline in infectious disease associated with improvements in living conditions in many countries, serious diseases such as meningitis, tuberculosis and food poisoning remind us of the continuing importance of infections and the need for vigilance and control. Timely information about cases of infectious diseases such as these is vital to the work of those responsible for control measures. In the UK, a system of notifying certain specified infectious diseases has been in operation for many years. The responsibility for notification rests with the doctor who makes the diagnosis, and this includes cases where the diagnosis is made by laboratory testing of blood or other samples. All diseases currently notifiable in the UK are listed in the box on the following page.

Not surprisingly, doctors do not always get round to completing the notification forms, especially for the less serious conditions. This means that the statistics tend not to be complete (not all cases are notified), and this is termed *under-reporting*. Despite this, levels of under-reporting remain fairly constant over time, so it is possible to look at trends with a fair degree of confidence. We will now look at three examples, food poisoning, meningitis and mumps.

Communicable diseases currently notifiable in the UK

Anthrax	Measles	Relapsing fever
Cholera	Meningitis	Scarlet fever
Diphtheria	Meningococcal	Smallpox
Dysentery	septicaemia	Tetanus
Acute encephalitis:	Mumps	Tuberculosis (all forms)
• infective	Ophthalmia	
• Post-infectious	neonatorum	Typhoid fever
Food poisoning	Paratyphoid fever	Typhus fever
Lassa fever	Plague	Viral haemorrhagic disease
Leprosy	Acute poliomyelitis:	Viral hepatitis
Leptospirosis	• paralytic	Whooping cough
Malaria	• non-paralytic	
	Rabies	Yellow fever
	Rubella	

Time trends in food poisoning

Table 2.2.2 shows the numbers of notified cases of food poisoning for England and Wales for each of the years 1984 to 2003, together with the population numbers.

Table 2.2.2 Cases of food poisoning, and population (thousands), England and Wales 1984–2003

Year	Number of cases[1]	Population (1000s)[2]	Crude rate/1000/year
1984	20 702	49 713.1	0.416
1985	19 242	49 860.7	0.386
1986	23 948	49 998.6	0.479
1987	29 331	50 123.0	0.585
1988	39 713	50 253.6	0.790
1989	52 557	50 407.8	1.043
1990	52 145	50 560.6	1.031
1991	52 543	50 748.0	1.035
1992	63 347	50 875.6	1.245
1993	68 587	50 985.9	1.345
1994	81 833	51 116.2	1.601
1995	82 041	51 272.0	1.600
1996	83 233	51 410.4	
1997	93 901	51 559.6	
1998	93 932	51 720.1	
1999	86 316	51 933.5	
2000	86 528	52 140.2	
2001	85 468	52 360.0	
2002	72 649	52 570.2	
2003	70 895	52 793.7	

Source: [1] Statutory Notifications of Infections Diseases (NOIDS) available at http://www.hpa.org.uk
[2] Table T03 available at http://www.statistics.gov.uk/statbase

Self-Assessment Exercise 2.2.3

1. Calculate the crude incidence rates for 1996 onward expressed per 1000 population per year, and enter these in the column provided.

2. Plot the data (by MS Excel or on graph paper).

3. Comment briefly on the trend. What explanations for this trend can you think of?

Answers in Section 2.8

Seasonal and age patterns in meningitis

Like food poisoning, meningitis is another infectious disease that has received a lot of media attention in recent years, and is greatly feared by the public. This fear results from the seemingly unpredictable and sporadic way in which the disease spreads, and the high mortality rate (*case fatality*) associated with meningococcal meningitis (infection of the linings of the brain) and septicaemia (infection of the blood). As we shall see, children and young people are particularly vulnerable, which adds to the sense of concern. Table 2.2.3 shows the numbers of notifications of (a) meningitis and (b) mumps for each week of 2004 in England and Wales.

 Self-Assessment Exercise 2.2.4

1. Examine the data (Table 2.2.3) for meningitis and mumps, and briefly describe any trends that you see for the two diseases. You may wish to plot these data on a graph to help you to see the patterns.

2. Make a list of possible explanations for these variations, indicating which are likely to explain the variations in (a) meningitis and (b) mumps.

Answers in Section 2.8

Table 2.2.3 Numbers of cases of meningitis (all) and mumps for each week of 2004, England and Wales

Month	Week beginning	Meningitis (all)	Mumps
January	2	54	37
	9	57	115
	16	24	74
	23	37	110
	30	35	83
February	6	27	107
	13	31	83
	20	37	85
	27	29	98

March	5	29	117
	12	24	89
	19	31	124
	26	20	130
April	2	30	127
	9	17	122
	16	26	131
	23	37	162
	30	12	227
May	7	20	181
	14	27	291
	21	19	241
	28	27	306
June	4	20	257
	11	22	217
	18	18	288
	25	18	251
July	2	26	219
	9	13	298
	16	28	278
	23	16	333
	30	14	323
August	6	24	308
	13	22	248
	20	24	253
	27	16	234
September	3	14	162
	10	17	295
	17	15	211
	24	20	280
October	1	11	220
	8	18	276
	15	24	372
	22	24	395
	29	26	475
November	5	23	537
	12	22	702
	19	19	756
	26	20	950
December	3	17	992
	10	18	988
	17	19	915
	24	33	956
	31	18	460
Total		1221	16489

Source: http://www.hpa.org.uk

As a final example from communicable diseases, we will examine the variations by age of meningitis. The data are shown in Table 2.2.4 below.

Table 2.2.4 Provisional notification rates per 100 000 for meningococcal meningitis, England and Wales 2004

Age group (years)	Males	Females
0–	576.92	361.80
1–4	101.37	71.29
5–9	21.99	23.71
10–14	14.23	16.20
15–44	18.56	18.48
45–64	10.24	9.37
65–74	8.53	9.82
75+	9.07	9.90

Source: http:// HPA Centre for Infections, CDSC, London.

 Self-Assessment Exercise 2.2.5

1. Examine the data in the table, and describe what they show.

2. Interpret your observations.

Answers in Section 2.8

We have now looked at three examples of variation by time in the incidence of communicable disease. In doing so, we have learned about how the diseases behave in the population, and have started to think about factors determining these variations. This emphasises again the value of simple *descriptive epidemiology*, and how it can be a useful first step in any investigation.

2.2.6 Illness seen in general practice

Although much illness (morbidity) is never brought to the attention of the health system, general practice (in the UK) represents a very comprehensive first point of contact between illness in the population and the opportunity to make and record a diagnosis. Thus, although it can never provide true population *incidence* and *prevalence*, information on contacts with general practice is an important resource of morbidity data.

Case study of asthma from the National Morbidity Studies

The UK, along with other developed countries, has seen an increase in the incidence (and prevalence) of asthma over the last 20 to 30 years. It might be thought that routine statistics should provide a simple enough explanation for this increase, but this is not the case. One problem with following trends in health data over a number of years is that the way a given condition is described can change. Changes in definitions may result from increasing knowledge about the condition and its relationship to other similar problems, or from a change in fashion about what is the proper term for a condition.

Changes such as these are certainly true for asthma. Over the last 20–30 years, the treatment of asthma has improved greatly. In the past, fear of this disease and the lack of adequate treatment led to unwillingness to discuss the diagnosis, especially for children. For young children, the term 'wheezy bronchitis' was often used.

As knowledge of asthma has increased, doctors have become more aware of the need to make a diagnosis earlier, institute effective treatment, and help the child and his/her parents to understand how to manage the condition in a way that minimises the adverse effects on the child's life and education. The term *diagnostic fashion* is used to describe how these various influences can change the way a disease or condition is described in medical practice over time, or between different places. Since quite a high proportion of asthma episodes are brought to the attention of general practice, the National Morbidity Studies provided a good opportunity to study trends in asthma, in conjunction with the other conditions with which it may have been confused over the years. Table 2.2.5, reproduced from data in the 1981 report, shows annual consultation rates per 1000 persons at risk of acute bronchitis, asthma and hay fever.

Table 2.2.5   Annual consultation rates per 1000 persons at risk

Condition	1955/56	1971/72	1981/82
Acute bronchitis	48.9*	59.1	58.2
Asthma	-**	9.6	17.8
Hay fever	-**	11.0	19.7

Source: Reproduced with permission from Third National Morbidity Study (1981), OPCS.
* Includes bronchitis unspecified. ** Data not available separately for these two conditions.

Even this source of information does not provide a full picture. For one thing, in the first (1955/56) report, data for asthma and hay fever were not available separately. Nevertheless, there is some important information here, which is examined through this next exercise.

 Self-Assessment Exercise 2.2.6

1. Make brief notes on the trends in consultation rates for the three conditions.

2. Does this help answer the question as to whether the change in asthma rates has resulted from a change in diagnostic fashion; that is, some cases of what used to be called acute (wheezy) bronchitis in the past are now (more properly) termed asthma?

3. In the light of your observations, what do these data suggest has happened to the true rates of asthma over the period studied?

Answers in Section 2.8

There are of course a lot of other issues to think about. We have looked here at consultation rates for all ages, and we would need to check rates in the various age groups, and whether these are consultations for a first or repeat episode. Most of this information is available in the reports. This example has illustrated that, for a given problem, any one routine data source can provide some answers, but some key issues remain uncertain and incomplete. Valuable though these routine data sources are, there is still often a need to examine the research question more specifically and precisely through the various study designs examined in subsequent chapters. However, simple descriptive epidemiological analysis can be very powerful. Section 2.6, on the health effects of the 'smogs' (air pollution) in London during the 1950s, provides a good example of this.

Summary

- The key to descriptive analysis is the presentation and interpretation of variations in measures of health and health determinants by time, place and person.

- When trying to understand the reasons for variations, it is useful to think whether the observed patterns are due to chance, artefact, or real effects.

- Good morbidity data are generally harder to come by than mortality data, but very useful information is nevertheless available from sources such as notification, cancer registration, and the GP morbidity surveys (and subsequent GP databases). Some other survey-based sources will be considered in Section 2.5.

2.3 Information on the environment

2.3.1 Air pollution and health

The influence of the environment on health is becoming an increasingly important social and political issue. In 1992, the United Nations convened the Rio Earth Summit, which examined the environmental threats, such as climate change, facing the world, and which led to the global programme on sustainable development known as Agenda-21. Air pollution is one such environmental concern, due to increased risk of respiratory and cardiovascular illness and death.

2.3.2 Routinely available data on air pollution

Local government environmental health departments in the UK have carried out air-quality monitoring for many years, and in Section 2.6 we shall look at some of the historical information recorded at the time of the serious 'smogs' (mixtures of smoke from coal fires and fog) that occurred in London in the early 1950s. The UK government has developed a National Air-Quality Strategy, one component of which is the development of accessible air-quality data on key pollutants, derived from national monitoring sites. These data are now available on the Internet at: http://www.airquality.co.uk/archive/index.php, where information is updated hourly (Figure 2.3.1).

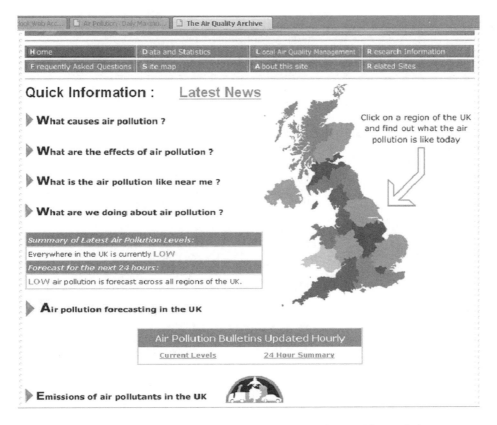

Figure 2.3.1 Example page from the Air Quality Archive website

The concentrations of a number of different pollutants are measured at various monitoring sites, which cover towns and cities in the UK. The pollutant we will look at is termed PM_{10}. This stands for particulate matter of aerodynamic diameter 10 microns or less (a micron is one-millionth of a metre). This pollutant, one of the most harmful components of smoke, is emitted by vehicle engines, burning of coal and other solid fuels in power stations, and other industrial processes. The importance of the size is that the smaller the particle, the further it can penetrate into the lungs.

The data in Table 2.3.1 are concentrations of PM_{10} recorded at each site at a particular point in time. The concentrations are measured in micrograms per cubic metre (one-millionth of a gram per cubic metre of air), written as $\mu g/m^3$. The locations are divided into rural and urban. There are only two rural locations, so we do not have much information about air pollution in rural areas. But what can the rest of the data tell us about levels of PM_{10} in urban areas? How do concentrations vary across the country? What is a 'typical' value? How can we compare PM_{10} concentrations from one time, or day, with another? We can gain some idea of the situation by looking at the individual data values listed, known as the ***raw data***, explored in the next exercise.

Table 2.3.1 Concentrations of PM_{10} in $\mu g/m^3$ from selected UK automatic monitoring sites at midday on a single day

Location	Concentration ($\mu g/m^3$)	Location	Concentration ($\mu g/m^3$)
Rural particulates (PM_{10})			
Northern Ireland	1.0	Rochester	22.0
Urban particulates (PM_{10})			
Edinburgh centre	0.4	Birmingham east	15.5
Glasgow centre	7.0	Birmingham centre	15.7
Newcastle centre	–	Thurrock	14.6
Belfast centre	14.3	London Bloomsbury	29.4
Middlesbrough	12.2	London Bexley	23.2
Leeds centre	18.0	London Hillingdon	30.7
Hull centre	15.6	London Brent	25.0
Stockport	–	Sutton Roadside	24.8
Bury Roadside	38.0	London Eltham	–
Manchester Piccadilly	16.6	London Kensington	24.9
Bolton	–	Haringey roadside	–
Liverpool centre	15.2	Camden kerbside	32.8
Sheffield centre	–	Swansea centre	23.0
Nottingham centre	13.0	Cardiff centre	15.0
Leicester centre	18.5	Port Talbot	20.1
Wolverhampton centre	16.2	Bristol centre	13.4
Leamington Spa	–	Southampton centre	30.0

 Self-Assessment Exercise 2.3.1

1. Find the locations with the lowest and highest concentrations.

2. Identify which locations did not record a level of PM_{10} at this time. What percentage of the urban locations is this?

Answers in Section 2.8

We can answer some of our other questions by picturing and summarising the data. This is worked through in the next section, where we will look at these air-pollution data in more detail.

2.4 Displaying, describing and presenting data

2.4.1 Displaying the data

In this section we will use the air-pollution data in Table 2.3.1 to introduce some basic statistical methods which are fundamental to the understanding and interpretation of information. Although we need the individual data values, also called ***observations***, or ***observed values*** of PM_{10}, to see the concentration of PM_{10} for any particular location, it is difficult to get the overall picture from a list of numbers. The first step in analysing the information in a data set is usually to picture the data in some way. Figure 2.4.1 shows one way of doing this.

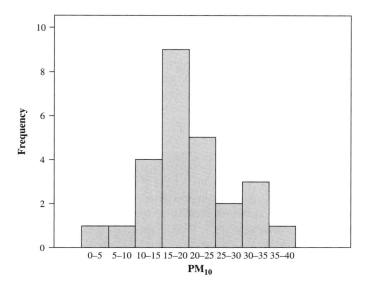

Figure 2.4.1 Histogram of the air-pollution data

This illustration is known as a ***histogram*** and presents the ***frequency distribution*** of the data. In this example the histogram shows the number (or ***frequency***) of air-pollution monitoring sites with PM_{10} concentrations in the intervals 0–5, 5–10, 10–15, and so on. Notice that there are no gaps between the bars representing frequency in the histogram. This is because PM_{10} concentration is a ***continuous*** measurement: theoretically, the concentration can be any value greater than or equal to 0, such as 0.5 or 23.65.

2.4.2 Calculating the frequency distribution

The frequency distribution is a table of numbers which shows how many of the data values are within each of a number of ***intervals***. The frequency distribution of PM_{10} concentrations that we displayed in the histogram is the number of measurements in each of the intervals 0–5, 5–10 and so on. The frequency distribution of a set of data is not unique, because the frequencies for each interval depend on how we choose the intervals. So to find the frequency distribution of a set of data, we first need to decide how to divide the data into intervals. Computer software can do this for you automatically, though you can also specify the intervals. To calculate the frequency distribution of the PM_{10} data by hand, the following procedure can be used.

Divide the PM_{10} scale into intervals

Between 5 and 20 intervals is a reasonable number to use. The smaller the number of observations, the fewer intervals we want (generally, not more than 10 intervals if we have fewer than 50 observations). The data values for the urban monitoring sites vary from 0.4 to 38.0 – a range of 37.6. To include all the data, we could start the first interval from 0.4, and, to achieve 10 intervals, each interval would have a width of $37.6/10 = 3.76$, or 4 to the nearest whole number. The intervals would then be

    0.4–4.4   4.4–8.4   8.4–12.4   . . . and so on

These are very messy numbers! We do not need to start at the smallest value, as long as the first interval starts at a smaller value. And dividing the data into any particular number of intervals, such as 10, is less important than having intervals of an 'easy' size, such as 5 or 10. So let's start again, with the first interval starting at 0 and each interval having width 5:

    0–5   5–10   10–15   15–20   20–25   25–30   . . . etc.

Count how many data values are within each interval

This is straightforward until we get to London Brent, which had a PM_{10} concentration of $25.0 \mu g/m^3$. Does this value fall in the interval 20–25 or 25–30? We can only count each value once – it cannot be in two intervals, so the intervals must not overlap. It is usual to define each interval to contain its lower boundary, but not its upper. So the interval from 20 to 25 includes 20.0, but not 25.0. Since the data are recorded to one decimal place, the largest value which can be included in 20–25 is $24.9 \mu g/m^3$. To emphasise this convention, the intervals may be written in one of the following alternative ways:

Alternative 1	0–	5–	10–	. . . etc.
Alternative 2	0–4.9	5–9.9	10–14.9	
Alternative 3	0–5–	5–10–	10–15–	

Seven urban locations do not have a value recorded, so we cannot include them in any of the intervals, but they should be noted. Now we can write down the complete frequency distribution as shown in Table 2.4.1. A frequency distribution is often just called a distribution.

Table 2.4.1 Frequency distribution of PM_{10} concentrations in 34 urban locations

PM_{10} ($\mu g/m^3$)	Frequency
0–5	1
5–10	1
10–15	5
15–20	9
20–25	5
25–30	2
30–35	3
35–40	1
Total*	27

*seven locations did not record PM_{10} at this time.

Summary: calculating a frequency distribution for continuous data

- Divide the range of the data into 5–20 <u>convenient</u> intervals of equal width.

- Avoid overlaps.

- Count how many observations fall within each interval.

 Self-Assessment Exercise 2.4.1

1. Calculate the frequency distribution of the urban-centre PM_{10} data using the intervals 0–4, 4–8, etc.

2. Draw a histogram of this distribution and compare it with the histogram with wider intervals, (Figure 2.4.1).

Answers in Section 2.8

Using too few intervals results in a histogram with few peaks and troughs which does not tell us very much about how the data values vary. Using too many intervals means that several of them may be empty, or contain only one observation. Although more detail can be seen, the histogram ceases to be a summary, and we do not get a very useful overall impression of the data. Choosing an appropriate number of intervals for the frequency may seem to be something of an art rather than a science. Experience and following the general rule of having between 5 and 20 intervals should result in a useful histogram.

2.4.3 Describing the distribution

We have seen that a list of raw data values is not very useful by itself. We generally want to summarise the data in a short description and a few numbers, so that we can present the important features of whatever we are measuring, or compare these data with another data set. We can summarise the information in a set of data by describing the *shape, location* and *spread* of the distribution.

Shape

We can see the *shape* from the histogram. We are interested in the overall shape, not the detail that results, for example, from having only a (relatively) small number of observations – we have only 34 monitoring sites.

You can imagine enclosing the histogram in a smooth curve, smoothing out the small ups and downs, to see the general shape. In Figure 2.4.2, this has been done (in SPSS) by fitting the normal distribution curve.

We describe the overall shape of the distribution in terms of how many peaks it has, whether it is approximately *symmetric* or *skewed* in one direction, and whether there are any marked deviations from the overall shape.

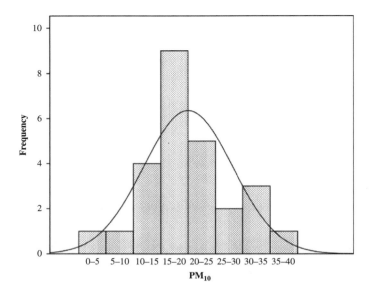

Figure 2.4.2 Distribution of PM_{10} (from Table 2.3.1, same as Figure 2.4.1), with normal curve fitted

Peaks are called ***modes***. A distribution with one distinct peak is called ***unimodal***; with two distinct peaks, it is called ***bimodal***. The distribution of the PM_{10} values we are studying is unimodal (Figure 2.4.2). The fact that the interval 30–35 has one more observation than the interval 25–30 is not important. It is sometimes difficult to decide whether a distribution is truly bimodal. It may help you to decide by knowing that most distributions of data are in fact unimodal, and that if a distribution really is bimodal, there is probably an explanation for this. For example, the histogram in Figure 2.4.3 illustrates the weights of a group of 92 students.

This distribution appears to have two distinct peaks. With the additional information that these are the weights of a mixed group of students (57 males and 35 females), we can be confident that this is a truly bimodal distribution: we would expect male students to be heavier than female students on average. In fact we have two overlapping (unimodal) distributions, one for female students and the other for male students.

The second feature of the distribution in which we are interested is whether it is symmetric or skewed (Figure 2.4.4). A distribution is ***symmetric*** if we can mentally divide it into two halves that are approximate mirror images. It is ***skewed*** to the right (also called ***positively skewed***) if the right tail (that is, the higher values) is much longer than the left tail. Again, we do not insist on exact symmetry in giving a general description of the shape of a distribution. Figure 2.4.4 shows two frequency distributions. The distribution of age at death is right skewed: the larger values are more spread out than the smaller values, giving a long right tail. The distribution of cholesterol levels is approximately symmetric. In both distributions, there is a gap: one interval does not contain any observations (age 60–65 and cholesterol level 312.5–337.5 mg/dl). These gaps are small and not important in describing the overall shape.

(a) Length of hospital stay (days) of a sample of 65 patients after minor surgery

(b) Height (centimetres) of a randomly selected sample of 45 men.

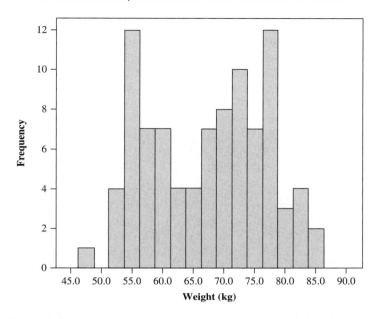

Figure 2.4.3 Histogram showing the distribution of student weights

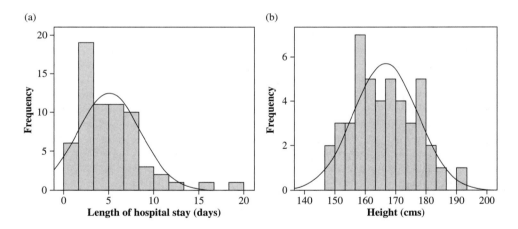

Figure 2.4.4 (a) a positively (right) skewed distribution and (b) a symmetric distribution

Most distributions of data are symmetric or right skewed. If the left tail is longer than the right tail, the distribution is *left skewed* (also called *negatively skewed*). Left and right refer to the sides of a histogram.

Lastly, in describing the shape of the distribution, we look for any marked deviations from the overall shape. Is there a large gap? Is there an isolated value (or values) far from the majority of data values? An individual observation that falls well outside the overall pattern of the data is called an ***outlier***. An outlier can arise in a number of ways. The value may have been measured or recorded incorrectly. Or it could be a correct value that is simply unusual, in which case it may be giving us important information. Apparent outliers should never be dismissed (see story of hole in the ozone layer, below). If possible, we should find out how the value arose.

In 1985, British scientists reported a hole in the ozone layer of the Earth's atmosphere over the South Pole. This is disturbing, because ozone protects us from cancer-causing ultraviolet radiation. The report was at first disregarded, because it was based on ground instruments looking up. More comprehensive observations from satellite instruments looking down showed nothing unusual. Then, examination of the satellite data revealed that the South Pole ozone readings were so low that the computer software used to analyse the data had automatically set these values aside as suspicious outliers, and not included them in the analysis. Readings back to 1979 were reanalysed and showed a large and growing hole in the ozone layer. Fortunately, although the outliers were omitted from the initial analysis, they were not discarded. It was therefore possible to reanalyse the data.

Reported in *The New York Times*

Here are some more data on student weights which illustrate another example of an outlier, and how this should be dealt with (Figure 2.4.5). Most of the data have an approximately symmetric

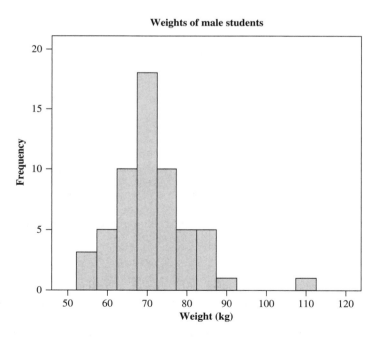

Figure 2.4.5 An outlier?

distribution, but one value (in the interval 107.5–112.5 kg) is far from the rest of the data. Is this the weight of a particularly heavy student, or has the value been recorded or input to the computer incorrectly? This value should be checked if possible, and any error corrected. In fact, a weight of around 110 kg is by no means impossible. Although it is much heavier than the other weights, this is not exceptionally heavy. If we cannot check the value, we should accept it as being correct. Outliers should never be dismissed, or ignored, simply because they spoil the look of the data!

Summary: describing the shape of a distribution

- Is the distribution unimodal or bimodal?

- Is it symmetric or skewed?

- Are there any large gaps or outliers?

 Self-Assessment Exercise 2.4.2

Look at Figure 2.4.1 (or the version in Figure 2.4.2) and describe the shape of the PM_{10} distribution.

Answers in Section 2.8

Location

We call the value around which a distribution is centred its location. We can roughly estimate this value from a histogram – this is easiest for an approximately symmetrical distribution. The central value of the distribution of PM_{10} values (Figure 2.4.1) is around $20 \, \mu g/m^3$. The central value of the distribution of cholesterol levels (Figure 2.4.4b) is around 235 mg/dl. Locating the centre of the distribution by eye is rather imprecise. To be more precise, we need to define what we mean by 'centre'. There is in fact more than one definition, resulting in different measures of location. These are the *mode, median* and *mean*.

Mode

We have already met one measure of location in describing the shape of the distribution: the *mode* is the value which occurs most frequently. We might say it is typical of the sorts of values that occur. When continuous data are grouped in a frequency distribution, the mode is the interval with the highest frequency, sometimes called the modal group – and this is the peak of the histogram. We can see from the histogram of the PM_{10} data (Figures 2.4.1 and 2.4.2) that most values lie between 15 and $20 \, \mu g/m^3$. The mode (or modal group) is $15–20 \, \mu g/m^3$. Note that the modal group will depend on how the intervals of the frequency distribution are chosen. The number of modes is important in describing the shape of a distribution, but the mode itself is not generally used to describe the location of a distribution of continuous values.

Mode: the mode of a distribution is the value, or group of values, which occur most often. The mode corresponds to the highest peak of a histogram.

Median

The simplest measure of location is literally the central, or middle, value of the distribution. This is called the ***median***, and half the observations fall above it and half below it. The median is often denoted by M. To find the median, we need to sort the data into ascending order. For example, the median of the values 12, 7, 6, 9 and 14 is 9.

> Median of five values:
> 6   7   **9**   12   14

We have 27 observations of urban PM_{10} concentration. The middle value of 27 is the 14th value (this is the $[(27+1)/2]$th value). Arranging the observations in ascending order and counting 14 from the smallest, we find the median concentration is $16.6 \mu g/m^3$, for Manchester Piccadilly:

Location	PM_{10}	Order	
Edinburgh centre	0.4	1	
Glasgow centre	7.0	2	
Middlesbrough	12.2	3	
Nottingham centre	13.0	4	
Bristol centre	13.4	5	
Belfast centre	14.3	6	
Thurrock	14.6	7	
Cardiff centre	15.0	8	
Liverpool centre	15.2	9	
Birmingham cast	15.5	10	
Hull centre	15.6	11	
Birmingham centre	15.7	12	
Wolverhampton centre	16.2	13	
Manchester Piccadilly	**16.6**	**14**	← **middle value is 16.6**
Leeds centre	18.0	15	
Leicester centre	18.5	16	
Port Talbot	20.1	17	
Swansea centre	23.0	18	
London Bexley	23.2	19	
Sutton Roadside	24.8	20	
London Kensington	24.9	21	
London Brent	25.0	22	
London Bloomsbury	29.4	23	
Southampton centre	30.0	24	
London Hillingdon	30.7	25	
Camden kerbside	32.8	26	
Bury roadside	38.0	27	

So if we have an odd number of observations, the median is the middle value. If we have an even number of observations, the median is defined to be halfway between the ***two*** middle values. For example, the median of the values 12, 7, 6, 9, 14 and 18 is halfway between 9 and 12; that is, 10.5.

$$6 \quad 7 \quad \mathbf{9} \quad \mathbf{12} \quad 14 \quad 18$$
$$\text{Median} = \frac{9+12}{2} = 10.5$$

Summary: median

The median M of a distribution is the middle value. To find the median:

1. Arrange the observations in order of size from smallest to largest.

2. If the number n of observations is odd, the median is the middle observation. This is the $(n+1)/2$th observation, counting from the smallest observation.

3. If the number n of observations is even, the median is halfway between the middle two observations. This is the average of the $n/2$th and $(n/2+1)$th observations.

The median is usually stated to the accuracy of the data, or to one more decimal place.

Although the *median* is the simplest measure of location, it is not the most commonly used. The most commonly used is the *mean*.

Mean

The *mean* is the arithmetic average of the observations, and is calculated by adding together all the observations and dividing by the number of observations. The mean of the urban PM_{10} observations (Table 2.3.1) therefore is:

$$\frac{0.4 + 7.0 + \cdots + 30.0}{27} = \frac{523.1}{27} = 19.37 \mu g/m^3$$

The mean is denoted by $\bar{x}$ (pronounced 'x bar'), and the individual observations by $x_1, x_2, \ldots$ and so on. For example, the first observation in the urban PM_{10} data set is 0.4, so $x_1 = 0.4$.

Summary: mean

If we denote n observations by $x_1, x_2, \ldots, x_n$, then the mean of the observations is

$$\bar{x} = \frac{1}{n}(x_1 + x_2 + \cdots + x_n)$$

This can also be written $\bar{x} = \frac{1}{n} \sum x_i$

The mean is usually stated to one more significant figure than the data.

The Greek letter $\sum$ (capital sigma) is shorthand for 'add up all the values'.

Self-Assessment Exercise 2.4.3

1. Use Table 2.3.1 to list the PM_{10} concentrations for the London locations. These include Sutton roadside, Haringey roadside and Camden kerbside.

2. Find the mean and median of these values.

Answers in Section 2.8

The median and mean compared

The median is just one observation (or the average of two observations) from the distribution. The other observations do not have a direct effect on the median; only their relative values are important. The mean, however, is calculated from **all** the observations: they all contribute equally to the value of the mean. The largest observed value of PM_{10} concentration was $38.0 \, \mu g/m^3$ at Bury roadside. Suppose this value was not $38.0 \, \mu g/m^3$, but $138.0 \, \mu g/m^3$ – an outlier. The median of the new distribution is still $16.6 \, \mu g/m^3$ – the middle value has not changed. However, the mean changes from $19.37 \, \mu g/m^3$ to $23.08 \, \mu g/m^3$, a substantial increase of almost 20 per cent. All the observations are included in the calculation of the mean, so it is **sensitive** to a few extreme observations.

In this example, we may exclude the outlier of $138.0 \, \mu g/m^3$ as atypical (the mean of the remaining 26 observations is $18.66 \, \mu g/m^3$; the median is $16.4 \, \mu g/m^3$). However, a skewed distribution with no outliers will also 'pull' the mean towards its long tail. So, for a right-skewed distribution, the mean will be greater than the median. If the distribution is left skewed, the median will be greater than the mean. Because the mean is sensitive to extreme observations – that is, it cannot resist their influence – we say that it is not a **resistant measure** of location. The median is a resistant measure. A resistant measure is not strongly influenced by outliers or by changes in a few observations, no matter how large the changes are.

Median or mean?

We have defined three measures of the location of a distribution, the mode, the median and the mean. We usually choose between the mean and the median. These are calculated in different ways, and as we have seen for the PM_{10} data, do not generally have the same value. They also have different properties: the median is resistant, whereas the mean is not. So which should we use to describe the central value of a distribution? The mean and the median both have the same value for symmetric distributions. In this situation, it does not really matter which we use. However, the mean is used in preference to the median for several reasons:

- It contains more information than the median (it is calculated from all the data values).

- The data do not need to be ordered to find the mean.

- The mean has useful mathematical properties.

For a skewed distribution, the mean and median will differ, and the stronger the skew, the greater the difference. In this case, the median is often used to describe the location of the distribution. This is because it is resistant to the extreme values, and thought to represent better the centre of the distribution. However, although the median is a useful summary measure, we shall see that, when we want to make comparisons between different distributions, we often use the mean even for skewed distributions, because of its mathematical properties.

Summary: measuring the location of a distribution

1. Location can be measured by the mean or median.

2. The mean is generally preferred to the median because of its mathematical properties.

3. The median may be a better measure of location for skewed distributions: it is resistant.

 Self-Assessment Exercise 2.4.4

1. Which of the following are correct statements? The shape of a distribution can be described by

   (a) a histogram

   (b) the mean

   (c) the mode

   (d) the number of modes.

2. Which **two** of the following are correct statements?

   (a) In a right-skewed distribution, the median is greater than the mean.

   (b) A skewed distribution is unimodal.

   (c) In a right-skewed distribution, most observations are less than the mean.

   (d) In a left-skewed distribution, the left tail is shorter than the right tail.

   (e) In a positively skewed distribution, the left tail is shorter than the right tail.

3. Figure 2.4.6 shows two distributions. In each case, at which point (a, b or c) does the mean lie, and at which point does the median lie?

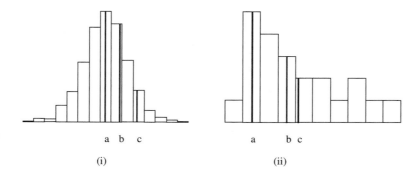

Figure 2.4.6 Mean and median

Answers in Section 2.8

Spread

Lastly, we summarise the information in a set of data by a measure of how variable the data are; in other words, how spread out. As well as the location of the distribution, it is important to know whether the values are bunched together or well spread out (Figure 2.4.7).

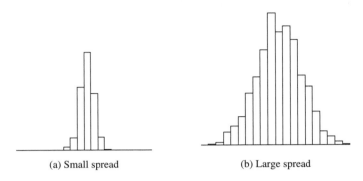

(a) Small spread   (b) Large spread

Figure 2.4.7   A distribution bunched together (a) or well spread out (b)

Again, there are several ways in which we can measure the distribution. The simplest measure is the *range*, which is simply the difference between the smallest and largest values. However, this is not a very useful measure. Because it is calculated from the two extreme values, it is not a resistant measure, and it does not tell us how spread out the majority of the data values are.

Interquartile range

An alternative measure that is resistant is the ***interquartile range*** (IQR). This is the range covered by the middle half of the data (Figure 2.4.8).

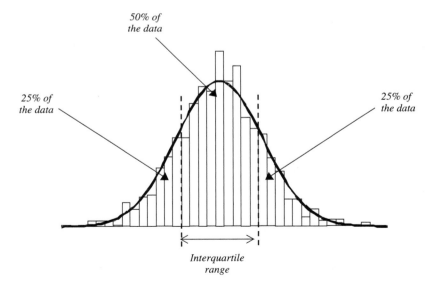

Figure 2.4.8   The interquartile range

One method for calculating the IQR is now described. The value below which 25 per cent, or one-quarter, of the data values fall is called the *first (or lower) quartile*. The value below which 75 per cent of the data falls (that is, one-quarter of the data are above this value) is called the *third (or upper) quartile*. The second quartile is the median. The first and third quartiles are usually denoted by Q_1 and Q_3, and the interquartile range IQR is the difference between the first and third quartiles, $IQR = Q_3 - Q_1$.

To find the quartiles, we need to sort the data into ascending order, as we did to find the median. Remember that the median is the middle value of the distribution; that is, 50 per cent of the values fall below it and 50 per cent are above it. So the first quartile is halfway between the smallest value and the median, and the third quartile is halfway between the median and the largest value. Here are the ordered PM_{10} data for urban monitoring sites again:

Location	PM_{10}	Order	
Edinburgh centre	0.4	1	
Glasgow centre	7.0	2	
Middlesbrough	12.2	3	
Nottingham centre	13.0	4	
Bristol centre	13.4	5	
Belfast centre	14.3	6	
Thurrock	**14.6**	**7**	← **first quartile is 14.6**
Cardiff centre	15.0	8	
Liverpool centre	15.2	9	
Birmingham east	15.5	10	
Hull centre	15.6	11	
Birmingham centre	15.7	12	
Wolverhampton centre	16.2	13	
Manchester Piccadilly	**16.6**	**14**	← **middle value is 16.6**
Leeds centre	18.0	15	
Leicester centre	18.5	16	
Port Talbot	20.1	17	
Swansea centre	23.0	18	
London Bexley	23.2	19	
Sutton roadside	24.8	20	
London Kensington	**24.9**	**21**	← **third quartile is 24.9**
London Brent	25.0	22	
London Bloomsbury	29.4	23	
Southampton centre	30.0	24	
London Hillingdon	30.7	25	
Camden kerbside	32.8	26	
Bury roadside	38.0	27	

There are 27 values, so the median is the 14th value. There are 13 values below the median and 13 values above, so the first quartile is the 7th value (the middle of 13), counting from the smallest, and the third quartile is the 7th value, counting back from the largest; that is, the 21st value. Using the ordered data given above, the first quartile is 14.6 and the third quartile is 24.9. The interquartile range is therefore $IQR = 24.9 - 14.6 = 10.3 \, \mu g/m^3$.

Summary: interquartile range

- The interquartile range is the difference between the first and third quartiles.

- The first and third quartiles (Q_1 and Q_3) are the values such that 25 per cent and 75 per cent, respectively, of the observations fall below them.

- To find the quartiles, first locate the median of the distribution. The first quartile is then the median of the values below the median, and the third quartile is the median of the values above the median.

- The interquartile range is $IQR = Q_3 - Q_1$.

Standard deviation

The most commonly used measure of the spread of a distribution is the **standard deviation**, or its square, the **variance**. This is not a resistant measure. It is a measure of how spread out the data are around the mean, so we only use the standard deviation as the measure of spread in conjunction with the mean as the measure of location. The variance is calculated by adding up the squared deviations from the mean (which are the differences between each observation and the mean value), and dividing by the number of observations less one. This gives the average squared deviation. For the PM_{10} data, the mean is $19.37\,\mu g/m^3$, and the deviations from the mean are $(0.4{-}19.37)$, $(7.0{-}19.37)$, $(14.3{-}19.37)$, and so on. The sum of squared deviations is therefore

$$(0.4 - 19.37)^2 + (7.0 - 19.37)^2 + (14.3 - 19.37)^2 + \ldots + (38.0 - 19.37)^2 = 1778.0119$$

and the variance is $1778.0119/(27 - 1) = 68.38507308 \approx 68.39$. The sum of squared deviations is shortened to **sum of squares**, and the number of observations less one $(n - 1)$ is called the **degrees of freedom** (see box below). So we have that

$$\text{variance} = \frac{\text{sum of squares}}{\text{degrees of freedom}}$$

If the observations are widely spread about the mean, the deviations will be large, and the variance will be large. If the observations are all close to the mean, the variance will be small. To calculate the variance, we square the deviations from the mean, so the variance does not have the same units of measurements as the data. Rather than measuring spread by the variance, we generally use the square root of the variance, called the **standard deviation**. The standard deviation measures spread about the mean in the original units.

Degrees of freedom

The term degrees of freedom (df) is a measure of the number of independent pieces of information on which the precision of an estimate is based. The degrees of freedom for an estimate equals the number of observations minus the number of additional parameters estimated for that calculation.

The standard deviation of the urban PM_{10} concentrations is $\sqrt{68.38507308} \approx 8.27\,\mu g/m^3$. The variance and standard deviation are usually stated to one more significant figure than the data. However, when calculating them, full accuracy should be retained for intermediate calculations, and only the final answer rounded. The variance is denoted by s^2 and the standard deviation by s.

 ### *RS - Reference section on statistical methods*

This section summarises the mathematical formula for variance and the relationship between variance and standard deviation. It also provides an easier alternative formula for standard deviation, for use with calculators. The variance of n observations $x_1, x_2, \ldots, x_n$, is

$$s^2 = \frac{1}{n-1}\left[(x_1 - \bar{x})^2 + (x_2 - \bar{x})^2 + \cdots + (x_n - \bar{x})^2\right]$$

This can also be written

$$s^2 = \frac{1}{n-1}\sum(x_i - \bar{x})^2$$

The standard deviation s is the square root of the variance. The variance and standard deviation are usually stated to one more significant figure than the data. Many calculators will calculate variance and standard deviation directly from the data. If you need to calculate them by hand, it is easier to use an alternative, but equivalent, formula, for the variance:

$$s^2 = \frac{1}{n-1}\left[\sum x_i^2 - \frac{1}{n}\left(\sum x_i\right)^2\right]$$

This formula uses the sum of all the data values ($\sum x_i$) and the sum of all the squared data values ($\sum x_i^2$). To calculate the variance of the PM_{10} data using this formula, we need the sum of all the values, which is 523.1 (we found this when we calculated the mean in Section 2.4.3), and the sum of all the squared values. This is

$$0.4^2 + 7.0^2 + \cdots + 38.0^2 = 11912.59$$

So the variance is

$$\frac{1}{26}\left[11912.59 - \frac{1}{27}(523.1)^2\right] = 68.38507123 \approx 68.39\mu g/m^3$$

as we found before. The slight difference in the unrounded value is because, when we first calculated the variance, we used the value of the mean rounded to two decimal places, not the exact value.

 ### *RS - ends*

Measures of spread for mean and median

We have seen that the interquartile range is related to the median (the quartiles are the medians of the two halves of the data, below and above the median), and that the standard deviation isrelated to the mean (it is a measure of variation about the mean). These measures of location and spread are always used in these combinations: *mean and standard deviation* or *median and interquartile range*. It does not make sense to mix them.

Summary: measuring the spread of a distribution

1. Spread can be measured by the standard deviation or the interquartile range.

2. The standard deviation is generally preferred.

3. The interquartile range may be more useful for skewed distributions. It is resistant.

4. The standard deviation is used when the mean is used as the measure of location.

5. The interquartile range is used when the median is used as the measure of location.

 Self-Assessment Exercise 2.4.5

1. Find the interquartile range of the PM_{10} concentrations for the London locations that you listed in Exercise 2.4.3.

2. Use a calculator (if you wish to try calculating this yourself) or computer to find the standard deviation.

Answers in Section 2.8

Summary: describing the distribution of a set of data

- We describe a distribution by its shape, location and spread.

- The shape indicates whether the distribution is unimodal or bimodal, symmetric or skewed in one direction, and whether there are any gaps or outliers.

- The location is the value around which the distribution is centred. This is measured by the mean or median. The median is resistant to extreme values and outliers.

- The spread is how variable the values are. This is measured by the standard deviation or the interquartile range. The interquartile range is a resistant measure.

- We use the mean and standard deviation to summarise the location and spread of an approximately symmetric distribution. We may use the median and interquartile range to summarise the location and spread of a skewed distribution.

An example of 'summarised' data

This lengthy explanation of how we describe a distribution may lead you to think that summarising and describing data is a lengthy task. We should, however, be able to summarise the important features of a set of data quite briefly – otherwise it is not a summary! Here is a summary of the data on PM_{10} concentrations, drawn together from the text and exercises.

The concentration of PM_{10} in the air was recorded at 27 urban locations at a particular point in time. No data were available for a further seven locations with monitoring equipment.

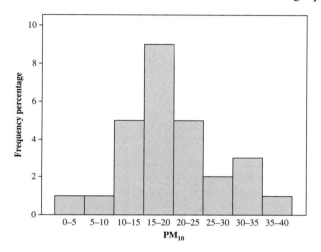

The histogram shows the distribution of the data. The distribution is unimodal and slightly right skewed, with no outliers. The mean PM_{10} concentration is $19.37 \, \mu g/m^3$, and the standard deviation $8.27 \, \mu g/m^3$.

Remember that throughout this section we have been dealing with **continuous** data: measurements that can take any value within some range (such as any value greater than zero). Later we will meet other types of data which can take only particular values, such as number of children of a partnership (0, 1, 2, etc.) and blood group (one of four groups). We will use different techniques to describe and summarise this type of data. For now, in the next section, we will look at another useful way of displaying continuous data – the *relative frequency distribution*.

2.4.4 The relative frequency distribution

Histograms may be used to display the *relative frequency distribution* instead of the frequency distribution. The relative frequencies are the percentages or proportions of the total frequency which are in each interval. For example, for the PM_{10} data (Table 2.4.1), there is one observation (Edinburgh $0.4 \, \mu g/m^3$) in the interval $0–5 \, \mu g/m^3$. This is one out of 27 observations; that is, 3.7 per cent of the observations. We say that the relative frequency of the $0–5 \, \mu g/m^3$ interval is 3.7 per cent (Table 2.4.2). Similarly, the relative frequency of PM_{10} values in the interval $15–20 \, \mu g/m^3$ is $(9/27) \times 100\% = 33.3\%$:

Figure 2.4.9 is identical to our original histogram of the frequency distribution in Figure 2.4.1 apart from having a different scale on the vertical axis (percentage, instead of frequency/number).

Table 2.4.2 Relative frequency distribution of PM_{10} concentrations in 34 urban locations at a particular point in time

PM_{10} ($\mu g/m^3$)	Frequency	Relative Frequency (%)
0–5	1	3.7
5–10	1	3.7
10–15	5	18.5
15–20	9	33.3
20–25	5	18.5
25–30	2	7.4
30–35	3	11.1
35–40	1	3.7
Total*	27	99.9

* Seven locations did not record PM_{10} at this time.

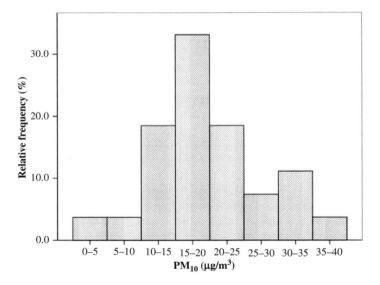

Figure 2.4.9 Relative frequency distribution of PM_{10} data

So what use is it? Relative frequency histograms are useful if we want to compare two or more distributions with different numbers of observations.

For example, if we want to compare the age distribution of Liverpool with that of England and Wales, the frequency histogram for the latter towers over the one for Liverpool and the bars of the histogram for Liverpool can barely be seen, Figure 2.4.10(a).

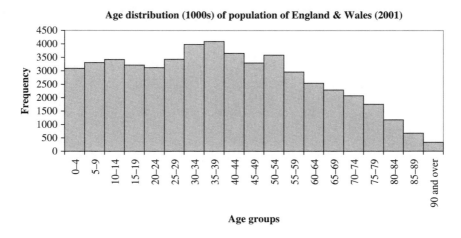

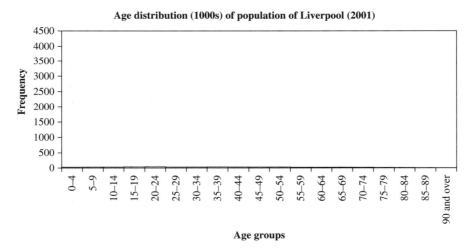

Figure 2.4.10(a)   Frequency histograms for (i) England and Wales, and (ii) Liverpool

However, if both histograms have a vertical scale which is a percentage (relative frequency), we can more easily compare the shapes of the two distributions, Figure 2.4.10(b). We can see that the age distributions of Liverpool and England and Wales were very similar in 2001, although Liverpool had a larger proportion of young adults.

Exercise on displaying, describing and presenting data

In this exercise you will have the opportunity to practise the techniques that have been introduced in this section, using another set of air-pollution data. The data are PM_{10} concentrations recorded at urban monitoring sites some 5 hours after the data we have been studying (Table 2.3.1) were recorded.

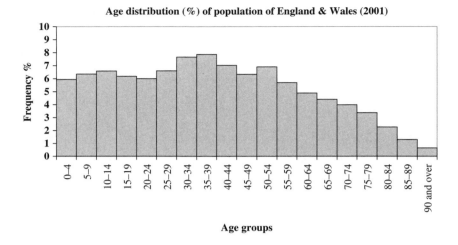

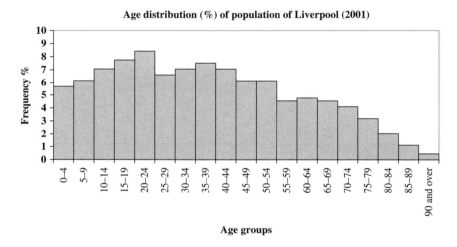

Figure 2.4.10(b)   Relative frequency histograms for (i) England and Wales, and (ii) Liverpool

 Self-Assessment Exercise 2.4.6

1. Using the data in Table 2.4.3, calculate the frequency distribution in intervals of width $5\,\mu g/m^3$, and present the distribution in a table.

2. Prepare a histogram (draw or use a computer) of the frequency distribution and describe its shape.

3. Use a calculator (if you wish to try calculating this yourself) or computer to find the mean and standard deviation of the data.

Table 2.4.3 Concentrations of urban PM_{10} from UK automatic monitoring sites at 5 pm, 5 hours after concentrations previously recorded

Location	Concentration ($\mu g/m^3$)	Location	Concentration ($\mu g/m^3$)
Edinburgh centre	29.0	Birmingham east	31.0
Glasgow centre	43.0	Birmingham centre	31.0
Newcastle centre	33.0	Thurrock	28.0
Belfast centre	49.0	London Bloomsbury	34.0
Middlesbrough	–	London Bexley	25.0
Leeds centre	164.0	London Hillingdon	25.0
Hull centre	39.0	London Brent	28.0
Stockport	28.0	Sutton roadside	32.6
Bury roadside	–	London Eltham	23.6
Manchester Piccadilly	37.0	London Kensington	27.2
Bolton	–	Haringey roadside	33.5
Liverpool centre	34.0	Camden kerbside	46.3
Sheffield centre	45.0	Swansea centre	29.0
Nottingham centre	51.0	Cardiff centre	42.0
Leicester centre	33.0	Port Talbot	2.0
Wolverhampton centre	38.0	Bristol centre	42.0
Leamington Spa	32.0	Southampton centre	25.0

4. Write two or three sentences comparing the distribution of PM_{10} concentrations at 5 pm with that at midday (see Section 2.3.4 for an example of how to summarise data).

Answers in Section 2.8

2.4.5 Scatterplots, linear relationships and correlation

We have been studying measurements that vary from one location, or time, to another. A quantity that varies is called a *variable*. Thus, PM_{10} concentration at a particular time is a variable (it varies from location to location); blood pressure is another variable (it varies from person to person). These are both examples of *continuous variables*: the values they can take form a continuous range.

Two variables are said to be related, or associated, if knowing the value of one variable provides some information about the value of the other variable. For example, knowing a person's height tells us something about what their weight might be: weight and height are related. It is not a perfect relationship of course – knowing someone's height does not tell us exactly how much they weigh. In this section, we shall look at how to display and summarise the relationship between two continuous variables, each measured for the same individuals (people, locations, countries, or whatever). Table 2.4.4 shows the gestational ages and birthweights for 24 babies.

Table 2.4.4   Gestational age and birthweight for 24 babies

Gestational age (weeks)	Birthweight (kg)	Gestational age (weeks)	Birthweight (kg)
40	2.968	40	3.317
38	2.795	36	2.729
40	3.163	40	2.935
35	2.925	38	2.754
36	2.625	42	3.210
37	2.847	39	2.817
41	3.292	40	3.126
40	3.473	37	2.539
37	2.628	36	2.412
38	3.176	38	2.991
40	3.421	39	2.875
38	2.975	40	3.231

Scatterplots

We have a set of gestational ages and a set of birthweights for the same babies – the two values in each half-row are linked by the fact that they correspond to the same baby. We would like to display and summarise the data, just as we did with a set of values of one variable. We begin by picturing the information we have. We could construct a histogram of ages and a histogram of birthweight, but we would then lose the vital information that the measurements are linked. The appropriate picture is a *scatterplot* (Figure 2.4.11).

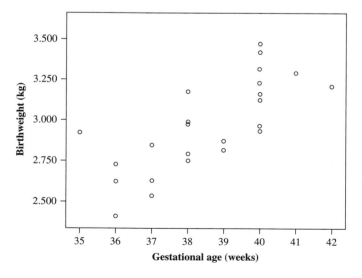

Figure 2.4.11   Birthweight and gestational age of babies

Each point on the scatterplot corresponds to one baby. Note that the scales on the two axes do not start at zero. It is not necessary for scales to start at zero, but they should always be clearly labelled, and show the units of measurement as well as the values. If we started at zero, the plot would include a lot of empty space, and the data, the vital information that we are interested in, would be squashed up and less clear (Figure 2.4.12).

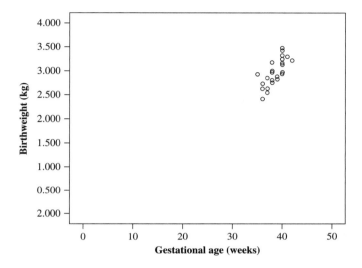

Figure 2.4.12 An uninformative scatterplot

The babies' gestational ages and birthweights are clearly related, despite a lot of variation in birthweight for any particular gestational age. Overall, high values of one are associated with high values of the other. We describe the relationship between the variables in terms of the *form* of the relationship, the *strength* of the relationship, and whether it is *positive* or *negative*.

Linear and non-linear relationships

The simplest form of relationship between two variables is a *linear* relationship. This means that the overall pattern of the data can be described by a straight line. It does not mean that the points in the scatterplot lie exactly on a straight line. This would be a perfect linear relationship, which is rarely observed in practice. In our example, we do not expect gestational age and birthweight to have a perfect relationship, because gestational age is only one of a number of factors which may affect birthweight. Even when a relationship is governed by an exact physical law (such as the relationship between voltage and current for fixed resistance), we would not expect to get a straight line plot from measurements of voltage and current. This is because there would be errors in our measurements.

What we are looking for is whether the points on the scatterplot are roughly grouped around a straight line, without showing any obvious non-linear pattern such as is seen in the following example of road casualties that show a cyclical pattern (Figure 2.4.13).

We can describe the relationship between gestational age and birthweight as approximately linear: there is no obvious non-linear pattern. If the points in a scatterplot lie close to a straight line,

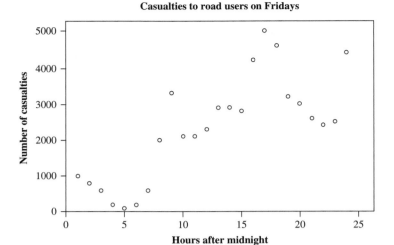

Figure 2.4.13 A non-linear relationship

we say there is a strong linear relationship. Conversely, if they are widely spread, the relationship is weak (Figure 2.4.14).

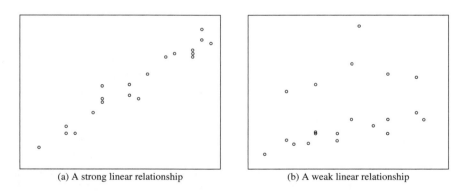

(a) A strong linear relationship   (b) A weak linear relationship

Figure 2.4.14 Strong and weak linear relationships

Finally, we need to say whether the relationship is positive or negative. In a positive relationship, high values of one variable are associated with high variables of the other (and low values of the two variables are associated). In a negative relationship, high values of one variable are associated with low values of the other (Figure 2.4.15).

We can therefore describe the relationship between gestational age and birthweight for the babies in Table 2.4.4 as a fairly strong, positive, linear relationship.

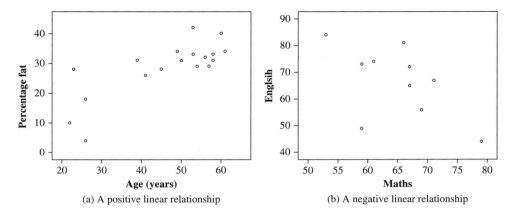

Figure 2.4.15 (a) A positive linear relationship between age and the percentage of body fat, and (b) a negative linear relationship between exam scores for maths and English

 Self-Assessment Exercise 2.4.7

The scatterplot shows the percentage of births attended by trained health personnel (1983–90) and the under-5 mortality rate (1990) for 33 countries. Describe the relationship between under-5 mortality and the percentage of births attended.

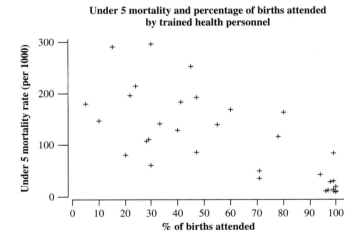

Source: The State of the World's Children (1992).

Answers in Section 2.8

The correlation coefficient

A scatterplot shows the direction, form and strength of any association, and is an important first step in investigating the data. However, the interpretation of a scatterplot by eye is subjective. For example, changing the scale or the amount of white space on the plot affects our perception of a linear, or any other, pattern. We can summarise the strength of a linear relationship with a single number, the *correlation coefficient*. This is a measure calculated from the data, and it has an objective interpretation.

The value of the correlation coefficient always lies between -1 and $+1$, with -1 corresponding to a perfect negative relationship (the points lie on a straight line sloping from top left to bottom right), and $+1$ corresponding to a perfect positive relationship (the points lie on a straight line sloping from bottom left to top right). For any relationship that is not exactly linear, the correlation coefficient lies somewhere between -1 and $+1$. A positive relationship has a positive correlation coefficient, and a negative relationship a negative coefficient. A value of zero means that there is no *linear* association between the two variables (but note that it is possible for variables with a correlation coefficient of zero to be non-linearly related).

The correlation coefficient calculated from a set of data is usually labelled r. Here are some sets of data with their correlation coefficients (Figure 2.4.16).

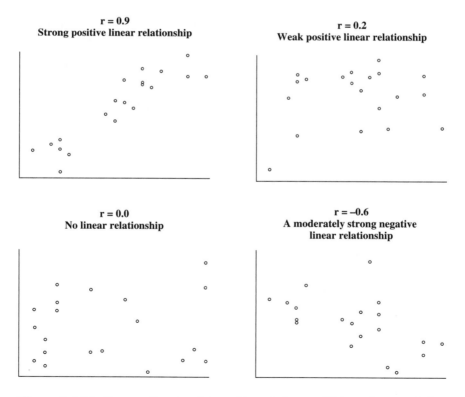

Figure 2.4.16 Range of scatterplots and correlation coefficients for association with strength varying from none to strong, and direction from positive, through none, to negative

RS - Reference section on statistical methods
Calculation of the correlation coefficient

To show how to calculate the correlation coefficient, with an example, we will label the values of one variable x and the other y. In our example, we may call the gestational ages of the babies x and the birthweights y. If we have n pairs of values (x, y), ($n = 24$ for the babies), then the correlation coefficient is defined as follows:

$$r = \frac{\sum (x - \bar{x})(y - \bar{y})}{\sqrt{\sum (x - \bar{x})^2 \sum (y - \bar{y})^2}}$$

where $\bar{x}$ and $\bar{y}$ are the means of the x and y values. The terms $(x - \bar{x})$ and $(y - \bar{y})$ are deviations from the means of the two sets of values. Many calculators will find the correlation coefficient directly, without the need to use the above formula. Correlation coefficients are also calculated by many computer spreadsheets and statistics packages. To find the correlation coefficient with a calculator which does not have statistical functions, it is easier to use an alternative, but equivalent, version of the formula:

$$r = \frac{\sum xy - (\sum x)(\sum y)/n}{\sqrt{\left[\sum x^2 - (\sum x)^2/n\right]\left[\sum y^2 - (\sum y)^2/n\right]}}$$

The expression $\sum xy$ means 'multiply each x value by the corresponding y value and then add them all together'. We can set out the calculation in a table. To calculate the correlation coefficient between gestational age and birthweight (Table 2.4.4), we need the following values:

Gestational age x	Birthweight y	x^2	y^2	xy
40	2.968	1600	8.809024	118.720
38	2.795	1444	7.812025	106.210
40	3.163	1600	10.004569	126.520
35	2.925	1225	8.555625	102.375
36	2.625	1296	6.890625	94.500
37	2.847	1369	8.105409	105.339
41	3.292	1681	10.837264	134.972
40	3.473	1600	12.061729	138.920
37	2.628	1369	6.906384	97.236
38	3.176	1444	10.086976	120.688
40	3.421	1600	11.703241	136.840
38	2.975	1444	8.850625	113.050
40	3.317	1600	11.002489	132.680
36	2.729	1296	7.447441	98.244
40	2.935	1600	8.614225	117.400
38	2.754	1444	7.584516	104.652
42	3.210	1764	10.304100	134.820
39	2.817	1521	7.935489	109.863

(Continued)

	Gestational age x	Birthweight y	x^2	y^2	xy
	40	3.126	1600	9.771876	125.040
	37	2.539	1369	6.446521	93.943
	36	2.412	1296	5.817744	86.832
	38	2.991	1444	8.946081	113.658
	39	2.875	1521	8.265625	112.125
	40	3.231	1600	10.439361	129.240
Total	**925**	**71.224**	**35727**	**213.198964**	**2753.867**

So the correlation coefficient is

$$r = \frac{2753.867 - 925 \times 71.224/24}{\sqrt{(35727 - 925^2/24)(213.198964 - 71.224^2/24)}} = 0.74$$

(Remember, in any mathematical calculation, always complete multiplication and division before addition and subtraction.)

The correlation coefficient is positive, showing that, on the whole, birthweight increases as gestational age increases. The value of 0.74 is closer to 1 than to 0 and indicates a fairly strong linear relationship between birthweight and gestational age.

  RS - ends

  ## Self-Assessment Exercise 2.4.8

The following data are population and total daily water consumption for 10 Scottish regions in 1995.

Region	Population (thousands)	Water consumption (megalitres/day)
Borders	105	32
Central	273	218
Dumfries and Galloway	148	76
Fife	351	146
Grampian	528	166
Highland	207	95
Lothian	754	284
Orkney and Shetland	43	22
Tayside	395	123
Western Isles	29	12

1. Draw a scatterplot of these data with water consumption on the vertical axis and describe the relationship between water consumption and population.

2. Using the information and formulae provided in the reference section (above) or a computer, we find the correlation coefficient between water consumption and population to be 0.89. (If you wish to try calculating the coefficient with the above formulae, the answer and explanation are provided in Section 2.8.) Interpret this result as fully as you can.

Answers in Section 2.8

Remember that the correlation tells us only about the strength of a *linear* association. Variables with a small correlation coefficient may have a strong non-linear relationship (Figure 2.4.17). This shows the importance of *picturing* the data on a scatterplot before calculating a correlation coefficient. For the examples in Figure 2.4.17, it is clearly inappropriate to calculate a measure of the strength of linear association.

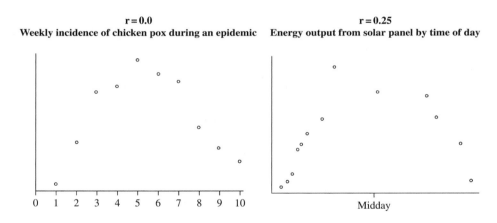

Figure 2.4.17 Non-linear relationships, and their respective correlation coefficients

Coefficient of determination

The correlation coefficient which we have defined is sometimes called the ***product moment correlation coefficient*** or the ***Pearson correlation coefficient***. This is because there are other correlation coefficients which can be defined to summarise the strength of association between variables which are not continuous (the most commonly used of these is the non-parametric Spearman rank correlation, which is described in Chapter 11). When the term 'correlation coefficient' is used on its own, it nearly always means the correlation coefficient between two continuous variables as defined here.

Note also that a useful interpretation of the numerical value of r is provided by the value r^2, termed the ***coefficient of determination***. It can be thought of as the amount of the total variation in one variable which can be 'explained' by the variation in the other variable.

In our example of birthweight and gestational age, it makes sense to try to explain birthweight in terms of gestational age, but not vice versa. We have already seen in the scatterplot how the birthweights varied for different gestational ages, and how the correlation coefficient $r = 0.74$ implied a fairly strong positive linear relationship between the two variables. If we now calculate $r^2 = 0.74 \times 0.74 = 0.55$, we get an idea of how much of the total variation in birthweight can actually be explained by the variation in the ages. In fact, only 55 per cent of the total variation in birthweight is explained by the variation in gestational age; the remaining 45 per cent of the variation is left unexplained and must be due to other factors which have not been considered in the analysis, or which are unknown.

Summary: the relationship between two continuous variables

- The values of two continuous variables, each observed for the same individuals, can be displayed in a scatterplot.

- The scatterplot shows the form, strength and direction of any relationship between the variables.

- The strength and direction of a linear association between continuous variables can be summarised by the correlation coefficient.

- The correlation coefficient has a value between -1 and $+1$. A value of -1 indicates a perfect negative relationship, $+1$ a perfect positive relationship, and 0 that there is no linear relationship between the variables.

- The correlation coefficient is commonly stated to two decimal places, but there is no general rule.

- Useful interpretation of the strength of a relationship is provided by the coefficient of determination, r^2.

2.5 Summary of routinely available data

2.5.1 Introduction

The examples of routinely available data we have looked at so far cover death statistics, infectious disease, illness episodes seen in general practice, and environmental pollution data. These sources cover a wide range of data, including legally required registration and notifications, health service records, and measurements made completely outside the health-care system. This emphasises the great variety of information routinely available about health and disease, and also the many factors which influence public health. These data are a valuable resource, but in using these data sources it is always important to remember their limitations, and to ask the following questions:

- What can I find out about how this information was collected and prepared?

- What is the nature and extent of any error or bias that has occurred in the data collection and preparation?

- If there are errors and bias, how much does it matter for the purposes I intend to use these data?

The next section reviews the nature, uses and limitations of some of the key routine data sources commonly used in health research.

2.5.2 Classification of health information sources

Routine data can be classified into three types:

- Demographic data: these data describe populations and therefore the number or characteristics of people at risk of ill health or mortality. Such information is required to interpret morbidity and mortality data.

- Health (disease) events data: these data describe health-related or disease events recorded through contact with health services.

- Population-based health information: these data include information on lifestyle and other aspects of health status that is not reliant on contact with health services. This kind of information is often one of the most useful in health-related research but is less easily identified through routine sources.

Routine data sources share a number of strengths and weaknesses, listed in Table 2.5.1. Table 2.5.2 gives examples of these different types of routinely available data sources in the UK.

Table 2.5.1 Strengths and weaknesses of routine data sources

Strengths	Weaknesses
• Readily available data; regularly updated.	• Often incomplete with a risk of imprecision and bias.
• Repeated analysis over time allows for assessment of trends.	• Limited details on some determinants of health such as ethnicity.
• Useful for baseline description of expected levels of disease and to identify hypotheses.	• Accessible but may be presented in a form that is difficult to interpret.
	• Many health services data are primarily intended for health services management rather than investigation of health status.

Table 2.5.2 Classification of routine data

Types of data	Examples
Demographic data	• National population census • Vital registration (births, marriages and deaths) • Continuous registration (e.g. registration with a GP) • Sample surveys (e.g. National Statistics Longitudinal Study)
Health (disease) event data	• Mortality data (death certification) • Hospital systems (morbidity data, hospital episode statistics, Körner data) • Community and GP systems (registers, audit data, vaccination data, family planning returns) • National disease registers, including cancer and congenital malformations

(Continued)

Table 2.5.2   *(Continued)*

Types of data	Examples
	• Communicable disease surveillance
	• EPACT (prescribing data via the NHS prescribing database)
Population-based health information	• Health surveys (e.g. General Household Survey, Health Survey for England)
	• Secondary data sets (e.g. Public Health Common Data Set)
	• Other health-related information (deprivation measures, local government data on transport, the environment, education, etc.)

2.5.3   Demographic data

Demography is the study of the size and structure of populations. Population size is affected by fertility, death and migration. Population structure includes consideration of age, sex, ethnicity, socio-economic status and geographical location. Key routine sources of data include the national population census, vital registration (births and deaths), population estimates and projections, and geographic location.

The national population census

Census data offer a reference-standard population estimate for analysis of population trends and are used to provide essential statistical information for epidemiology, to enable planning and funding of public services, and to support research and business.

The census provides extensive socio-economic data collected across the whole country at one point in time, data that can also be compared with previous censuses. Completion of the census is a legal requirement, so coverage of households (but not travelling populations) is good, with less than 0.5 per cent of households missed. (In 2001, a census coverage survey was undertaken to estimate the level of undercount and identify the characteristics of individuals or households missed by the main census.) Questions on the census form are piloted to minimise errors due to ambiguity in phrasing, and internal audit mechanisms aim to maximise the quality of data collation and analysis.

However, the census is expensive, time-consuming and an immense administrative task. In the UK (as in many countries), the census is carried out once every 10 years, and subnational population estimates in the run-up to the next census date may be inaccurate. This is because estimates can adjust for births, deaths and migration in and out of the country, but cannot accurately account for internal migration. There is also consistent undercounting of certain subgroups of the population, including young men, armed forces personnel, the homeless and travelling communities.

Data collection is dependent on self-report, and this may lead to inaccuracy and possible bias. Moreover, when forms are submitted, they are electronically read, so inaccurate completion of the form may lead to coding errors. In terms of trend analysis, the introduction of the poll tax negatively affected coverage rates in 1991 (and possibly 2001) with substantial undercounts among certain subgroups of people. Some changes in the wording of questions over time also affects the interpretation of longitudinal data. Important gaps in data collection, however, are being addressed. For example, questions on ethnicity were added in 1991.

Vital registration: births and deaths

Registration of births and deaths contributes to updating estimates of population size between census dates. Registration is a legal requirement, and a network of superintendent registrars and local registrars exists in the UK to oversee the process and report to National Statistics. The qualified informant (usually the nearest available relative) is responsible for notification.

Registration of births

It is a legal requirement to register a birth within 42 days. Information recorded includes the name, sex, and date and place of birth of the child; the name, date and place of birth, occupation, usual address, and number of previous children of the mother; and (if registered) the name, date and place of birth, and occupation of the father. Completeness of registration is good, as it is a legal requirement, but some of the accompanying information, such as the occupation, or place and date of birth of parents, may be less accurate.

Mortality statistics

Collection of mortality data is described at the beginning of this chapter. Mortality data are considered an extremely important routinely available data source. As with birth data, completeness is virtually 100 per cent, since registration is required before a body can be disposed of and death is an unequivocal event.

If information on the cause of death is not available at the time, the registrar can indicate that it will be available at a later date. This further information can then be added to the statistical system later, but will not be included in the public record. As we saw, there are clear guidelines on reporting deaths to the coroner for further investigation if the cause of death is unclear. The coroner is responsible for following this up by post-mortem examination (autopsy) and inquest if necessary. Cause of death is coded according to an international classification system (the International Classification of Disease (ICD)). Once the cause is coded, it is relatively straightforward to analyse data by cause of death.

Nevertheless, inaccuracies can be introduced at all stages in the process of collating mortality data, including clinical diagnosis of cause of death, completion of the death certification, coding of data and interpretation of statistics. Death certification is not a priority for many working clinicians, and coding relies entirely on data obtained from the certificate. In addition, death certification is becoming increasingly complex with multifactorial causes of death; as a result, accuracy of diagnosis varies between subgroups of the population. For example, cause of death in children is more likely to be investigated and correctly diagnosed than in the elderly. We have also seen how diagnostic fashions and 'less acceptable' causes of death, such as suicide, also influence what is entered on the certificate.

As noted earlier, ICD coding undergoes periodic revision, which has implications for analysis of disease trends, and bridging tables are produced to allow any necessary adjustments to be made. Finally, some of the data categories on a death certificate may be recorded less reliably than others. For example, occupational mortality data rely on the accuracy of information provided by informants about the type of employment and position held, which is not always reported accurately or systematically.

Population estimates and projections

Estimates of population size and distribution between census dates are produced with knowledge of births, deaths and migration. While registration of births and deaths is a legal requirement, migration is more complex. External migration (in and out of the UK) is relatively accurately recorded, although the effects of illegal immigration are hard to quantify. However, internal migration, that is, migration within the UK, can only be estimated from local knowledge; for example, the building of new housing estates and creation of new jobs. Thus, when we calculate mortality rates at a small area level, the accuracy of the data is affected by the effect of internal migration on census data.

Some short-term population projections can be quite accurate (for example, the expected numbers of 65–74-year-olds in 20 years' time: based on the present number of 45–54-year-olds and expected mortality rates). However, the number of schoolchildren in 30 years' time is harder to predict, as fertility rates may change. Population projections therefore often include a *sensitivity analysis*, giving a range of estimates for different assumptions of fertility rates.

2.5.4 Data which describe health events

Health events that trigger routine recording of data include:

- Death data: certain causes of death such as suicide and maternal mortality are subject to additional routine investigation (Confidential Enquiries).

- Hospital episode data: hospital episode statistics (HES) provide data which are relatively accurate and complete but capture only a small proportion of illness occurring within a community.

- General practice data: primary care data cover a wider spectrum of health episodes, but data collection is less well developed than in secondary care.

While HES and general practice data provide useful additional information on health and disease that we cannot obtain from mortality data alone, there are a number of problems with these data sources. Traditionally, most data collection focuses on analysis of process (for example, number of bed days per patient stay or completed consultant episodes) rather than treatment outcomes. This is because data collection systems were originally designed for service monitoring rather than evaluation or planning.

Mortality data for specific causes: Confidential Enquiries

Deaths from certain causes where preventative measures or better clinical management could reduce death rates undergo additional routine investigation. These so-called Confidential Enquiries fall under the remit of the National Institute for Health and Clinical Excellence (NICE) and include:

- The National Confidential Inquiry into Suicide and Homicide (NCISH), which examines suicide and homicide by people using mental health services.

- The Confidential Enquiry into Maternal and Child Health (CEMACH), which includes routinely published data on infant and maternal mortality.

- The National Confidential Enquiry into Patient Outcome and Death (CEPOD), which examines deaths following medical or surgical intervention.

Annual reports on these different causes of death are used to inform health service practice in the hope of reducing deaths from these causes in the future. However, the reports often focus on individual subcategories each year, limiting the scope for analysis of trends. Further information can be found on the NICE website: **http://www.nice.org.uk.**

Morbidity data from hospital systems

Mortality data do not, of course, provide an adequate assessment of the extent and nature of health need within a population. Morbidity (illness) data are clearly preferable when measuring health need, but collection of morbidity data brings new challenges in terms of completeness and accuracy. Currently, most morbidity data are collected through records of contact with health services, often reflecting more serious morbidity, although many factors other than nature of the disease influence hospital use. No single data source exists for morbidity data, and routine data within secondary care has largely been established to monitor service management rather than monitor morbidity for epidemiological purposes and health-care planning. This is apparent in the way that the data are collected and limits their utility from a population health perspective.

Hospital episodes statistics (HES)

HES include data on every episode of inpatient care (including day case interventions) in NHS hospitals in England since 1989. An episode of care is defined as a period of treatment under a particular consultant. In the NHS system, data collected include details of:

- the hospital, primary care trust (PCT) and GP

- the patient (age, sex, NHS number, postcode)

- the process of arrival and discharge

- the process of care, including number of consultant episodes and treatment received

- outcomes including disease diagnosis (by ICD code) and final outcome (death, discharged, etc.).

The information is routinely collected via the Patient Administration System. The simplicity of collection contributes to the data set being relatively complete. However, since it contains patient-identifiable information, for reasons of confidentiality the database cannot be accessed directly, but analyses can be requested.

Although the focus of these data is service management, ICD codes are available. While this is useful in terms of analysing data by clinical diagnosis, there are concerns with the accuracy of coding of diagnoses. This is because coding is based on finished consultant episode, not admission and discharge. For example, a patient admitted to hospital, having attended the accident and emergency department, will be registered under a particular consultant. Subsequently, their care may be transferred to another consultant – for example, a specialist in cardiology. These will be recorded as two separate episodes, since episodes are defined as periods of care under one consultant. As medical teams in hospitals become increasingly specialised, this may happen more often and add further complexity to interpretation of the data. Further information on hospital statistics can be obtained from the HES website at http://www.hesonline.nhs.uk.

Körner data

This is the main system for recording health service activity in hospital and community services for anything other than inpatient care. This includes accident and emergency attendance, ambulance attendance, diagnostic testing (including radiology and laboratory work), outpatient clinics, health visitors and community clinics. Returns are made quarterly or annually and provide data for human resources and financial planning. Published summaries are presented by broad clinical specialty.

National disease registers, such as the National Cancer Register

The National Cancer Register is collated by the National Cancer Intelligence Centre (NCIC) at National Statistics and is a secondary data set routinely collecting data on all cases of cancer diagnosed in the UK. The data set includes patient details (name, address, postcode, sex, NHS number, date of diagnosis, date of death); tumour details (type, stage, site, histology); treatment (what and when); and details of death (date, cause, place). The NCIC provides reports on regional and national cancer incidence, prevalence and survival. Information on risk factors for cancer, monitoring quality and effectiveness of cancer care, and evaluation of cancer screening programmes (e.g. breast, cervix), is also available for research.

Morbidity data from general practice

A high proportion, approximately 95%, of the population is registered with a GP, and 90 per cent of problems presented to primary care are dealt with in primary care. Knowledge of what happens here gives insight into 'minor illness', early stages of the natural history of disease, and, increasingly, chronic disease management. Data collection in primary care is therefore becoming progressively more important. Practice records contain a wealth of data. Nevertheless, problems arise in the quality and consistency of these data, and in accessing them. It is hoped that the recent introduction of a new contract for general practices in the UK will contribute to improvements in data collection. Sources of data within primary care include:

- In-practice systems: disease registers, age-sex registers and audits.

- Service data: returns to PCTs on immunisation, screening, family planning and other disease-related data.

- Prescribing data known as Electronic Prescribing and Financial Information for Practices (ePFIP).

- The General Practitioner Research Database (GPRD), and the preceding GP National Morbidity Surveys (see Section 2.2.6 of this chapter).

General Practitioner Research Database (GPRD)

The GPRD provides data from 1987 onwards from over 300 practices (accounting for 5–6 per cent of the population of England and Wales). Participating practices must follow agreed guidelines on recording and returning anonymised data on prescriptions, significant morbidity and important consultation outcomes for all patients. Quality-control mechanisms aim to maximise the accuracy of the data. It is primarily a research data set, but useful information is becoming available on health services, such as chronic disease management.

Disease registers

The new GP contract (together with requirements of National Service Frameworks) requires that practices establish disease registers for patients with, for example, coronary heart disease or asthma. Practice registers are used to promote delivery of standardised and quality health care, and at a national level the registers provide useful information for health-service planning and research. A disease register must (a) identify and record data on individuals with a given disease or health problem, (b) provide longitudinal information through a systematic mechanism for updates and follow-up, and (c) be based on a geographically defined population (thus enabling calculation of rates of disease). Such registers are potentially resource intensive and thus require clearly defined aims and objectives, identification of adequate resources from the outset, and skilled organisation to set up and maintain the register. Accuracy is vital and requires dedicated and motivated staff to run the register. Nevertheless, disease registers provide a good source of data for audit and research, can help with service delivery and patient care, and are important in planning services through identification of disease incidence and prevalence. Potential problems with disease registers include selective registration and ascertainment bias (the most serious cases or patients who attend the GP more often may be registered), administrative problems of completeness and duplication, maintenance of confidentiality, and variation in data collection and quality across regions.

2.5.5 Disease surveillance

Disease surveillance is the 'systematic and ongoing collection, analysis and use of health information (about a disease or factors influencing disease) for the purpose of disease prevention and control'. In the UK, examples include laboratory reports of infectious disease, GP sentinel practices, drug misuse databases, adverse drug reactions, congenital anomalies, and home and leisure accidents. Notification systems are an approach to surveillance that requires the reporting of a particular disease or event to an official authority. Normally based on law or regulations, reporting is often patchy due to weak sanctions or rewards. Examples include the infectious diseases notification system (discussed in Section 2.2.5), legal abortion, and certain injures at work.

2.5.6 Population-based health information

In this section so far, we have looked at sources of information that rely on individuals with illness coming into contact with the health system. For some outcomes the condition is so unequivocal (e.g. maternal mortality) or serious enough (most cancers) that all – or virtually all – cases do reach the health-care system. But, for most illness, only a proportion does. Many different factors determine who does and does not reach the health system, including age, sex, ethnicity, language, illness severity, service access and quality, etc. Hence, data on disease frequency and determinants in the population are very important in 'filling the gap', but can only be obtained by going to the community with a survey, or by establishing data monitoring that captures all (or a sample, if possible representative) of events such as road traffic accidents.

Population-based health and related social, economic and other information includes routine surveys such as the General Household Survey (GHS) and the Health Survey for England (HSE), as well as information from a range of agencies, including local government and the police, on transport, road traffic accidents, the environment, education, etc.

The General Household Survey

The GHS surveys people from the general population, so it is not dependent on presentation to health services. It started in 1971, and is an annual survey of a representative sample of around 12 000 private households in Britain. It is interview based (adult members are asked about their children) and includes questions on many aspects of life, including housing, economic activity, leisure, education, and health. Health questions include acute and chronic health problems experienced during the last two weeks, health in the last year, presence of chronic disease, consultations with doctors, visits to hospital, risk factors such as smoking and alcohol consumption, and use of spectacles. Considerable resources are invested in planning, training and data quality, and the results are timely and considered to be relatively accurate although (unlike the census), since the survey is non-statutory, the response rate is around 70–80 per cent.

The Health Survey for England

The HSE has run annually since 1991, using a random sample of 16 000 adults in private households. Since 1995, it has also included children aged 2–15 years. Data are collected by (i) a health and socio-economic questionnaire; (ii) physical measurements of height, weight, waist:hip ratio and blood pressure; and (iii) a blood sample for measurement of haemoglobin, cholesterol and ferritin. Key topics are repeated annually, allowing comparison of trends. Specific issues, such as coronary heart disease or accidents, are also covered in greater depth at periodic intervals.

Office of National Statistics (ONS) Longitudinal Study

Established in 1971, the primary purpose of the ONS Longitudinal Study is to provide more accurate information on occupational mortality. It follows up a small sample taken from the 1971 census, babies born on census day 1971, and immigrants with this birthday. It relies on linkage of records for these individuals with other ONS and NHS Central Register information (the NHS Central Register contains details of all NHS-registered patients). Events recorded include deaths of a study member or their spouse, births to women in the cohort, infant deaths, cancer, immigration and emigration. Data are not released directly to the public but are available in the form of reports describing how the topics included in the study vary by occupation. A particular advantage of the ONS Longitudinal Study in the investigation of work and health is that health status can be determined in advance of changes in employment status, and vice versa, and the timescale is also known. It is therefore possible to untangle a problem that beset many studies of work and health; that is, knowing whether poor health led to loss (or change in type) of employment, or whether the type of work led to the observed health status. This temporal advantage of longitudinal (prospective) studies in studying causal relationships is explored in more detail in Chapter 5 on cohort studies.

2.5.7   Secondary data sets

Secondary data sets are routinely published analyses of primary data sources. Examples include Public Health Annual Reports and the Public Health Common Data Set (PHCDS). The PHCDS includes data on demography, fertility, morbidity, mortality and provision of health care in England. Data have been collated since the 1980s and provide numbers and standardised rates or ratios for geographical areas in a conveniently accessible form (see chapter 3). The Neighbourhood Statistics Database arose as part of the National Strategy for Neighbourhood Renewal. It is a database run by National Statistics, which gives small-area data that can inform local and national policy initiatives. This electoral ward-level data set includes the Index of Multiple Deprivation (see 2.5.8), and the underlying data are organised into themes. In due course, it is expected that the data set will include other census data at ward level.

2.5.8   Deprivation indices

Socio-economic deprivation and its contributing factors are recognised to be very important determinants of health. Measures of deprivation are now well established, and a number are in common use. All of these indices assess the proportion of individuals or households in a socially or geographically defined area that have poor living conditions. It should be noted, however, that not all people living in an area with a high deprivation score are deprived, and vice versa. This issue, a feature of group-based (or 'ecological') analyses, is discussed further in Section 2.6.2 of this chapter.

Deprivation indices provide a summary measure of key social, economic and environmental factors which together have a very substantial impact on health

Deprivation indices were developed for different purposes, and care should be taken when selecting them for other uses. Examples include:

- The Townsend Material Deprivation Score. This was originally based on information from the 1991 census with four measures – unemployment, no car ownership, households not owner occupied, and overcrowding. Equal weight is given to all four variables. It is a measure of material deprivation and is available at enumeration district (ED), ward, and local authority (LA) levels.

- The Jarman Underprivileged Area Score. Originally developed as a measure of GP workload, it combines measures of the proportion of elderly living alone, children under 5, lone parent households, unskilled, unemployed, overcrowding, ethnic minorities, and mobility of the population. Scores are available at ED, ward, and LA levels.

- The Indices of Multiple Deprivation (IMD) 2004. This provides a ward-level score made up of an overall Index of Multiple Deprivation and seven individual domains (income deprivation, employment deprivation, health deprivation and disability, education skills and training, barriers to housing and services, living environment deprivation, and crime). Each ward is given a score and a national ranking. More information can be found on the website of the Department for Communities and Local Government (DCLG): http://www.communities.gov.uk.

2.6 Descriptive epidemiology in action

2.6.1 The London smogs of the 1950s

In this example we will see how investigation of severe episodes of air pollution in London during the 1950s contributed to the introduction of new legislation to control the burning of solid fuels in urban areas.

Contemporary descriptions of these 'smogs', a mixture of smoke and fog, tells of the streets being so dark that vehicles had to use lights in daytime, and people being barely able to see a few feet in front of them. This is how serious the air pollution had become in London during the early 1950s.

The smoke arose mainly from domestic use of coal for heating and cooking, so the pollution was worse in the coldest months of the year. The fog was associated with temperature inversions, with cold, still air trapped in the bowl of the Thames Valley. Serious pollution episodes caused by coal burning no longer occur in London due to regulatory control of coal use (only 'smokeless' types can be used), and the wide availability of clean fuels such as electricity and natural gas. Air pollution is still a problem, but the main source now is motor vehicles.

We will start by looking at health and air-pollution data for this now infamous episode, using descriptive epidemiological methods, and consider what can be discovered from interpretation of variations by time, place and person. Table 2.6.1 below shows data for Greater London on deaths (all causes), air temperature, and air pollution for each day over the period 1–15 December 1952.

Table 2.6.1 Deaths, air temperature, and air pollution in London 1–15 December 1952

Variable	Date (period 1–8 December)							
	1st	2nd	3rd	4 th	5th	6th	7th	8th
Deaths								
– central London	112	140	143	120	196	294	513	518
– outer London	147	161	178	168	210	287	331	392
Air temperature:								
– daily mean (°F) at Kew[1]	36.9	34.2	39.0	36.5	29.5	28.9	28.9	31.5
Air pollution:								
– smoke ($\mu g/m^3$) Kew[1]	340	340	190	420	1470	1750	870	1190
– smoke ($\mu g/m^3$) County Hall[2]	380	490	610	490	2640	3450	4460	4460
– Sulphur dioxide (ppm)	0.09	0.16	0.22	0.14	0.75	0.86	1.34	1.34
Deaths								
– central London	436	274	255	236	256	222	213	
– outer London	362	269	273	248	245	227	212	
Air temperature:								
– daily mean (°F) at Kew[1]	36.6	43.3	45.1	40.1	37.2	35.2	32.0	
Air pollution:								
– smoke ($\mu g/m^3$) Kew[1]	470	170	190	240	320	290	180	
– smoke ($\mu g/m^3$)	1220	1220	320	290	500	320	320	
County Hall[2] – Sulphur dioxide (ppm)	0.47	0.47	0.22	0.23	0.26	0.16	0.16	

[1] Kew is southwest London, about 6 miles from the centre of the city (Westminster).
[2] County Hall is on the south bank of the Thames, opposite the Houses of Parliament (Westminster).

Self-Assessment Exercise 2.6.1

1. Plot the data for all variables in a way that allows you to compare the variations of each across the period under study (1–15 December 1952).

2. Describe the findings for the deaths occurring in central London and outer London.

3. Describe the findings for smoke pollution (Kew and County Hall), and for sulphur dioxide (only County Hall data available).

4. Describe the findings for temperature (Kew). Do you think that these temperature data are representative of the whole city?

5. Interpret the information you now have on variations in these atmospheric variables and the deaths, paying careful attention to the timing of the variations.

6. Do we have information by person, time and place (all three)? What additional information would you like to have had for this investigation?

Answers in Section 2.8

The Clean Air Act

This legislation was passed in 1956, in part because of this and other episodes of severe air pollution which resulted in substantial loss of life. The Act established smokeless zones and controlled domestic smoke emissions for the first time. It resulted from the action of the National Society for Smoke Abatement, a pressure group consisting of MPs and some Medical Officers of Health, and led to a marked decline in smoke emissions, which were reduced by around 65 per cent between 1954 and 1971. Sulphur dioxide emissions continue to fall.

In this section we have looked at an example of how descriptive epidemiology has contributed to national public health policy. The focus on environmental data also illustrates the value of information from outside the health services.

2.6.2 Ecological studies

Introduction

Ecological studies are a type of descriptive epidemiological study design that we have already encountered. An *ecological study* or analysis is essentially one that examines association between units of grouped (or *aggregated*) data, such as electoral wards, regions, or even whole countries.

There are many examples of this approach; for instance, a scatterplot of socio-economic condition by electoral ward, versus the percentage of smokers in each ward. The point is that the data are for the group (in this case a ward), and this is in contrast to surveys, cohort and case-control studies, where we will look at information on exposures and outcomes for every individual. The following example (Figure 2.6.1) shows the ecological association between a measure of fat consumption in a number of countries, and the incidence rate for breast cancer in each country.

 Self-Assessment Exercise 2.6.2

This ecological study demonstrates a very clear association, and it is tempting to think this is *causal* – that is, higher fat consumption increases the risk of breast cancer. Can you think of any reasons why this type of analysis could be misleading?

Answers in Section 2.8

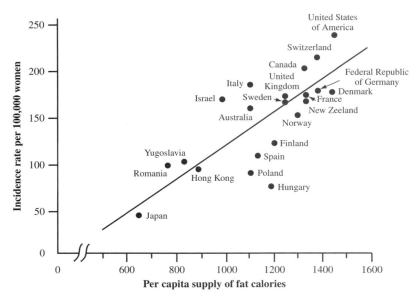

Figure 2.6.1 An ecological association: measure of fat consumption and breast cancer incidence

Source: Reproduced with permission from Leon Gordis (derived from Prentice *et al.*, 1988).

The ecological fallacy

As we have seen, aggregate measures tell you nothing for certain about individuals. This gives rise to the possibility of an *ecological fallacy*. This occurs when we ascribe to members of a group one or more characteristics they do not possess as individuals. The consequence of an ecological fallacy can be that an association seen between aggregated data does not exist at the individual level, and is in fact explained by other associated factors. If the association is seen at the ecological level, but not at the individual level, it cannot be causal.

The risk of encountering the ecological fallacy does not mean that such analyses are unhelpful, but that they need to be used with caution. As an initial step in studying disease causation, this is a useful means of exploring associations worthy of further investigation at the individual level.

Summary

- Ecological studies are a useful initial stage in the epidemiological investigation of association and causation.

- Ecological studies are carried out at an aggregated level.

- There is an implicit assumption that the characteristics of the aggregated group apply to the individuals that make up the group. If this is wrong, an ecological fallacy will arise.

2.7 Overview of epidemiological study designs

In this chapter on descriptive epidemiology, based as it has been mainly on routine data sources, we have seen how relatively simple analyses by *time, place* and *person* have actually been remarkably informative. At least some of our examples, however, have raised more questions than were answered, leaving us with questions such as these:

- OK, so people with greater socio-economic deprivation have higher mortality, but why? We do not have the detailed and specific kind of information about these people's lifestyles, views, experiences, etc., that we need in order to explain the findings, nor to advise what should be done to alleviate the problems.

- How can we be sure that the factors we found to be associated with death rates actually cause the disease? Some of the apparent associations could easily be caused by other factors about which we have little or no information.

- If we are planning to publish our research findings and develop public health and health-care policies based on them, surely it is not going to be sufficient to say, for example, that air pollution seems to be associated with asthma. We need to be able to show what levels of specific pollutants cause how much disease, and what benefit can be expected from feasible reductions in these pollutants. We need to be able to measure these effects, and to state what the margins of error are.

These and other questions, which we will discuss throughout the book, will return again and again in research. They are, if you like, the crux of why we need more sophisticated research methods, and give an idea of what these methods have to offer. Descriptive epidemiology has been a good starting point, to set the context, to open up ideas about explanations and causes, and to help us in handling and presenting information. What we need now, however, are more powerful and focused research designs: methods which can answer questions in ways that can really advance our understanding of causation, or measure the effects of health care and prevention in ways that are useful to those who carry out the work, as well as to those who have to manage ever more restricted budgets.

Table 2.7.1 presents a summary of the main types of health studies, including case studies (which we will not consider further) and epidemiological studies (which are the main focus of the book). We have dealt with the first of these epidemiological designs, descriptive studies, in this part of the book. We will look at the next design, surveys, in Chapter 4. The main purpose of surveys is to collect information, from individuals, that was not available from routine sources. Here we are setting out to explore the first of a series of increasingly focused and rigorous scientific research methods that can provide the tools to address our unanswered questions.

Table 2.7.1   An overview of research study designs

(a) Case studies

Study type	Nature of investigation	Comment on research design
Case studies		
• *case reports*: descriptions of one or more cases (of disease), together with circumstances of interest. • *case series*: as above, but a consecutive series of cases.	A good way of getting ideas about what might be causing, or predisposing to, a health problem. We can call this hypothesis generation.	As a research method, this approach is very weak. For example, we have no way of knowing for sure whether people without the disease are any different from those with it.

Table 2.7.1   (Continued)

(b) Epidemiological study designs

Study type	Nature of investigation	Comment on research design
Descriptive epidemiology Studies of patterns of disease in populations, and variations by time, place and person.	With this design, we are beginning to test ideas on cause and effect, but still largely dependent on routinely available data.	Stronger than case studies, as formal comparisons between population groups can be made.
Surveys So-called cross-sectional studies, often using samples, designed to measure prevalence, and more particularly to study associations between health status and various (possibly causal) factors.	In contrast to working with routinely available data, surveys are designed to collect information exactly as we specify, from the individuals that we are especially interested in.	More focused than descriptive studies, and as a result a more powerful means of investigating associations. The inclusion of information on a range of factors means that some allowance can be made for these in studying causal links.
Case-control studies In these studies, people with a disease ('cases') and people without ('controls') are investigated, essentially to find out whether 'exposure' to a factor of interest differs between cases and controls.	A focused research design that allows measurement of the strength of the association between a disease and its possible cause, or factors (such as health interventions) that can afford protection. The most appropriate and practical study design for less common diseases.	A valuable and widely used study design, but one that is rather subject to bias. Careful design is vital, but even so there is often room for a lot of debate about the interpretation. Compared to cohort studies and trials (see below), this design is relatively quick and cheap to carry out.
Cohort studies By first surveying, and then following up, a sample of people (a 'cohort'), it is possible to measure by how much the incidence of disease differs between those who were exposed to a factor of interest (at the time of the survey) and those who were not exposed, or exposed less.	This design also provides a good measure of the strength of association, and is far less open to bias than the case-control design. This major advantage is, however, gained at the expense of time, cost and complexity. In contrast to case-control studies, cohort designs are not suitable for uncommon conditions due to the time it would take for enough cases to arise.	A valuable and widely used design. Cohort studies, as a result of their design, provide true estimates of incidence, and are less subject to bias than case-control studies due to the opportunity to measure exposure before the disease occurs. The information about temporal relationships (that is, that exposure preceded the disease) helps in assessing whether the association seen between exposure and outcome is causal.
Intervention trials By taking a sample of people, and intervening (e.g. with a medication, operation or preventative measure) among some (the 'intervention' group), but not others (the 'control' group), we can assess how much the level of health or incidence of disease has been altered by the intervention.	In many respects the ultimate research design, because of the control we have over who does (and does not) have exposure to the factor we wish to test. Where the allocation to intervention and control is random, all other factors that can influence the outcome are equally distributed across the two groups.	Evidence from trials is powerful, especially if the study is randomised, controlled and blinded (that is, neither investigators nor subjects know who was in intervention or control groups). It can be appreciated, however, that there are many situations where allocating some people to receive a health-care intervention or be exposed to a risk factor, and others not, would be impractical and/or unethical.

Some reassurance

Do not worry if you find it difficult to understand all the terms and concepts included in Table 2.7.1 at this stage. These will become clearer as we progress through each study design, and at this point you should just try to understand the general ideas. As we work through these study designs, you will see how each successive method gains in 'quality'. Stronger research design means that questions can be answered with greater certainty, especially when we are dealing with causation, and when trying to measure (quantify) the effects of risk factors, health-care interventions, etc. This greater strength generally comes with a price though. The more rigorous the study design, the more difficult, time-consuming and expensive it usually is to carry out. All designs have their place and value, however, and you will appreciate this better as you become more familiar with the strengths and limitations of each. You may find it useful to refer back to this table as we start to look at each new study design.

Natural experiments

One final design, which in some respects is like an intervention study but may draw on other study designs, is the ***natural experiment***. This might be used, opportunistically, when some substantial natural or man-made event or policy change takes place. A good example of such an event was the nuclear reactor explosion at Chernobyl, which provided the opportunity (and duty) to study the effects of radiation exposure. Such studies may provide sometimes unique opportunities to study high-risk exposures, such as radiation or toxic chemicals. We will not look further at natural experiments as a specific study design in this book, but many aspects of other designs and epidemiological methods in general would be relevant in designing and carrying out such a study.

2.8 Answers to self-assessment exercises

Section 2.1

Exercise 2.1.1

1. Certification

The correct answer is the hospital doctor. Death certificates must be completed by a registered medical practitioner. As explained in the story, there was no need to involve the coroner's office in this death, as the death was not sudden and Mrs Williams' mother was under the care of the hospital. The circumstances in which the coroner should be involved are discussed in more detail shortly.

3. Quality of information

(a) In this case the information is likely to be accurate, as a diagnosis of lung cancer had already been confirmed by investigation (chest radiography, bronchoscopy and biopsy).

(b) The autopsy probably would not make a difference in this case. If the lung cancer had not been confirmed (by confirmation of the type), it is possible that the original site of the cancer may have been found to be elsewhere, from which it spread to the lung. Only a minority of deaths in the UK go to autopsy, however (about 25 per cent in England and Wales, and 15 per cent in Scotland), with the lowest percentage in the 65+ age group.

Exercise 2.1.2

1. Reason for verdict

Even though it may seem to us that this was obviously a suicide, the coroner did not return a verdict of suicide because the evidence was not strong enough. If the verdict can be challenged (e.g. by relatives), the coroner will tend to return an open verdict, or a verdict of accidental death.

2. Proportion receiving verdict of suicide

In the UK, true suicides receive verdicts of suicide, open (injury undetermined), and (some) accidental death. When studying suicide, we often use the numbers of suicide and open verdicts combined, as this represents the best easily available estimate of the true suicide rate. In England and Wales in 2003, there were 3287 suicide verdicts and 1540 open verdicts, making a total of 4827. On this basis, 68 per cent ($3287 \div 4827$) of our estimate for all suicides actually received an official verdict of suicide. Thus, only two-thirds of suicides may be recorded as such, and the true proportion may be even lower than this. This example illustrates well how social, legal and other factors can influence the recorded cause of death.

Exercise 2.1.3

1. Plot of data for men:

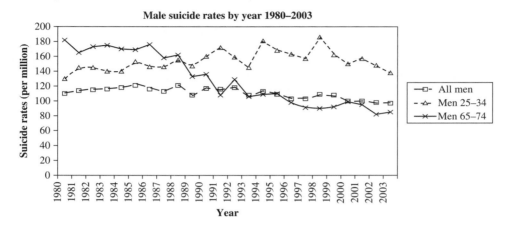

This is called a line graph. The graphical presentation of data will be covered in more detail in Section 2.4 of this chapter.

2. The main observation from these data is that while the rates for older men (65–74) have fallen, those for young men (25–34) increased and were higher in 2003 than they were in 1980. There has, however, been a fall since 1998, but it may be wise to await more data before concluding that this is a genuine reversal in the trend. The rate for all men shows little change, emphasising how rates for all ages (or very wide age bands) can mask very different trends within key age subgroups.

Exercise 2.1.4

1. Combined male and female suicide rates:

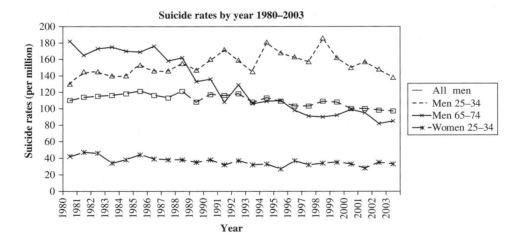

2. Interpretation

The rates for young women (25–34) are very much lower than those for men of the same age group, and appear to have stayed constant (perhaps have even declined a little). This is a striking contrast to the clearly increasing rates in young men over the same period.

Before moving onto the next section, you might find it useful to spend a little time exploring the National Statistics website and familiarising yourself with the many different types of health data available. It can be found at http://www.statistics.gov.uk/.

Exercise 2.1.5

1. The group 7: group 1.1 IMR ratio is $6.58/2.95 = 2.23$

2. Infants born to families in the lower social classes may be more vulnerable for the following reasons:

- Higher proportion of low birthweight (that is, less than 2500 g), as these babies are more at risk of infections and other problems.

- Lower uptake of antenatal care.

- Poorer access to high-quality health services, due to location, language barriers for ethnic minorities, etc.

- Higher rates of maternal smoking and drug use during pregnancy.

- Higher rates of parental smoking in the home environment during the first year of life.

- Poorer home circumstances, including housing quality (damp, cold), risk of accidents, etc.

Section 2.2

Exercise 2.2.1

1. The data for Austria and Ireland are for the years 2000 and 1999, respectively: since underlying trends in lung cancer change only slowly, this 1-year difference does not prevent us making a valid comparison. The numbers of deaths among women aged 65–74 is greater in Austria, but the rates are higher in Ireland because Ireland has a much smaller population (denominator). The rate for Ireland is around twice as high as Austria.

2. When considering the reasons for differences, you should always consider the following three possibilities:

- *Chance*; that is, it is due to random variation where relatively small numbers are concerned.

- *Artefact*; that is, the difference is not real, but the result of how the information is collected, coded or presented.

- *Real*; that is, the rate for lung cancer really is higher in Ireland.

We will look at chance and artefact more in due course (artefact is in the next exercise). In thinking about the possible explanation for a real difference, we need to consider the known causes of lung cancer, which are smoking (by far the most important), and other exposures, including radon gas (a natural radioactive gas which permeates from the ground into houses, mainly in areas where there is granite), air pollution, and asbestos exposure. The difference in these country rates is almost certainly due to smoking, as the individual risk and exposure patterns for the other causes could not account for such a large difference. One aspect of smoking to consider among women of this age is country differences in the time period at which women began smoking. These women would have been in their early twenties around the time of the Second World War (1939–45), which is very likely to have had a major influence on patterns of smoking among young women in the two countries.

Exercise 2.2.2

1. The systems are really very similar, with the exception of the percentage of deaths going to autopsy. This information does not, however, tell us anything about how underlying or predisposing causes of death are coded in practice; for instance, whether a women with lung cancer, but dying eventually of pneumonia or heart failure precipitated by the cancer, would be handled the same way by certifying doctors and coding staff in the two countries.

2. A higher autopsy rate should lead to greater accuracy of diagnosis in this age group, but given the nature of lung cancer and the high chance of intensive contact with the health services for treatment and care, the diagnosis will often be made before death.

3. Although there is a substantial difference in the autopsy rate, this is unlikely to explain much of the difference in lung cancer death rates. We do not have information about certification and coding rules, and it would be useful to find out about these in making international comparisons. Nevertheless, the difference in death rates is so great that these explanations relating to artefact are unlikely to alter our overall conclusion.

Exercise 2.2.3

1. Food poisoning rates per 1000 population

Table 2.2.2 Cases of food poisoning, and population (thousands), England and Wales 1984–2003

Year	Number of cases	Population (1000s)	Crude rate/1000/year
1996	83 233	51 410.4	1.619
1997	93 901	51 559.6	1.821
1998	93 932	51 720.1	1.816
1999	86 316	51 933.5	1.662
2000	86 528	52 140.2	1.660
2001	85 468	52 360.0	1.632
2002	72 649	52 570.2	1.382
2003	70 895	52 793.7	1.343

2. Plot of food poisoning rates

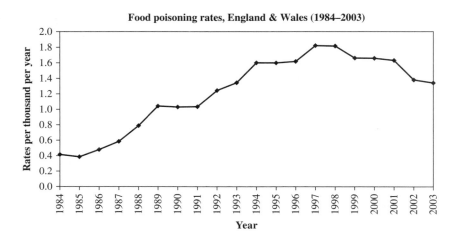

Food poisoning rates, England & Wales (1984–2003)

3. Comment and possible explanations

There has been a steady rise in the rate over the period 1984–1998, during which time there was an almost fourfold increase. However, rates have dropped slightly from 1999 onwards. Again we should think about *chance, artefact* and *real* change.

- **Chance**: given the numbers involved, and the progressive nature of the change, this cannot be a chance increase (we will look at how we quantify the range of chance variation in due course when considering confidence intervals).

- **Artefact**: could this be due to improvements in the proportion of cases being recognised and notified, termed *case ascertainment*? The evidence is that, although there is under-notification, this generally runs at about the same level, so that trends in notifications in this country can be interpreted with a fair degree of confidence.

- **Real increase**: there is a range of possible explanations, including the increase in fast-food outlets, less home cooking, more pre-packed foods, problems with food production (salmonella in eggs and poultry), and so on.

Exercise 2.2.4

1. Trends

Meningitis peaks in the winter months, falling from a high in January and February, to its lowest level during the summer, and rising again towards the end of the year.

In contrast, recorded cases of mumps were quite low at the beginning of the year and subsequently showed a gradual increase through to October, when the number of cases rose dramatically. By the beginning of December, the number of cases was much higher than at the beginning of the year, illustrating the beginning of a national mumps outbreak.

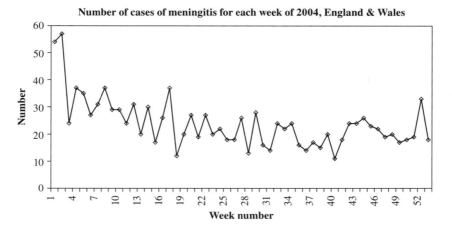

Number of cases of meningitis for each week of 2004, England & Wales

2. Possible explanations for variations

Meningitis	Mumps
• Overcrowding (more people together indoors) • Concurrent respiratory infections • Transmission is increased in winter due to one or more of the above situations	• More detailed investigation reveals that the increase in cases largely occurred among teenagers and young adults who were too old to have been offered the MMR vaccine routinely (MMR vaccine was introduced in 1988). • Since this increase occurred, the Health Protection Agency has launched an MMR vaccination programme aimed at increasing vaccination coverage among 16–23-year-olds.

Exercise 2.2.5

1. Meningitis rates by age and sex

The age-specific rates are approximately the same for females as for males, although lower among females in the youngest age groups. For both sexes, the rates decline progressively with increasing age. Infants (children under 1 year of age) are most vulnerable to meningitis, with rates around five times those for children aged 1–4 years.

2. Interpretation

Although the rates for boys less than 5 years are higher than those for girls, the age patterns are otherwise very similar. Age is a very strong determinant of susceptibility to meningitis, and being male also appears to carry some additional risk in young children. Given the severity of this illness, it is unlikely that the age patterns are the result of more complete notification in young children than older people. The consistency of the trends with age (we do not have the numbers in this table to assess precision, but these data are for the whole country) strongly suggests that this pattern is not due to chance.

Exercise 2.2.6

1. Trends

We cannot be very certain of the trends without a more thorough examination of how consistently data have been recorded, and of the margins of random error. For the current purpose, however, we can note that the numbers of cases are quite substantial, and that considerable effort has been made to ensure reasonable comparability of the data recording over time. With this in mind, we observe that:

- Acute bronchitis increased between 1955/56 and 1971/72, and thereafter remained stable. There is certainly no evidence to suggest a marked reduction.

- Asthma, for which we have no separate data in 1955/56 (a reflection perhaps of how the condition was viewed at that time), has almost doubled between 1971/72 and 1981/82.

- Hay fever, again with no separate data for 1955/56, has also increased in line with the asthma rates.

2. Change in diagnostic fashion?

This appears to show that, as asthma increased, acute bronchitis has remained stable. If the recorded increase in asthma was due to change in diagnostic fashion (and was simply a relabelling of acute bronchitis cases), the true rate of acute bronchitis in the population would also have had to have increased. We do not know whether or not this has happened, but the data here show that acute bronchitis has not decreased, and are therefore consistent with the view that the increase in asthma is not simply due to change in diagnostic practice.

3. What has happened to rates of asthma?

Although there is some uncertainty about what is happening, it appears that rates of asthma really have increased.

Section 2.3

Exercise 2.3.1

1. Edinburgh centre has the lowest concentration of PM_{10} ($0.4 \mu g/m^3$). Bury roadside has the highest concentration ($38.0 \mu g/m^3$).

2. The locations which did not record a level of PM_{10} are as follows:

Newcastle centre	Stockport
Bolton	Sheffield centre
Leamington Spa	London Eltham
Haringey roadside	

These are 7 out of the total of 34 urban locations. The percentage is

$$\frac{7}{34} \times 100\% = 20.6\%$$

About 20 per cent, or one in five, of the urban monitoring sites did not record a level of PM_{10} at this time.

Section 2.4

Exercise 2.4.1

1. Frequency distribution

A convenient way of finding the frequency distribution (in the absence of a computer) is to tally the data, write down the intervals, and then go through the data in the order they are given and make a tally mark for each value next to the appropriate interval. It is then simple to count up the number in each interval to get the frequency distribution. (It is also easy to make mistakes with this method, so check your results.) Remember not to include the values at the upper limit of each interval.

PM_{10}	Tally	Frequency
0–4	/	1
4–8	/	1
8–12		0
12–16	///// /////	10
16–20	////	4
20–24	///	3
24–28	///	3
28–32	///	3
32–36	/	1
36–40	/	1
Total		27

2. Histogram

Your histogram should look like this.

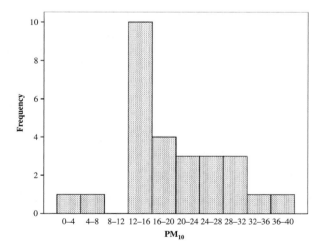

It is important that the axes are labelled and have scales marked on them. The vertical axis can be labelled frequency, or number, or count. There is now a gap in the histogram: there are no values in the range $8–12\,\mu g/m^3$. There are two values on their own, followed by a peak for the interval $12–16\,\mu g/m^3$. Then it is downhill all the way. This histogram gives the impression of the data being bunched up at lower values and then slowly tailing off towards the higher values.

The histogram in Figure 2.4.1 does not show this so clearly. In that picture, the patterns of data each side of the peak $(15–20\,\mu g/m^3)$ look more similar to each other.

Exercise 2.4.2

The distribution of PM_{10} values is unimodal with some right/positive skew. There are no gaps or outliers in the distribution. If you said that the distribution is approximately symmetric, rather than right skewed, that is a good enough approximate description, as the skewing is not marked.

Exercise 2.4.3

1. PM_{10} concentrations for the London locations

London Bloomsbury	29.4	London Bexley	23.2
London Hillingdon	30.7	London Brent	25.0
Sutton roadside	24.8	London Eltham	-
London Kensington	24.9	Haringey roadside	-
Camden kerbside	32.8		

2. Mean and median

The concentration of PM_{10} was recorded at seven locations in London. The mean concentration is found by adding up the seven values and dividing by 7:

$$\frac{29.4 + 23.2 + 30.7 + 25.0 + 24.8 + 24.9 + 32.8}{7} = \frac{190.8}{7} = 27.25714286$$

The mean concentration of PM_{10} is $27.26 \mu g/m^3$. The data are recorded to one decimal place, so the mean is stated to two decimal places. Any sensible degree of accuracy will do, such as one, two or three decimal places, but eight decimal places is not sensible. The accuracy of the data do not justify it. To find the median, we need to order the data:

23.2 24.8 24.9 **25.0** 29.4 30.7 32.8

There are seven values. The middle value is the fourth. The median PM_{10} concentration is therefore $25.0 \mu g/m^3$.

Exercise 2.4.4

1. (a) Yes. This is a picture of all the data, and shows the shape.

   (b) No. The mean tells us where the distribution is located, but not its shape.

   (c) No. The mode is the peak of the distribution.

   (d) No. This is part of the description of the shape, but is not sufficient. We also want to know whether the distribution is symmetric or skewed, and whether there are any outliers.

2. (a) No. The mean is greater than the median because the high values in the long right tail of the distribution all contribute to the value of the mean.

   (b) No. Skewed distributions are not necessarily unimodal, although they usually are, because most distributions are unimodal.

   (c) Yes. The mean is greater than the median, so more than 50 per cent of the observations are less than the mean.

   (d) No. The definition of left skewness is that the distribution has a long left tail.

(e) Yes. Positive skewness is an alternative name for right skewness, which means the right tail is longer than the left.

The two correct statements are (c) and (e).

3. (i) The mean and median are both at point (a).

The distribution is approximately symmetric, so the mean and median have about the same value. This is in the middle.

(ii) The mean is at (c) and the median is at (b).

The distribution is right skewed, so the mean is greater than the median. Fifty per cent of the data are less than the median, so half the area of the histogram must be to the left of the median.

Exercise 2.4.5

1. Interquartile range

There are three observations each side of the median. So the quartiles are the 2nd and 6th values:

$$Q_1 = 24.8; \, Q_3 = 30.7$$

The interquartile range is therefore IQR $= 30.7 - 24.8 = 5.9 \, \mu g/m^3$.

2. Standard deviation

The alternative formula for calculating the variance of the observations is

$$s^2 = \frac{1}{n-1} \left[\sum x_i^2 - \frac{1}{n} \left(\sum x_i \right)^2 \right]$$

We need to calculate the sum of the observations and the sum of the squared observations.

x_i	x_i^2
23.2	538.24
24.8	615.04
24.9	620.01
25.0	625.00
29.4	864.36
30.7	942.49
32.8	1075.84
$\sum x_i = 190.8$	$\sum x_i^2 = 5280.98$

The number of observations is $n = 7$, so

$$s^2 = \frac{1}{6} \left(5280.98 - \frac{(190.8)^2}{7} \right) = 13.38619$$

and

$$s = \sqrt{13.38619} \approx 3.66 \mu g/m^3 \text{ (to one more decimal place than the data).}$$

Exercise 2.4.6

1. Frequency distribution

PM_{10}	Frequency
0–5	1
5–10	0
10–15	0
15–20	0
20–25	1
25–30	9
30–35	9
35–40	3
40–45	3
45–50	3
50–55	1
. . . .	0
160–165	1
Total*	31

* Three locations did not record a value of PM_{10}.

You can tally the data to obtain the frequency distribution. You do not need to include all the empty intervals between the outlier and the rest of the data, but make sure it is clear that there is a gap, as shown in the table below.

2. Histogram

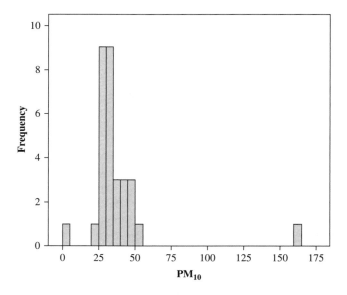

Urban PM_{10} concentrations at 5 pm

The distribution of PM_{10} concentrations is unimodal and right skewed. Most of the data fall within the range 20–60 μg/m^3, but there are two outliers with concentrations in the intervals 0–5 μg/m^3 and 160–165 μg/m^3.

3. Mean and standard deviation

The sum of the 31 values is $\sum x_i = 1160.2$ so the mean is $\dfrac{1160.2}{31} = 37.43$ μg/m^3.

The sum of the squared values is $\sum x_i^2 = 62608.5$, so the variance is

$$s^2 = \frac{1}{n-1}\left[\sum x_i^2 - \frac{(\sum x_i)^2}{n}\right]$$

$$= \frac{1}{30}\left[62608.5 - \frac{(1160.2)^2}{31}\right]$$

$$= 639.5693118$$

and the standard deviation is $s = 25.29$ μg/m^3. Since the distribution is skewed, we could have chosen to describe the location and spread with the median and interquartile range. This is perfectly acceptable, but here we will use the mean and standard deviation to make comparisons with the PM_{10} values recorded at midday. Note that the outlying value of 164.0 greatly affects the mean and standard deviation, and so these measures could be misleading. If we omit 164.0 from the calculations, the mean is 33.21 μg/m^3 and the standard deviation dramatically reduces to 9.53 μg/m^3.

4. Comparison of PM_{10} concentrations at midday and 5 pm

Concentrations tend to be higher at 5 pm than at midday (the mean is 37.43 μg/m^3, compared with 19.37 μg/m^3 at midday), and they are more spread out (standard deviation of 25.29 μg/m^3 compared with 8.27 μg/m^3).

The concentrations at 5 pm are more clearly right skewed than those recorded at midday. Most of the data lie between 23.6 μg/m^3 and 51.0 μg/m^3. There are two outliers of 2.0 μg/m^3 and 164.0 μg/m^3. The very high value will inflate the mean and standard deviation. However, it is clear from the histogram that even without this high value, concentrations are higher, on average, at 5 pm than at midday.

Exercise 2.4.7

- The relationship is approximately linear (there is no obvious non-linear pattern).

- It is a negative relationship – under-5-year mortality decreases with increasing percentage of births attended.

- The relationship between under-5-year mortality and percentage of births attended is moderately strong.

Exercise 2.4.8

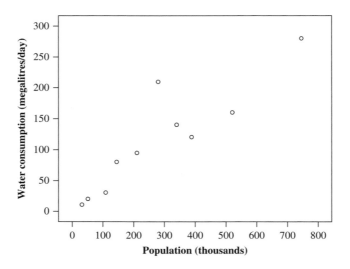

Water consumption and population for Scottish regions, 1995

There is a strong, positive, approximately linear relationship between water consumption and population.

Calculation of correlation coefficient is provided for reference. Labelling population x and water consumption y, we have

$$\sum x = 2833 \quad \sum x^2 = 1279523 \quad \sum y = 1174$$
$$\sum y^2 = 208634 \quad \sum xy = 496696$$

The correlation coefficient is therefore

$$r = \frac{496696 - 2833 \times 1174/10}{\sqrt{(1279523 - 2833^2/10)(208634 - 1174^2/10)}} = 0.89$$

The high value (close to $+1$) confirms that the relationship is strong and positive. You may have noticed that all the points on the scatterplot except one (Central Region) lie very close to a straight line. A point which is distant from the rest of the data and does not follow the general pattern is called an **_outlier_**. This is the same definition as for data on one variable (see Section 2.4.3). There is no reason to think that the values for Central are in error (they are almost certainly correct). It may be of interest to investigate why water consumption in Central does not follow the same pattern as in the rest of the Scottish regions.

The presence of an outlier reduces the correlation between the variables. If we calculate the correlation coefficient again, excluding Central, we obtain a value of 0.98 – representing an almost perfectly linear relationship. Note that this calculation is for illustration only – if we are interested in the relationship between water consumption and population, we should not exclude the outlier.

Section 2.6

Exercise 2.6.1

1. Plots of data

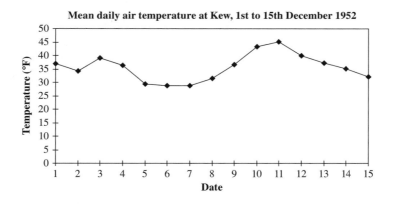

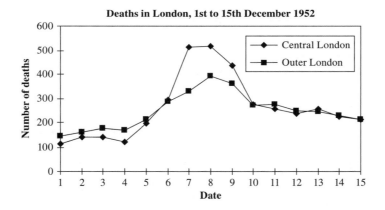

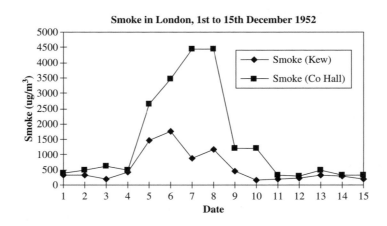

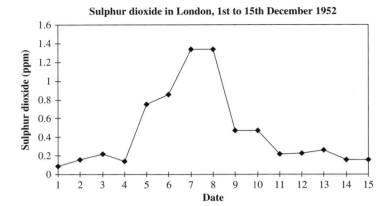

2. Findings: deaths

- Outer London: Steady at around 150–180 deaths per day until 4 December, and thereafter steady rise to peak of about 400 on 8 December, and then gradually falls to a little over 200 per day by the end of the observation period.

- Central London: Steady at around 110–140 deaths per day until 4 December (*below* level for outer London), then steep increase to peak of over 500 on 7–8 December (considerably *above* level for outer London), and thereafter falling to similar level as outer London.

3. Findings: pollution

- Smoke: County Hall levels began rising on 4–5 December, reaching a peak on 7–8 December, falling rapidly on 9 December, and returning to initial level by 12 December. The initial rise on 4–5 December was very rapid, and appeared to occur a day in advance of the equivalent rise (and fall) in deaths. The Kew data show a very similar time pattern, but at rather lower levels. Note that these values of smoke concentration (up to $4460 \mu g/m^3$) are very high indeed.

- Sulphur dioxide (SO_2): County Hall levels mirror the smoke changes very closely, apart from the less steep increase on 5–6 December.

4. Findings: temperature

At the same time as the pollution increased after 4 December, the temperature fell below freezing ($32 \,^\circ F$), as expected with the climatic conditions associated with smogs (cold, trapped, still air). The temperature began rising again on 8 December, before the pollution began to fall, consistent with the fact that the change in climatic conditions allowed the polluted air to disperse. It can be seen how quite warm air then appeared on the scene over the next few days. Although the temperature data were reported only for the one site (Kew), it seems unlikely that there would have been any substantial variation in air temperature across the city.

5. Interpretation

How can we interpret these findings? We know a number of facts now:

- Deaths began increasing on 4 December, though mainly from 5 December, and increased most in central London.

- The pollution levels increased at the same time, and there is some evidence that the steep rise occurred a day or so in advance of the rise in deaths (especially for smoke), and fell a day or so in advance of the decline in deaths.

- The pollution reached much higher levels in central London, although levels were very high by modern standards in both parts.

- The temperature fell at the time that the pollution increased.

This information strongly suggests that the air conditions could have led to the increase in deaths. Was smoke, SO_2, or temperature responsible, or was it a combination of these? The spatial pattern (central/outer London) and the time sequence (pollution changes precede changes in deaths), are supportive of this being a real and probably causal association.

6. **What other information?**

We have information on place (different parts of London) and time, but not on person (for example, age, sex, etc.). We could strengthen our conclusions with additional information, as follows:

- Break down the deaths by age, sex and cause to see whether those most likely to be affected by air pollution (e.g. respiratory and heart conditions such as heart failure) showed the most dramatic increase.

- Obtaining additional information on hospital admissions (morbidity) could add numbers and detail.

- It would be useful to see whether a fall in temperature, not associated with marked increases in pollution, led to increased deaths (in fact, it does, but not on the scale seen here: what happened in London in 1952 was a combined effect with a major contribution from the pollution, mainly due to the smoke component).

Exercise 2.6.2

A problem can arise because we are assuming that just because the fat consumption (average per capita) is high for a country, it is also high for those individual women in that country who develop breast cancer. For all we know, these women could be the ones with average, or even lower-than-average fat consumption in that country. Without data on the actual fat consumption of women with and without breast cancer, we cannot say whether or not this is the case.

3

Standardisation

Introduction and learning objectives

Standardisation is a very important and commonly used technique that effectively allows you to make more valid comparisons between sets of data than would otherwise be possible. We are going to explore this method, and you will learn how to carry it out, by reference to comparisons of mortality data from two very different parts of Merseyside in northwest England.

Learning objectives

By the end of this chapter, you should be able to do the following:

- Describe the purpose of standardisation.

- Describe direct and indirect methods of standardisation, and calculate and interpret examples of each.

- Describe the concept of a confidence interval, and calculate and interpret this for a standardised mortality ratio.

- Describe the main characteristics of direct and indirect approaches to standardisation and use these to select the most appropriate method for a given data set.

3.1 Health inequalities in Merseyside

3.1.1 Socio-economic conditions and health

For a variety of reasons, including the allocation of resources and monitoring of health status, it is very important to be able to quantify levels of ill health within a local health system administrative unit such as the primary care trust (PCT), as well as variations between PCTs. We will now explore

Quantitative Methods for Health Research   Nigel Bruce, Daniel Pope and Debbi Stanistreet
© 2008 John Wiley & Sons, Ltd

this through the example of *all-cause mortality* among men in two of Merseyside's most contrasting areas, the PCTs of Central Liverpool (high levels of unemployment and poverty) and Southport and Formby (quite affluent).

Liverpool, like all other cities, contains areas of poverty and wealth. These social inequalities are, however, very great, and the reasons lie principally in the history of the city's economic growth and decline. The growth of Liverpool was based on maritime trade, the industries that grew up in the Merseyside area processing raw materials brought in from overseas, such as sugar and tobacco, and manufacturing industry such as shipbuilding. The decline of this maritime trade, combined with the general loss of the manufacturing industry in the UK, hit Liverpool particularly badly, with the result that, historically, unemployment has been extremely high. More recently, Liverpool has attracted considerable investment through European Union funding and also as a result of its successful bid to become European Capital of Culture (2008). However, the legacy of high levels of unemployment, poverty and lack of opportunity has been high levels of morbidity and mortality from common conditions such as heart disease and lung cancer.

Southport and Formby PCT, on the other hand, is a more affluent and rural community on the coast north of Liverpool. It is a popular retirement area and a well-known seaside resort for residents of northwest England.

3.1.2 Comparison of crude death rates

If we wish to compare the mortality in Central Liverpool PCT and Southport and Formby PCT, either with each other or with the region or country, we could simply do so with the *crude death rates*. Based on data for the year 2003, the all-cause crude death rate for Central Liverpool PCT was 11.39 per 1000/year, and that for Southport and Formby PCT was 13.59 per 1000/year. This appears to suggest that mortality is higher in Southport and Formby PCT, although this is not what we would expect given the socio-economic circumstances of the two areas. Let's now consider the consequences of one PCT having a higher proportion of older people than the other. We would expect that this factor alone would result in a higher overall death rate in the PCT with the older population. We know that Southport and Formby is a popular retirement area, so this is a reasonable explanation. Table 3.1.1 shows the *age distributions* for the two PCTs in 2003.

Table 3.1.1 Populations of Central Liverpool PCT and Southport and Formby PCT 2003

PCT (2003)	Central Liverpool PCT		Southport and Formby PCT	
Age group	Population (1000s)	(%)	Population (1000s)	(%)
0–4	12.7	5.4	5.5	4.8
5–14	27.5	11.6	14.0	12.1
15–24	47.0	19.8	11.9	10.3
25–34	33.9	14.3	11.6	10.0
35–44	33.3	14.0	16.6	14.3
45–54	27.6	11.6	15.4	13.3
55–64	22.3	9.4	15.2	13.1
65–74	18.5	7.8	13.0	11.2
75–84	11.0	4.6	9.3	8.0
85 and over	3.3	1.4	3.2	2.8
Total	**237.1**		**115.7**	

Source: http://www.statistics.gov.uk

Self-Assessment Exercise 3.1.1

1. Examine these data, and comment on the age distributions of the two PCTs. You may find it helpful to plot the data in a histogram.

2. What are the implications of your observations for any comparison of crude death rates between the PCTs?

Answers in Section 3.5

3.1.3 Usefulness of a summary measure

The analysis of the age distribution for the two PCTs shows how important it is to examine *age-specific death rates*. We shall do this shortly, but for many purposes it is very useful to have a summary measure of mortality for all age groups (or perhaps a wide band of age groups that we may be interested in). For example, if we wish to look at mortality for all PCTs in one region of the country, imagine how cumbersome it would be to try to do so with many tables of rates for each age group, especially if all of these were to be included in a report.

What we are looking for is a summary measure of mortality that takes account of the differences in age distribution of the two areas. This is provided by a technique called *standardisation*, and there are two methods:

- The *indirect* method, which provides the *standardised mortality ratio (SMR)*, and *indirectly standardised rates.*

- The *direct* method, which provides *directly standardised rates*.

We will look at the *indirect* method first. Using Central Liverpool PCT as an example, we will first work through the calculation and interpretation of the *SMR*. You will then have the opportunity to try this out with the Southport and Formby PCT data.

Summary: why standardise for age?

- If two populations differ in their age structure, a simple comparison of overall disease or death rates is misleading.

- This is because age is a powerful determinant of disease and death rates.

- Standardisation provides a means of 'adjusting' for these differences in age distribution, and hence of making a more valid comparison.

3.2 Indirect standardisation: calculation of the standardised mortality ratio (SMR)

3.2.1 Mortality in Central Liverpool PCT ward

Table 3.2.1 provides all of the data that we require for carrying out the standardisation, and calculating the SMR:

- The population in Central Liverpool PCT in each age group in 2003.

- The age-specific annual death rates for a 'standard' population; in this case, England and Wales, for 2003.

The table also provides the number of deaths that occurred in each age group in Central Liverpool PCT for the year 2003. While it is not necessary to have information on the numbers of deaths in each age group in order to calculate the SMR, we have included these in the table so that you can calculate and compare the local and national mortality rates.

Table 3.2.1 Deaths, population and death rates (Central Liverpool PCT), and death rates (England and Wales), for 2003

Age group	Deaths: Central Liverpool PCT 2003 'observed'	Population: Central Liverpool PCT 2003 (thousands)	Central Liverpool PCT: age-specific mortality rate per 1000/year	England and Wales 2003: mortality rate per 1000/year	Deaths 'expected' in Central Liverpool PCT 2003
0–4	22	12.7	1.73	1.29	16.38
5–14	5	27.5	0.18	0.12	3.30
15–24	15	47.0		0.46	
25–34	28	33.9		0.71	
35–44	99	33.3		1.28	
45–54	151	27.6		3.16	
55–64	284	22.3		7.72	
65–74	591	18.5		21.25	
75–84	875	11.0		59.98	
85 plus	632	3.3		172.93	
Total	**2702**	**237.1**			

Source: http://www.statistics.gov.uk.

 Self-Assessment Exercise 3.2.1

1. We will look first at the *age-specific rates* for Central Liverpool PCT. For age 0–4, this has been calculated as 22 (deaths) divided by 12 700 (population), and multiplied by 1000 (to express as a rate per 1000 per year). This comes out at 1.73 deaths per 1000 population per year.

(a) Calculate the rate for the age group 5–14 and ensure that you obtain the correct value of 0.18 per 1000 per year.

(b) Now calculate the missing values for the remaining age groups, and check these against the answers (Section 3.5).

2. Compare the age-specific rates for Central Liverpool PCT with those for England and Wales. What do you notice?

It has been useful to calculate age-specific mortality rates for Liverpool so that we can compare rates with those of England and Wales, but we do not need to do this in order to calculate an SMR for Central Liverpool PCT. In fact, we do not need to know how many deaths occurred in each age group in Central Liverpool PCT, but only the overall number of deaths.

3. We now need to calculate the numbers of deaths that would have occurred in Central Liverpool PCT, in each age group, if the England and Wales death rates had applied. This is in the last column, and is termed the **expected** deaths. So, for the 0–4 age group, we multiply the national rate (1.29 per 1000/year) by the local population in the same age group (12 700), and obtain 16.38 **expected deaths**:

$$\frac{1.29 \times 12700}{1000} = 16.38$$

Of course, we cannot really have fractions of deaths! This is not a problem here though, since we are dealing with a hypothetical situation of *'how many deaths would you expect if national rates applied to the local population?'*

(a) Check now that you can calculate the correct number for the 5–14 age group (3.30 deaths).

(b) Finally, calculate the numbers for the other age groups, and check your results with the answers.

4. To calculate the SMR, we need the total expected deaths. This is calculated by adding up all the age-specific expected deaths $(16.38 + 3.30 + \ldots)$. Note, it is *not* calculated by multiplying the total Central Liverpool population by the all-age ('crude') mortality rate for England and Wales.

5. We are now in a position to calculate the SMR. This is defined as:

$$\frac{\text{Total number of } \boldsymbol{observed} \text{ deaths}}{\text{Total number of } \boldsymbol{expected} \text{ deaths}} = \frac{2702}{1990.95}$$

It is usually expressed as if it were a percentage, and therefore multiplied by 100. So for Central Liverpool PCT, the SMR is 2702 (observed) divided by 1990.95 (expected), multiplied by 100, which comes out at 135.7, or 136 rounded to the nearest whole number.

Answers in Section 3.5

Summary: calculating the SMR

- An SMR is calculated by the indirect method of standardisation.

- To do this, we need to select a 'standard population' (e.g. the country) and know the rates for each category of the variable we wish to standardise for (in this case age).

- Standardisation is achieved by applying these standard category-specific rates to the category-specific population in the area to be standardised. This yields expected cases.

- The SMR is calculated by adding up all the expected cases, and presenting the ratio of observed to expected, usually as a percentage.

3.2.2   Interpretation of the SMR

The SMR was calculated by using the England and Wales rates as a standard. In other words, we are comparing the actual (observed) numbers of deaths in Central Liverpool PCT with the number that would have occurred (expected) if the local population experienced these national mortality rates in each age group. An SMR of 136 therefore means that, independently of the influence of the age distribution in Central Liverpool PCT, the overall mortality in that PCT is 36 per cent higher than that in England and Wales. We are not yet in a position to make any comparison with Southport and Formby PCT, but we will come to that shortly.

3.2.3   Dealing with random variation: the 95 per cent confidence interval

It can be appreciated that the exact number of deaths occurring in Central Liverpool PCT in a given year is determined by the level of mortality in that population, but will inevitably vary from year to year. This variation is essentially due to *chance* (random), so that in one year there may be 2735 deaths, in the next year 2681, in the following year 2700, and so on. This random variation is separate from systematic effects such as a *trend* over time, which may show a gradual increase or decrease in the level of mortality. It is also distinct from variation due to changes in the population numbers or age distribution.

The result of this chance, year-to-year variation is that the SMR is subject to *random error*. This error is greater if the numbers of deaths are small, as with a small population and/or a less common cause of death. So we have an SMR of 136 but we also know that this *estimate* could, by chance, be too high or too low. The question is, how much random variation might there be? That is, can we quantify this random variation? The way to answer this very important question is by calculating a *confidence interval (CI)*. We will be exploring the uses and calculation of CIs a good deal more in later chapters, so at this stage we will focus mainly on the purpose and interpretation. We will, however, calculate the CI for the SMR in this exercise, to allow a more complete understanding of the interpretation of an SMR. The 95 per cent CI for the SMR for a given population can be defined as follows:

The 95 per cent CI for an SMR is the range in which we can be 95 per cent confident that the true mortality value for the population lies.

The calculation of this 95 per cent CI is quite straightforward by the following method (which is adequate for most purposes):

$$\text{Upper limit of 95\% CI for SMR} = SMR + 1.96 \times \frac{SMR}{\sqrt{observed\ deaths}}$$

$$\text{Lower limit of 95\% CI for SMR} = SMR - 1.96 \times \frac{SMR}{\sqrt{observed\ deaths}}$$

The upper limit is therefore

$$136 + \left[1.96 \times \frac{136}{\sqrt{2702}} \right] = 136 + 5.128 = 141.128$$

The derivation of the 1.96 multiplication factor will be covered in Chapter 4 (Surveys). There is no point being too precise with the confidence limits, so we will round this to 141. The lower limit therefore is 136–5.128 = 130.874, which we will round to 131.

The term in the formula (SMR/$\sqrt{}$number of observed deaths) is known as the ***standard error*** (SE) of the SMR. The SE is a measure of the precision of an estimate, and this applies whether we are talking about an SMR, a mean, a proportion, a measure of risk, etc. We will look at SE in more detail when thinking about the precision of means derived through sample surveys in Chapter 4. At this stage, it is sufficient to understand the concept of SE as being a measure of how big the margin of random error is around something measured in a sample.

We have now determined that the Central Liverpool PCT SMR is 136, with a 95 per cent CI of 131–141. If we fit these figures into the definition given above, we can be 95 per cent confident that the true SMR lies between 131 and 141, or 31–41 per cent above the national level of mortality. It is clear, then, that mortality in Central Liverpool PCT, independent of age distribution, is still some way above the national average.

3.2.4 Increasing precision of the SMR estimate

We have been able to estimate the precision of the SMR quite accurately, as Central Liverpool PCT includes quite a large population. However, this would not necessarily be true if we were dealing with electoral ward level data, where the population would be considerably smaller. In this situation we may find that our estimate is very imprecise with a wide CI. In this case, the best way to reduce this imprecision is to increase the numbers. We usually do this by calculating the SMR for a longer period of time, say, 3 or 5 years.

Summary: 95 per cent CI for the SMR

- The SMR is subject to year-on-year random variation.

- It is very helpful to be able to quantify this variation, and this is provided by the 95 per cent CI.

- The statistical derivation of the CI, the reason for choosing a 95 per cent CI, etc., will all be discussed in later chapters.

3.2.5   Mortality in Southport and Formby PCT

Now it is your turn to calculate the SMR for the more affluent PCT, Southport and Formby. Work through the data provided in Table 3.2.2, and the questions which follow. Once we have completed this stage, we will look at how to compare the results for the two wards.

Table 3.2.2   Deaths, population and death rates (Southport and Formby PCT), and death rates (England and Wales), for 2003

Age group	Deaths: Southport and Formby PCT 2003 'observed'	Population: Southport and Formby PCT 2003 (1000s)	Southport and Formby PCT: age-specific mortality rate per 1000/year	England and Wales 2003: mortality rate per 1000/year	Deaths 'expected' in Southport and Formby PCT 2003
0–4	2	5.5		1.29	
5–14	2	14.0		0.12	
15–24	3	11.9		0.46	
25–34	13	11.6		0.71	
35–44	15	16.6		1.28	
45–54	45	15.4		3.16	
55–64	99	15.2		7.72	
65–74	273	13.0		21.25	
75–84	537	9.3		59.98	
85 plus	583	3.2		172.93	
Total	**1572**	**115.7**			

   Self-Assessment Exercise 3.2.2

1. Calculate the age-specific mortality rates for Southport and Formby PCT, and put these into the table. Comment on how these rates compare with those for Central Liverpool PCT (Table 3.2.1).

2. Calculate the expected numbers of deaths from the 2003 England and Wales age-specific rates, and put these into the table.

3. Calculate the SMR for Southport and Formby PCT.

4. Calculate the 95 per cent CI for the Southport and Formby PCT SMR.

5. Interpret the results you now have for Southport and Formby PCT (do not compare with Central Liverpool PCT yet).

Answers in Section 3.5

3.2.6 Comparison of SMRs

It might be tempting to make a direct comparison between the two SMRs, and say that Central Liverpool PCT mortality is $136 \div 98 = 1.38$ times higher than for people in Southport and Formby PCT. This, however, would be incorrect, as SMRs should not be compared directly in this way. What we can say, based on the single year of data for 2003, is that mortality in Central Liverpool PCT is 31–41 per cent higher than the national average. For Southport and Formby PCT, mortality lies between 6 per cent lower, and 3 per cent higher; that is, it does not differ significantly from the national level (the 95 per cent CI includes 100). The reason why we cannot make a direct comparison between the two SMRs is that the age-specific rates used for the standardisation have been applied to two different populations.

In Section 3.4, we will look at *direct standardisation*. One characteristic of this method is that it does allow a simple comparison between standardised rates.

3.2.7 Indirectly standardised mortality rates

If we wish to express the mortality in Central Liverpool PCT or Southport and Formby PCT as an overall rate (equivalent to the crude rate, but standardised), it is derived as follows:

$$\text{Indirectly standardised rate} = \frac{\text{SMR} \times \text{ crude rate for the Standard population}}{100}$$

The crude death rate for the standard population (England and Wales) in 2003 was 10.2 per 1000/year.

- For Central Liverpool PCT, the male *indirectly standardised rate* $= 1.36 \times 10.2$ per 1000/year $= 13.9$ per 1000/year.

- For Southport and Formby PCT, the male *indirectly standardised rate* $= 0.98 \times 10.2$ per 1000/year $= 10.0$ per 1000/year.

Compare these with the unstandardised crude rates for each PCT, of 11.4 per 1000/year and 13.6 per 1000/year, respectively, to see how much difference the age-standardisation has made.

3.3 Direct standardisation

3.3.1 Introduction

We have noted that there are two main ways of standardising, *indirect* and *direct*. In both methods, the underlying principle is that we break the data down into categories of the factor we wish to standardise for (e.g. age, social class, ethnic group), and apply category-specific rates to category-specific population numbers to find out how many events to expect if those rates had applied. The difference between the two methods is as follows:

- With the **indirect** method, we used age-specific rates from another 'standard' population (England and Wales), and applied these to the population numbers (in the same age bands) for the group we intended to standardise (often referred to as the **index** population).

- With the **direct** method, we will use the age-specific rates from the group we intend to standardise (the **index** population), and apply these to the numbers of people (in the same age bands) in a standard population.

3.3.2 An example – changes in deaths from stroke over time

Suppose that we are helping to plan and develop stroke services in a PCT with a relatively high proportion of older residents. In the background review, we looked at the **crude death rates** for women aged 65 and over for the last 20 years, and were surprised to find that these had increased from 10 per 1000 per year in 1985 to 12.8 per 1000 per year in 2005. We are aware that the population has been ageing (that is to say, there is now a higher proportion of older people in the population when compared to 1985) and that it is a popular area for retirement, and we therefore wonder whether this might be the explanation, or at least part of it. The data are as shown in Table 3.3.1.

Table 3.3.1 Population and observed deaths from stroke for hypothetical population, 1985 and 2005

Age group	1985			2005		
	Population	Deaths observed	Age specific rate/ 1000 per year	Population	Deaths observed	Age specific rate/ 1000 per year
65–74	5000	25		4100	15	
75–84	3500	35		3000	31	
85+	1500	40		2900	78	
Total	**10 000**	**100**	**10.0**	**10 000**	**124**	**12.4**

 Self-Assessment Exercise 3.3.1

We are going to standardise the 2005 data to find out the expected deaths in 2005, using the 1985 population:

1. First of all, study the data in Table 3.3.1 carefully and describe what has happened to the population numbers and the observed numbers of deaths from stroke.

2. The first step in direct standardisation is to calculate and study the category-specific death rates (in this case age-specific rates for 2005). Put these rates into the table in the spaces provided.

3. What do you notice about the age-specific rates?

4. You will now standardise the 2005 rate to the 1985 population. To do this,

(a) Transfer your 2005 age-specific rates to the table below, and apply these to the 1985 age-specific population to calculate the expected numbers in each age group. Enter these results into the table:

Age group	Age-specific rate for 2005	Population 1985	Expected deaths for 2005
65–74		5000	
75–84		3500	
85+		1500	
Total		**10 000**	

(b) Add up the expected deaths to obtain the total.

(c) Divide the total expected cases by the total population in the standard (which is 1985 in this case) to obtain the age-standardised death rate.

5. Before checking the answers, have a go at interpreting the result you have obtained.

Answers in Section 3.5

3.3.3 Using the European standard population

In this example, we have standardised one group (2005) against the population of the other group (1985). Thus, 1985 has been taken as the standard, and this allows comparison between the standardised rates. As an alternative, we could have standardised both groups against another standard population, and this also allows comparison between the two groups. Although this gives essentially similar results, we will examine one example of how this is done, because it is a method that you are quite likely to encounter.

Table 3.3.2   The European standard population

Age group	Population	Age group	Population
0 – (infants)	1600	45–49	7000
1–4	6400	50–54	7000
5–9	7000	55–59	6000
10–14	7000	60–64	5000
15–19	7000	65–69	4000
20–14	7000	70–74	3000
25–29	7000	75–79	2000
30–34	7000	80–84	1000
35–39	7000	85 and over	1000
40–44	7000	**Total**	**100 000**

Source: World Health Annual of Statistics 1991.

So, what other population can we use as a standard? We could have used the national population, or one of a number of 'standard populations' available for this purpose. These are not real populations, but created to represent the population structure of the area we are dealing with. Thus, we will use the **European standard population**, but there are others, such as that for Africa, which has a much younger age distribution than that for Europe.

 ### Self-Assessment Exercise 3.3.2

1. Try standardising both the 1985 and 2005 data from the previous exercise (Table 3.3.1) to the European standard population, which is reproduced above. To do this, you will need to use the population numbers from the relevant age groups in Table 3.3.2, and apply (to these population data) the age-specific rates for 1985, and then those for 2005, to obtain the expected deaths for each year.

2. Does the use of this alternative 'standard' population make any difference to your conclusions?

Answers in Section 3.5

3.3.4　Direct or indirect – which method is best?

Having looked now at both indirect and direct standardisation, how do we decide which is the best method to use in any given situation? The following table summarises and compares the most important characteristics of the two methods:

Characteristic	Indirect method	Direct method
Age-specific rates in populations to be standardised ('index' populations)	Not actually required, as we need only the age-specific population data. Thus, this is the only method that can be used if the numbers of deaths (cases) in each age group are not available.	Age-specific rates in index population are required; hence, both the number of cases and the population in each age group must be available.
Precision	Generally more precise, since category-specific rates are those from a standard population which can be selected to be as precise as possible. This is especially true when numbers of deaths (cases) are relatively small in the categories of the index population.	Since we have to rely on category-specific rates in the index population, the result may be imprecise if these rates are based on small numbers.
Comparison of standardised rates	Direct comparison is not possible.	Direct comparison is possible.

In making a choice, the most important criterion is likely to be the precision, especially if we are dealing with small numbers, such as cause-specific mortality data at the level of a PCT or a smaller area such as an electoral ward. In these situations, the indirect method may be more appropriate.

3.4 Standardisation for factors other than age

In the examples used in this section, we have standardised death rates for age, but the method is equally applicable for any rate, such as incidence of disease, and for standardising for other factors that could affect a comparison that we wish to make (e.g. socio-economic classification, geographical area of residence, ethnic group).

Taking socio-economic classification as an example (see Chapter 2, Section 2.1.5), we would break down the data into categories of (group 1: large employers and higher managerial; group 1.2: higher professional; group 2: lower managerial and professional; group 3: intermediate,. . . through to group 8: never worked and long-term unemployed) in exactly the same way as we have used age categories (0–4, 5–14, etc.). Obtaining the category-specific rates and populations that we require may not always be as straightforward as for age, but the principle is the same as that we have worked through for age standardisation.

Summary

- Standardisation is done to adjust rates for the influence of one or more factors which could affect the comparison of those rates. These factors may include age, socio-economic classification, area of residence, ethnic group, etc.

- There are two main methods of standardisation: indirect and direct.

- Indirect standardisation applies category-specific rates from a standard population to the numbers of people in each category in the index population.

- Direct standardisation applies category-specific rates from the index population to the numbers of people in each category of a standard population.

- Indirect standardisation is generally more precise, does not require category-specific rates in the index population for its calculation (but see next point, below), and does not allow direct comparison with other indirectly standardised rates.

- It is always a good idea to check the category-specific rates in the populations being standardised, to see whether there are any important inconsistencies that should be highlighted, and which may be masked by an overall standardised rate, or standardised ratio.

One final word of caution regarding standardisation of rates for males and females. In the example based on Liverpool and Southport & Formby PCTs, we carried out standardisation for the whole population (males and females combined) because the pattern of male rates relative to female rates is more or less consistent. However, when it comes to looking at specific causes death, for example road traffic accidents, it would be very misleading to standardise using rates for persons (combined rates for males and females) as rates differ markedly at some age groups.

3.5 Answers to self-assessment exercises

Exercise 3.1.1

1. Population structures

These data show that Central Liverpool PCT has a younger population.

2. Implications

All other factors being equal, since Central Liverpool PCT has a younger population, we would expect a lower death rate. Our aim now is to find out how the two PCT areas compare, independently of the effects of this difference in age distribution.

Exercise 3.2.1

1. Age-specific rates

Age group	Deaths: Central Liverpool PCT 2003 'observed'	Population: Central Liverpool PCT 2003 (thousands)	Central Liverpool PCT: age-specific mortality rate per 1000/year	England and Wales 2003: mortality rate per 1000/year	Deaths 'expected' in Central Liverpool PCT 2003
0–4	22	12.7	1.73	1.29	16.38
5–14	5	27.5	0.18	0.12	3.30
15–24	15	47.0	**0.32**	0.46	
25–34	28	33.9	**0.83**	0.71	
35–44	99	33.3	**2.97**	1.28	
45–54	151	27.6	**5.47**	3.16	
55–64	284	22.3	**12.74**	7.72	
65–74	591	18.5	**31.94**	21.25	
75–84	875	11.0	**79.55**	59.98	
85 plus	632	3.3	**191.52**	172.93	
Total	2702	237.1			

2. Comparison of age-specific rates with England and Wales

For all but the 15–24 age group, the age-specific rates for Central Liverpool PCT are above those for the country. Note that for age groups where the number of deaths are small (such as the 5–14 age group), rates are highly influenced by just one additional death, illustrating well how unstable these rates are when we are dealing with small areas and numbers.

3. Expected numbers of deaths

Age group	Deaths: Central Liverpool PCT 2003 'observed'	Population: Central Liverpool PCT 2003 (thousands)	Central Liverpool PCT: age-specific mortality rate per 1000/year	England and Wales 2003: mortality rate per 1000/year	Deaths 'expected' in Central Liverpool PCT 2003
0–4	22	12.7	1.73	1.29	16.38
5–14	5	27.5	0.18	0.12	3.30
15–24	15	47.0	0.32	0.46	**21.62**

25–34	28	33.9	0.83	0.71	**24.07**
35–44	99	33.3	2.97	1.28	**42.62**
45–54	151	27.6	5.47	3.16	**87.22**
55–64	284	22.3	12.74	7.72	**172.16**
65–74	591	18.5	31.94	21.25	**393.13**
75–84	875	11.0	79.55	59.98	**659.78**
85 plus	632	3.3	191.52	172.93	**570.67**
Total	**2702**	**237.1**			**1990.95**

Exercise 3.2.2

1. SMR for Southport and Formby PCT

Age-specific rates are shown in the table below.

Age group	Deaths: Southport and Formby PCT 2003 'observed'	Population: Southport and Formby PCT 2003 (thousands)	Southport and Formby PCT: age-specific mortality rate per 1000/year	England and Wales 2003: mortality rate per 1000/year	Deaths 'expected' in Southport and Formby PCT 2003
0–4	2	5.5	**0.36**	1.29	
5–14	2	14.0	**0.14**	0.12	
15–24	3	11.9	**0.25**	0.46	
25–34	13	11.6	**1.12**	0.71	
35–44	15	16.6	**0.90**	1.28	
45–54	45	15.4	**2.92**	3.16	
55–64	99	15.2	**6.51**	7.72	
65–74	273	13.0	**21.00**	21.25	
75–84	537	9.3	**57.74**	59.98	
85 plus	583	3.2	**182.19**	172.93	
Total	**1572**	**115.7**			

The Southport and Formby PCT age-specific mortality rates are consistently below those for Central Liverpool PCT. This is important and reassuring, because it is unwise to standardise if there is a less consistent pattern: suppose, for example, that the Southport and Formby PCT rates for young/middle-aged people were higher than Central Liverpool PCT, while those for older people were lower. When calculating an SMR, it will 'mix' these two characteristics of the data, and the overall SMR would be misleading.

2. Expected deaths

Table 3.2.2 Deaths, population and death rates (Southport and Formby PCT), and death rates (England and Wales), for 2003

Age group	Deaths: Southport and Formby PCT 2003 'observed'	Population: Southport and Formby PCT 2003	Southport and Formby PCT: age-specific mortality rate per 1000/year	England and Wales 2003: mortality rate per 1000/year	Deaths 'expected' in Southport and Formby PCT 2003
0–4	2	5.5	0.36	1.29	**7.10**
5–14	2	14.0	0.14	0.12	**1.68**
15–24	3	11.9	0.25	0.46	**5.47**

Table 3.2.2   Continued.

Age group	Deaths: Southport and Formby PCT 2003 'observed'	Population: Southport and Formby PCT 2003	Southport and Formby PCT: age-specific mortality rate per 1000/year	England and Wales 2003: mortality rate per 1000/year	Deaths 'expected' in Southport and Formby PCT 2003
25–34	13	11.6	1.12	0.71	**8.24**
35–44	15	16.6	0.90	1.28	**21.25**
45–54	45	15.4	2.92	3.16	**48.66**
55–64	99	15.2	6.51	7.72	**117.34**
65–74	273	13.0	21.00	21.25	**276.25**
75–84	537	9.3	57.74	59.98	**557.81**
85 plus	583	3.2	182.19	172.93	**553.38**
Total	**1572**	**115.7**			**1597.18**

3. Calculation of SMR

The SMR is observed/expected $\times 100$; hence, SMR $= (1572 \div 1597.18) \times 100 = 98.4$.

4. Calculation of 95 per cent CI

Refer to Section 2.6 to check the formula for the CI. The SE $= 2.47$, so $(1.96 \times SE) = 4.84$, and the 95 per cent CI $= 93.6$ to 103.2 (94 to 103 rounded to nearest whole numbers).

5. Interpretation of SMR

We can be 95 per cent confident that the all-cause mortality for Southport and Formby PCT (2003) lies between 6% below the national level and 3 per cent above it. This range includes 100, which is the value for the standard population (England and Wales), and hence we have no evidence that the SMR for Southport and Formby PCT differs from that for the country.

Exercise 3.3.1

1. Change in population and deaths

The population has aged (there is now a higher proportion of people represented in the older age groups). The numbers of deaths have fallen in the 65–74 age group, are unchanged in the 75–84 age group, but have risen (substantially) in the 85+ year age group.

2. Calculation of age-specific death rates

Age group	1985			2005		
	Population	Deaths observed	Age specific rate/1000 per year	Population	Deaths observed	Age specific rate/1000 per year
65–74	5000	25	**5.0**	4100	15	**3.7**
75–84	3500	35	**10.0**	3000	31	**10.3**
85+	1500	40	**26.7**	2900	78	**26.9**
Total	**10 000**	**100**	**10.0**	**10 000**	**124**	**12.4**

3. **Changes in age-specific rates**

Between 1985 and 2005, the death rates have fallen in the youngest age group, but stayed almost constant (risen very slightly) in the older two age groups.

4. **Calculation of the standardised rate**

Age group	Age-specific rate for 2005	Population 1985	Expected deaths for 2005
65–74	**3.7**	5000	**18.5**
75–84	**10.3**	3500	**36.1**
85+	**26.9**	1500	**40.4**
Total	**9.5**	**10 000**	**95.0**

The age-standardised rate for 2005 is $(95.0/10\,000) \times 1000 = 9.5$ per 1000 per year. This is just a little lower than the crude rate for 1985 (10 per 1000/year). You can directly compare these, by dividing 9.5 per 1000/year by 10 per 1000/year, to get 0.95, or, expressed as a percentage, 95 per cent.

5. **Interpretation**

You will note that after standardisation of the 2005 rate to the 1985 population, far from being higher than the 1985 rate, the 2005 rate is actually a little lower. Thus, it appears that the changing population structure was the main reason for the rise in the crude rate. Please note, however, that the age-specific rates have changed in an inconsistent way, and if we had not examined these, we could have wrongly assumed that the situation had improved for all three age groups given that the 2005 standardised rate is 95 per cent of the 1985 crude rate.

Exercise 3.3.2

1. **Standardisation using the European standard population**

The directly standardised rates using the European standard population are as follows:

Age group	European population	1985		2005	
		Rate	**Expected**	**Rate**	**Expected**
65–74	7000	5.0	35.0	3.7	25.9
75–84	3000	10.0	30.0	10.3	30.9
85+	1000	26.7	26.7	26.9	26.9
Total	**11 000**		**91.7**		**83.7**

1985: $(91.7/11000) \times 1000 = 8.34$ per 1000/year
2005: $(83.7/11000) \times 1000 = 7.61$ per 1000/year
Ratio of rates (2005 : 1985) = 91.2 per cent.

2. **Does it make any difference**?

You will notice that the actual values of the rates are different when calculated with the European standard population, and the ratio of rates is a little lower, but the overall conclusion is similar. The different results are due to the standardising population being different, and, more specifically, the population structure being different; in the original example, the population was much more heavily weighted towards elderly people than the European standard, as this was a retirement area. Thus, it is important to check that the standard population used is appropriate to the study population, even though the process is fairly robust.

4

Surveys

Introduction and learning objectives

In Chapter 2 we saw that, although we can learn a great deal from the presentation and analysis of routinely collected data, we are inevitably limited to using the information that has been collected for purposes that, to a greater or lesser extent, often differ from our own. Not only may the information be different from what we are after, but it may have been collected in a way that does not meet the rigorous standards we seek. Surveys provide the opportunity to fill in these gaps; both in the nature of the information collected and in the means by which it is collected.

Learning objectives

By the end of this chapter, you should be able to do the following:

- Define concepts of population, sample and inference, and explain why sampling is used.

- Describe the main probability and non-probability sampling methods, including simple random, stratified, cluster, multistage, convenience, systematic and quota, giving examples of their uses.

- Define bias, and give examples relevant to sampling (selection bias).

- Define sampling error and describe its relationship with sample size.

- Define, calculate and interpret standard error for a mean and a proportion.

- Discuss the issue of sample size, in relation to precision of estimates from a sample.

(Continued)

Quantitative Methods for Health Research   Nigel Bruce, Daniel Pope and Debbi Stanistreet
© 2008 John Wiley & Sons, Ltd

- Define, calculate and interpret the confidence interval (CI) for a population mean and a population proportion.

- Calculate sample size for precision of a sample estimate, for continuous data (mean) and categorical data (proportion).

- Describe the principles of valid and repeatable measurement, with examples from interview and questionnaire material.

- Describe sources of bias in measurement and some of the ways in which good design can minimise bias.

- Prepare a simple questionnaire, employing principles of good design.

- Define categorical, discrete and continuous data types, providing examples of each type and present these by suitable display methods.

We will be studying survey methods, mainly using the example of the National Survey of Sexual Attitudes and Lifestyles (NATSAL), which was carried out to provide high-quality information not available from any other source.

The original survey was carried out in 1990 and subsequently repeated in 2000. For the purposes of this chapter, we will be looking mainly at the follow-up study (known as NATSAL 2000). However, we will also refer to the original study as this includes more detail on some important aspects of study design.

Resource paper for the NATSAL 2000 study

Paper A

Johnson, A. M., Mercer, C. H., Erens, B. *et al.* (2001). Sexual behaviour in Britain: partnerships, practices, and HIV risk behaviours. *Lancet* **358**, 1835–1842.

Resource paper for the NATSAL 1990 study

Paper B

Wellings, K., Field, J., Wadsworth, J. *et al.* (1990). Sexual lifestyles under scrutiny. *Nature* **348**, 276–278.

4.1 Purpose and context

4.1.1 Defining the research question

We saw in Chapter 1 how important it is to formulate a clear research question. So, one of the first jobs for the research team is to define the purpose of the study as clearly and concisely as possible. This is very important for those carrying out the research, but it is also important that anyone reading the published report is absolutely clear about what the research is trying to achieve. Any assessment you make of the methods, findings, interpretation and conclusions will be of limited value if the underlying purpose is not clear in your mind.

Please now read the following abstract and introduction taken from paper A.

Abstract

Background

Sexual behaviour is a major determinant of sexual and reproductive health. We did a National Survey of Sexual Attitudes and Lifestyles (Natsal 2000) in 1999–2001 to provide population estimates of behaviour patterns and to compare them with estimates from 1990–91 (Natsal 1990).

Methods

We did a probability sample survey of men and women aged 16–44 years who were resident in Britain, using computer-assisted interviews. Results were compared with data from respondents in Natsal 1990.

Findings

We interviewed 11,161 respondents (4762 men, 6399 women). Patterns of heterosexual and homosexual partnership varied substantially by age, residence in Greater London, and marital status. In the past 5 years, mean numbers of heterosexual partners were 3·8 (SD 8·2) for men, and 2·4 (SD 4·6) for women; 2·6% (95% CI 2·2–3·1) of both men and women reported homosexual partnerships; and 4·3% (95% CI 3·7–5·0) of men reported paying for sex. In the past year, mean number of new partners varied from 2·04 (SD 8·4) for single men aged 25–34 years to 0·05 (SD 0·3) for married women aged 35–44 years. Prevalence of many reported behaviours had risen compared with data from Natsal 1990. Benefits of greater condom use were offset by increases in reported partners. Changes between surveys were generally greater for women than men and for respondents outside London.

Interpretation Our study provides updated estimates of sexual behaviour patterns. The increased reporting of risky sexual behaviours is consistent with changing cohabitation patterns and rising incidence of sexually transmitted infections. Observed differences between Natsal 1990 and Natsal 2000 are likely to result from a combination of true change and greater willingness to report sensitive behaviours in Natsal 2000 due to improved survey methodology and more tolerant social attitudes.

You should not be concerned if you do not understand all the technical terms used in describing the study. We deal with all of these as we work through this chapter, and will only assume understanding of concepts and methods that have already been covered, or that are being introduced in the section to which the paper refers.

Introduction

Population patterns of sexual behaviour are major determinants of conception rates, sexually transmitted infections (STI) and HIV transmission, and other sexual health outcomes. Probability sample surveys have made a major contribution to understanding the diversity of human sexual behaviour.[1–6] In 1990–91, the first National Survey of Sexual Attitudes and Lifestyles (Natsal 1990) was done in Britain and focused on patterns of HIV risk behaviour, partnership formation, and sexual practices.[1,2,7] The results have been widely used to model the extent of the HIV epidemic in Britain and to plan sexual health services and preventive interventions.[6,8,9]

(Continued)

Since Natsal 1990 was undertaken, there have been substantial changes in public attitudes towards sexual matters, a decline in the intensity of public HIV education, but increased attention on school sex education and teenage pregnancy.[10] Surveillance data indicate higher STI incidence rates in 2000 than 1990 suggesting that sexual behaviours may have changed over time.[11] Advances in understanding the transmission dynamics of STIs have created demands for population estimates of new variables such as prevalence of monogamy and concurrency, social and sexual mixing (including age, ethnicity, and location), and rates of partner acquisition.[12]

In 1999–2001 we did a second survey (Natsal 2000) using similar questions to Natsal 1990 but with improved methodology, to provide updated estimates and to assess changes in reported sexual behaviour over time.[13] Our results are presented here.

 Self-Assessment Exercise 4.1.1

List the reasons given for carrying out the NATSAL 2000 study.

Answers in Section 4.8

Aim and objectives

The purpose of a study is usually described in terms of an *aim* and *objectives*. These can be defined as follows:

- *Aim(s)*: a summary statement of what is proposed and the purpose of the study;

- *Objectives*: more specific description of what the various stages and/or components of the research are being designed to achieve. The objectives should not be over-complex or too numerous.

The aim of the NATSAL 2000 study can be described as being 'to provide updated estimates and to assess changes in reported sexual behaviour over time'.

4.1.2 Political context of research

Most, if not all, health research has some political implications. This is important in thinking about how the findings of the research can be translated into policy, and how various groups in society will respond. Not surprisingly, sexual behaviour is a subject about which many people hold strong views, including the political establishment. The NATSAL study did not escape this, particularly in respect of funding:

Researchers on both sides of the Atlantic have encountered difficulties in obtaining funds to mount large-scale cross-sectional surveys of sexual behaviour. Fieldwork for the main stage of the British survey of sexual attitudes and lifestyles, set to begin in April 1989 . . . was delayed because of a much-publicised government veto on financial support. (Paper B)

Exercise for reflection

Look through some newspapers (print copy or websites) of your choice for articles based on some research of relevance to health. See whether you can identify some political issues relating to (a) funding, (b) the methods used, or (c) the implications of the results for policy.

As this is an exercise for reflection, no answers or commentary are provided in Section 4.8.

Summary

- In planning your own research, defining a clear aim and a set of objectives is very important.

- Equally, when studying research carried out by others, it is necessary to be clear in your own mind about their aim(s) and objectives.

- The original (1990) NATSAL study was carried out to provide accurate estimates of sexual behaviour and to assess changes in reported sexual behaviour over time. Little or no useful information could be obtained from routine data sources, and a survey was therefore necessary. The original study was designed to meet this need, and overcome the limitations of methods used in earlier surveys of sexual attitudes and lifestyles.

- The new (2000) NATSAL study was carried out to update this information and to study changes over the 10-year period.

- All research has a political context which can influence design, funding, reporting and implementation.

4.2 Sampling methods

4.2.1 Introduction

Two of the greatest challenges faced by researchers studying sexual attitudes and lifestyles were obtaining *accurate* information and ensuring that the information was *representative* of the general population. These two points essentially sum up what good study design is about – first, is the information accurate, and, second, is it possible to infer from sample results to the population of interest, in this case the British population? We will examine these two issues by looking first at how the team obtained the *sample* (Sections 4.2–4.5), and second at how they developed methods for obtaining accurate information about the relevant attitudes and behaviours (Sections 4.6 and 4.7).

4.2.2 Sampling

What is a *sample*, and why do we need one? A sample is a group of individuals taken from a larger population. The *population* is the group of people in whom we are interested, and to whom we wish the results of the study to apply. A sample is required because, in most instances, it is not practical or necessary to study everyone in the population. Clearly, then, in taking a sample, it is absolutely vital that it be representative of the population. It is worth remembering that if the sampling is not representative, little can be done about it once data collection is complete. Over the next few sections, we will examine how to (a) select and contact a sample, and (b) check how well it represents the population. There are essentially two ways in which a sample may be inadequate:

- It may be too small, and its characteristics are therefore likely to differ substantially from those of the population simply due to chance. This is called *sampling error*, and it can be reduced by increasing the sample size. These issues will be examined in more detail in Section 4.4.

- It may have been selected in such a way as to under- or over-represent certain groups in the population. For example, a survey carried out by telephone will inevitably exclude people who do not have telephones. Another example was noted by the NATSAL 1990 research team in reviewing previous studies of sexual attitudes and lifestyles: many of these studies had been carried out on volunteers, who would almost certainly be atypical of the general population. This type of systematic misrepresentation of the population is called *selection bias*, and cannot be removed by increasing the size of the sample. Selection bias can be avoided only by representative sampling (although adjustment by weighting can be used to reduce bias to some extent – as was done in NATSAL 2000).

Bias is a systematic error in sampling or measurement that leads to an incorrect conclusion.

Turning now to the NATSAL 2000 study, the researchers developed an interview questionnaire which was implemented by trained staff using a combination of face-to-face interviews and computer-assisted self-interview techniques (CASI). The *population* was all men and women aged 16–44 years in Britain (England, Wales and Scotland), and the task was to obtain a representative *sample* of these people.

Please now read the following excerpt from paper A: methods, participants and procedure. This account of the sampling is quite complex and includes descriptions of 'over-sampling' and 'weighting', which we have not covered. For now, try to gain a general understanding of the approach to sampling: we will discuss the various methods used during the rest of this section.

Methods, participants and procedure

A stratified sample of addresses was selected from the small-user postcode address file for Britain, using a multistage probability cluster design with over-sampling in Greater London, where prevalence of risk behaviours was expected to be higher.[15] Sampling ratios were 3·5 in Inner London and 1·8 in Outer London relative to the rest of the country.

Interviewers from the National Centre for Social Research visited all selected addresses between May, 1999, and February, 2001. At each address, residents aged 16–44 years were enumerated, and one was randomly selected and invited to participate. Interviews took place in respondents' homes. Interviewers were present for the CASI* component of the interview to provide assistance if required, but were not permitted to view responses, which were locked inside the computer after the module was completed so that interviewers could not access the data.

The data were weighted to adjust for the unequal probabilities of selection—ie, residence in inner London, outer London, and rest of Britain, and number of eligible residents in the household. After selection weighting, the sample was broadly representative of the British population although men and London residents were slightly under-represented as were those aged 25–29 years (compared with 1999 population estimates).[16,17] To correct for differences in gender, age group, and government office region between the achieved sample and population estimates, we applied a non-response post-stratification weight. Comparison with the 1998 Health Survey for England[18] showed that after application of the final weights, there were no major differences in sample structure by marital status, social class, and the proportion of households with children.

*CASI = Computer aided self interview.

The key to achieving good representation of the population is ***random*** sampling. This means that it is purely a matter of chance whether or not each member of the population is chosen to be in the sample – their selection does not depend on their particular characteristics. An important consequence of this is that random sampling ensures that any differences between the sample and the population are due to chance alone. Random sampling and variants of this are the most important and commonly used sampling methods in health research, but not the only ones. The following table lists the sampling methods that we will review in this section.

Overview of sampling methods

- Simple random sampling
- Systematic sampling
- Stratified sampling
- Convenience sampling
- Cluster sampling
- Sampling of people who are hard to contact
- Multistage sampling
- Quota sampling

Before looking further at these methods, however, we need to discuss ***probability***, which is how we quantify chance.

4.2.3 Probability

Probability is a numerical measure of chance. It quantifies how likely (or unlikely) it is that a given event will occur. The probability of an event has a value between 0 and 1 inclusive.

Probability

- If an event is impossible, its probability is 0.
- If an event is certain, its probability is 1.
- Any event which is uncertain but not impossible has a probability lying between 0 and 1.
- The probability that each of us will die is 1 (a certain event).
- The probability that a person weighs $-10\,kg$ is 0 (an impossible event).

Suppose we are interested in a population which consists of 10 people. If we choose one person at random (for example, by putting all their names into a hat and selecting one), then each of the

10 people has the same probability of being selected. The probability is 1 in 10, or 0.1. Suppose now that four of the population are men and six are women. What is the probability that the person chosen at random is a woman? The probability of selecting a person with a particular characteristic is

$$\frac{\text{Number of people in the population with that characteristic}}{\text{Total number in the population}}$$

So the probability of selecting a woman is $6/10 = 0.6$. Choosing a sample by random sampling means that we can apply **probability theory** to the data we obtain from the sample. As we work through this chapter, you will see how this enables us to estimate the likely difference between the true characteristics of the population and those of the random sample, that is to say, to estimate how precise our results are.

 Self-Assessment Exercise 4.2.1

In a Primary Care Trust (PCT) with a population of 100 000, there are 25 000 smokers, 875 of whom have experienced (non-fatal) ischaemic heart disease (IHD) in the past 5 years. Of the non-smokers, 750 have also suffered IHD in the same period. If a person is chosen **at random** from this PCT,

1. What is the probability that this person is a smoker?

2. What is the probability that this person has had (non-fatal) IHD in the last 5 years?

3. What is the probability that this person is a smoker *and* has suffered (non-fatal) IHD?

Answers in Section 4.8

4.2.4 Simple random sampling

This is the simplest method of random sampling, and is illustrated diagrammatically in Figure 4.2.1. Let's say that we want to sample 10 people from a total population of 60. Each of the 60 people

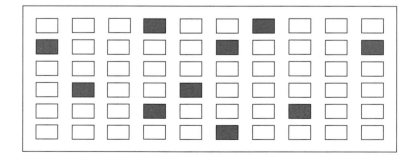

Figure 4.2.1 An example of simple random sampling of 10 subjects from a population of 60 (see text)

in the population (Figure 4.2.1) can be given an identifier (e.g. a number from 01 to 60), and then 10 numbers can be selected at random, usually by a computer. The most important principle of simple random sampling is that everyone in the population has an equal chance of being selected. This is because each person is chosen independently of the others – if person number 42 is chosen, this does not alter the chance of any other person being selected.

Simple random sampling works well because, of all possible samples, most are reasonably representative of the population. However, simple random sampling does not always produce a representative sample: by chance, we may be unlucky and choose a sample which does not represent the population very well.

4.2.5   Stratified sampling

Moving on from the simple random sampling example, imagine that we wish to study alcohol consumption habits in a population of 10 000 adults from a small town, 10 per cent of whom (1000 people) are from an ethnic minority group (for simplicity we will assume only one ethnic minority group). If a 2 per cent simple random sample is taken, it would contain a total of 200 people (2 per cent of 10 000), about 20 of whom would be from the ethnic minority group and 180 others.

We are interested to know whether the *prevalence* of heavy drinking differs between the ethnic minority group and other people. While 180 people may be enough to estimate prevalence among the majority group with reasonable precision, 20 people from the ethnic minority group is far too few. We could simply take a 20 per cent sample of the whole population, thus obtaining 200 ethnic minority subjects, but we will also then have to survey 1800 others – far more than necessary and therefore inefficient. A better alternative is to use a *stratified sampling* method, whereby the population is divided into groups (strata), and sampling is carried out within these strata. In this case, although *simple random sampling* is carried out within both strata, a much larger *sampling fraction* is taken from the ethnic minority group than from the others (20 per cent versus 2.2 per cent), as shown in Table 4.2.1.

Table 4.2.1   Example of stratified sampling

Strata	Total in population	Sampling fraction (%)	Number selected
Ethnic minority	1000	20%	200
Others	9000	2.2%	200

This procedure, known as *over-sampling*, allows us to measure the prevalence of heavy drinking with similar *precision* in both groups.

Stratified sampling may also be used with a constant sampling fraction to increase the precision of our sample estimate. By carrying out random sampling within strata, say, of age, we can be more confident that the sample is representative of the population with respect to age than if we just randomly select from the whole population. The key principle of stratified sampling is that the strata are defined by factors thought to be related to the subject under investigation. In the alcohol consumption example, the strata were defined by ethnicity ('minority' and 'other') because we want to know whether the prevalence of heavy drinking differs between these two groups. In the example of stratifying by age group, we may be investigating an age-related disease. A stratified sample should lead to a more representative sample than a simple random sample of the same size, and to more reliable results. That is, *sampling error* is reduced compared with simple random sampling. Stratification was carried out in the NATSAL study, and this will be explored further in the section on *multistage sampling*.

4.2.6 Cluster sampling

Suppose we wish to study the knowledge and views about nutrition and health among school-children aged 7/8 years (Year 3), in a given town. By far the easiest way to contact and survey these children is through their schools. An example is illustrated in Figure 4.2.2.

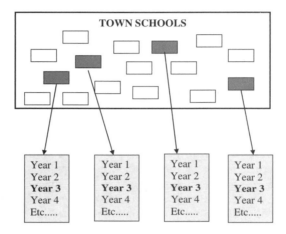

Figure 4.2.2 An example of cluster sampling of Year 3 children in a town. From the 16 primary schools (clusters) in the town, four have been selected. Within each of the selected schools, the children from Year 3 can be surveyed (see text).

Let's say that there are 480 children in the relevant age group in the town, attending 16 primary schools. If we require a sample of 120 children, a simple random sample would present us with the prospect of surveying seven or eight children from each of 16 schools. Would it not be more practical to study whole classes from a representative selection of fewer schools? In fact, a total of four schools would provide the necessary number (with 30 children per class, we require just four schools to achieve a sample of 120), and this would clearly be far more cost-effective. This method is known as *cluster sampling*, in which the schools (clusters of children) are selected as part of the sampling process.

Ideally, the schools should be selected randomly, although it may be better to *stratify* prior to random selection, for example by religious denomination.

Cluster sampling reduces the costs and time required for the study, but the penalty is increased *sampling error* compared with a simple random sample of the same size. This is because individuals in the same cluster tend to be more similar than individuals in the population as a whole. As well as the savings in time and money, cluster sampling has the advantage of not requiring a list of everyone in the population from which to sample. There is not, for example, an easily available list of all UK schoolchildren, so we could not easily select a simple random sample. There is, however, a list available of all schools. So we can select schools (clusters) from the list, and then obtain from each selected school a list of pupils from which to sample.

4.2.7 Multistage sampling

This describes a sampling method that is carried out in stages. To return to the example of the school survey, an alternative way of obtaining the 120 children is to randomly select more schools, say, eight, and then randomly select 50 per cent of the children from the specified class (Year 3) in each of those eight schools. This is multistage sampling: the first stage is to sample eight schools out of a total of 16, and in the second stage 50 per cent of children in Year 3 are selected. Multistage sampling was used in the NATSAL 2000 study.

4.2.8 Systematic sampling

Simple random sampling, as in the first example, requires giving each subject an identifier (such as a serial number), allowing the random selection to be made. There may be situations where this is very difficult to do. Imagine we wish to extract information on a representative selection of 250 subjects from a total of 10 000 health records, time is short, and there is no overall list. Simple random sampling would be ideal, but there is no list available to assign serial numbers. We could make such a list, but it would be much quicker to select every 40th record. This is called a *systematic sample*, and although it should be fairly random, there is potential for bias. If we are unlucky, the selection process may link into some systematic element of the way the records are sorted, with the result that we might select a disproportionate number with some characteristic related to the topic under study. The trouble with this kind of bias is that we will probably have no idea that it has occurred.

4.2.9 Convenience sampling

Where time and resources are very short, or there is no structured way of contacting people for a given study, it may be satisfactory to use what is known as a *convenience sample*. For example a study of patients' attitudes to a particular health service might be gathered from people in a waiting room simply by approaching whoever was there and had the time to answer questions and who did not leave while the interviewer was busy with someone else. While this type of procedure can be used to gather information quickly and easily, it is unlikely to be representative.

4.2.10 Sampling people who are difficult to contact

Suppose we wish to study the health of homeless men. Although some will stay in hostels, and be known to various agencies and care groups, others will be living on the street or in no regular place. Any list of such people is likely to be very incomplete. Moreover, many could be hard to contact or unwilling, for a variety of reasons, to take part in a study. Simple random sampling of names either for a postal questionnaire or interview visits, starting from the approach of a conventional sampling frame, would surely be doomed to failure. In this type of situation, it may be preferable to use an alternative approach that, although not random, is nevertheless likely to identify more of the people we want to contact. *Snowball sampling* is an example of this, and involves finding people from the population (in this case homeless men and people who care for them) who can use their networks and contacts to find other people who fulfil the selection criteria.

In addition to the advantage that these contacts know best where to find more 'snow' for the 'snowball', they will also be in a better position to gain the confidence of the people concerned.

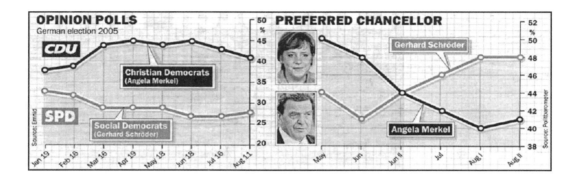

4.2.11   Quota sampling

Quota sampling is another sampling method of convenience, used extensively by market research organisations for obtaining views on products, political opinion polls such as we looked at in Chapter 1 (see example above), and so on. The following example will illustrate how it works.

A new male contraceptive pill is about to be launched, and we decide to study the views of men and women aged 15–34 about this product. It is important that the sample be representative of the different age groups among the general population in the area, but as the information is required quickly, there is insufficient time to conduct a random sampling procedure. An alternative, which requires no numbered list of names and addresses, is known as **quota sampling** and is carried out as follows. First of all, we must work out the number of people required in the sample for each subgroup of the population, in this example defined by age and sex. This would typically be done using information from the census or some other source on local demography. These numbers are called **quotas**, and, having determined these, we can then survey people until the required total in each group is obtained. For example, if we require a sample of 500 people aged 15–34 and the local population is as shown in the table below, then a quota of 75 men aged 15–19 (30 per cent of the 250 men) is needed.

	Men		Women	
Age group	% in population	Number required	% in population	Number required
15–19	30%	75 (30% of 250)	32%	80
20–24	28%	70	28%	
25–29	22%	55	22%	
30–34	20%	50	18%	
Totals	100%	250	100%	250

Although quota sampling is relatively simple and quick, how well the sample represents the population is entirely dependent on the skill with which the survey team identifies the people (respondents) for each *quota*. Here are some questions to help you think more about this sampling method:

 ### Self-Assessment Exercise 4.2.2

In the above example:

1. What size quota is required for women aged 20–24 years?

2. What would happen if the interviewers fulfilled their quota of women aged 20–24 solely by calling on homes during the working day (9 am to 5 pm)?

3. What could be done to ensure that the quotas are more representative of the population?

Answers in Section 4.8

Sampling in NATSAL 2000

Having reviewed the different approaches that are available for sampling, we will now look again at what was done in the NATSAL study. Bear in mind that the overall aim is to obtain a representative sample of the population aged 16–44 years in Britain, with the additional objective of ensuring sufficient precision of information about important risk behaviours – particularly in some areas of the country such as London. Although the sampling method seems complex, it is in essence a combination of the methods we have discussed. We will work through the sampling method, referring again to the excerpt from the methods section of paper A (see Section 4.2.2). Some of the details of the sampling described here are drawn from other NATSAL study reports.

1. For the first stage, postcode sectors (the first part of the postcode) were stratified by region and a number of socio-demographic factors: population density, demographic structure and socio-economic status. Postcode sectors were therefore the 'clusters' in this sampling method.

2. From all of these postcode sectors, 466 were selected randomly, but with a probability proportional to the number of postal addresses, so that a sector with 3000 addresses would be twice as likely to be selected as one with 1500.

3. From each of these postcode sectors, 84 (90 in London) addresses were selected, making a total of 39 828 addresses.

4. Finally, one eligible adult aged 16–44 was randomly selected from each household.

Addresses in Greater London were over-sampled; that is, the sample was stratified and a larger sampling ratio was used for the addresses in Greater London, 3.5 times as many in inner London, and 1.8 times as many in outer London. This was because the prevalence of HIV risk behaviours had been shown to be higher in London than elsewhere in Britain, yet they were still comparatively rare. By taking a larger sample, it would be possible to obtain a more precise estimate of the prevalence of risky sexual behaviours.

The team also wanted to obtain a larger sample of ethnic minority groups, so they selected a second sample for the study. For this second sample, they stratified postcode sectors by proportion of ethnic minority residents and then randomly sampled sectors with a higher proportion of ethnic minority residents. They then screened addresses within the selected sectors to identify eligible respondents.

Weighting

The over-sampling procedure requires that account be taken of this in estimates derived for the whole sample, such as the proportion of males in Britain reporting a specific behaviour. This is carried out by weighting. The next exercise should help clarify how weighting, which is an important technique, operates.

 Self-Assessment Exercise 4.2.3

Area	Number in sample*	Sampling ratio*	Respondents reporting the behaviour of interest	
			Number	Percentage
Inner London	900	3.0	225	25%
Outer London	1000	2.0	200	20%
Rest of Britain	9000	1.0	630	7%
Total	10 900		1080	

*The numbers in this exercise are modified from NATSAL for simplicity in this exercise.

1. If we use the data in the 'Total' line of the above table and ignore the sampling ratios, what is the overall percentage of people in the sample reporting the behaviour of interest?

2. Why is this result incorrect?

3. How many people would be in the inner London sample if the sampling ratio had been the same as for the rest of Britain?

4. How many people from the inner London sample would have reported the behaviour if the sampling ratio had been the same as for the rest of Britain?

5. Try working out the percentage reporting the behaviour in the country, after allowing for the over-sampling.

Answers in Section 4.8

This final exercise in this section should help consolidate the ideas and techniques we have covered so far on sampling methods.

Self-Assessment Exercise 4.2.4

Which sampling method would be most appropriate for:

1. A general population study of cardiovascular disease risk factors in men and women aged 20–59 years resident in a primary care trust (PCT)?

2. A study of patterns of drug treatment among people aged 75 and over living in residential care homes in a city?

3. A study of the health-care needs of female, intravenous drug users who are also single mothers living in an inner-city area?

Answers in Section 4.8

Summary

- The single most important principle of sampling is that the sample be representative of the population.

- Random selection is generally the best way of obtaining a representative sample.

- In some situations, random selection is not possible or practical within the constraints of time and resources, and other methods may give a useful sample. In experienced hands, methods such as quota sampling are very effective.

4.3 The sampling frame

4.3.1 Why do we need a sampling frame?

After we decide on the type of sample required, it is necessary to find a practical method of selecting and then contacting the people concerned. Ideally, we would like an accurate list of all the people in the population of interest, which includes various characteristics such as age and gender – indeed, this information is vital if we wish to stratify the sample (see Section 4.2.4). We also need contact details such as address and telephone number. This type of list is called a *sampling frame*.

 Self-Assessment Exercise 4.3.1

1. What potential sampling frames can you think of?

2. What are the advantages and disadvantages of the sampling frames you have identified?

Answers in Section 4.8

4.3.2 Losses in sampling

Despite our best efforts, the sampling frame may not comprise the entire population of interest. Some individuals may not be included in the sampling frame because, for example, they are not registered to vote or with a GP. There may also be individuals in the sampling frame who are not members of the population: for example, people who have recently moved to another part of the country but have not yet been removed from the old GP list. The following example summarises the various stages of selecting and contacting a sample, and the ways in which people can be lost. In this study of the prevalence of pain among older adults in North Staffordshire, the sampling frame comprised all those aged 50 years or more who were registered with three GP practices (Source: Thomas, E. *et al.* (2004), *Pain* **110**, 361–368).

Population to sample	Number in sample	Comments
Population of interest	Not stated*	Adults over 50 years in North Staffordshire.
Sampling frame	11 309	All adults over 50 years at three GP practices in North Staffordshire.
Eligible sample	11 230	GPs made 79 exclusions, as patients were considered unsuitable to take part in study.
Available sample	11 055	45 deaths or departures from practice. 105 questionnaires returned by postal service as 'not at this address'. 25 with comprehension or memory problems.
Sample on whom data were obtained	7878	255 people declined to participate. 109 stated ill health prevented participation. 2813 people from whom no response was received.

* Although population numbers are available from mid-year population estimates, it may not be easy to relate area-based population data to GP practice populations, which do not usually have geographically discrete catchment areas.
Source: Thomas, E. *et al.* (2004), *Pain* **110**, 361–368.

Starting from a total of 11 309 on the sampling frame, the investigators ended up with 7878 respondents, having lost the remainder for a variety of reasons, including, of course, that some people did not wish to take part in the study. In terms of the sampling process, it is notable that 45 were known to have died or left the practice, but a further 105 invitations were returned by the post office. Presumably, these people had moved (or died), but this information was not correct on the GP list (sampling frame). Problems such as these are inevitable with any sampling frame.

If we take the 'available sample' as the denominator, then $7878 \div 11\ 055$ responded, a response rate of 71.3 per cent. One marked advantage of using the GP list for this study is that the characteristics of responders and non-responders can be compared by using a range of information available to the practices. This will facilitate the assessment of ***response bias***, an important issue that we will return to shortly.

Summary

- The sampling frame must provide enough information about the population to allow sampling, and to contact the people selected.

- No sampling frame is without its problems, including inaccurate information on who is in the population, as well as the information required to contact those selected (e.g. addresses).

- It is very important to obtain and record details of losses in sampling, so that a judgement can be made about how representative the sample is.

4.4 Sampling error, confidence intervals and sample size

4.4.1 Sampling distributions and the standard error

Any quantity calculated from the sample data, such as a proportion or a mean, is a statistic. If we randomly select several samples of the same size from a population and calculate the value of the same statistic from each one, we expect, by chance, to obtain different values, and that these values will tend to differ from the population value. This variation is the ***sampling error*** introduced in Section 4.2.1 – the difference between the ***sample*** and ***population*** that is due to chance. Each possible random sample of a given size that could be selected from the population results in a value of the statistic. All these possible values together form the ***sampling distribution*** of the statistic, which tells us how the value of the sample statistic varies from sample to sample. The following example should help explain this.

Suppose our friends A, B, C, D and E obtain the following percentage marks in their end-of-module assessment:

$$35 \quad 52 \quad 65 \quad 77 \quad 80$$

The five friends are the population, so the mean mark of the population is:

$$\frac{35 + 52 + 65 + 77 + 80}{5} = 61.8\%$$

Now suppose that we do not know the marks for all five students in the population, but we want to estimate the population mean mark from a random sample of two students. If the sample chosen has marks of 35 and 65 per cent, the sample mean is 50 per cent – some way from the population mean of 61.8 per cent. If, however, we happen to choose a sample of students with marks 52 and 77 per cent, the sample mean is 64.5 per cent – quite close to the population value we want to estimate. This shows how our estimate of the population mean from a single sample is determined by the play of chance: rather a poor estimate for the first sample, but quite good for the second one. It is as well to remember at this point that in carrying out research (a) we only take one sample and (b) we have no way of knowing whether we were lucky or unlucky with that single sample. Returning to our example, there are 10 possible samples of size 2, and the marks and sample mean for each of these are as follows:

Sample marks	Sample mean mark
35, 52	43.5
35, 65	50.0
35, 77	56.0
35, 80	57.5
52, 65	58.5
52, 77	64.5
52, 80	66.0
65, 77	71.0
65, 80	72.5
77, 80	78.5

The values in the right column (all possible values of the mean which can be calculated from a sample size of two) form the ***sampling distribution*** of the sample mean mark. We can display this distribution in a frequency table or a histogram:

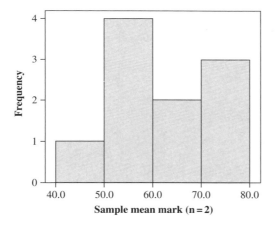

Sample mean mark	Frequency
40.0–49.9	1
50.0–59.9	4
60.0–69.9	2
70.0–79.9	3
Total	10

The mean of this distribution is $\dfrac{43.5 + \cdots + 78.5}{10} = 61.8\%$.

That is, the mean of the sample means exactly equals the population mean, though, note, this is only the case because we have taken all possible samples.

4.4.2 The standard error

The spread of all possible values of the sample mean is measured by the standard deviation of the sampling distribution. This is called the ***standard error*** of the sample mean. This term distinguishes the standard deviation of the sample means from the standard deviation of the population itself, but it is not a new concept: it simply tells us how spread out the sample means are. In this case, the standard error is 11.4 per cent. The possible values of the sample mean are spread out around the population mean. The smaller the standard error is, the more closely bunched the sample means are around the population mean. This means that it is more likely that the mean of any particular sample we choose will be close to the population value; that is, will be a good estimate of the population mean. A smaller standard error is therefore desirable. We will now look at how this can be achieved by increasing the sample size.

Reducing the standard error

Now suppose we increase the sample size to three in order to estimate the population mean mark. There are 10 possible samples that could be chosen, and the sampling distribution of the sample means is as follows:

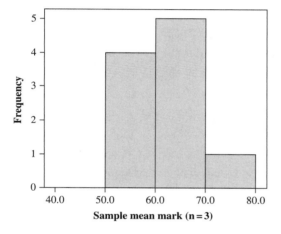

Sample mean mark	Frequency
40.0–49.9	0
50.0–59.9	4
60.0–69.9	5
70.0–79.9	1
Total	10

The mean of the sampling distribution is again 61.8 per cent, and the standard error is now 7.6 per cent, considerably less than the value of 11.4 per cent with a sample size of only two. So this distribution is less spread out – the sample means are bunched more closely around the population mean.

This example has illustrated that the larger the sample, the closer the sample mean is likely to be to the population mean: the standard error decreases with increasing sample size. The standard error of the mean also depends on the standard deviation of the population. This makes sense intuitively, since we would expect that the more spread out the population values are, the more spread out the sample means will be. The formula for calculating the standard error for the mean is as follows:

$$\text{Standard error of the sample mean} = \frac{\text{standard deviation of the population}}{\sqrt{n}}$$

for a sample of size n

If you try calculating this for the exam marks example, you will find that the answers differ from the standard errors quoted earlier. This is because the formula above applies strictly to random sampling from an infinitely large population – and the examples given are corrected for a large *sampling fraction* by using what is termed the finite population correction factor (see reference section below). The sampling fraction is the proportion that the sample is of the whole population – in the case of our sample of three marks, this is 3/5 (×100) = 60 per cent, which is a very large sampling fraction. Fortunately, in most practical situations, we can consider our population of hundreds or thousands or millions to be, in effect, 'infinite' without incurring any significant error, provided the sampling fraction is relatively small. If the sampling fraction is no more than about 10 per cent, or we are sampling with replacement (that is, after selection a subject goes back into the population and could in theory be selected again), there is no need to make any adjustment to the standard error.

 ### RS - Reference section on statistical methods

The finite population correction factor allows for the fact that, in reality, populations are not infinite, and in some cases may not be very large compared to the size of the sample. We achieve the correction by multiplying the standard error of a sample mean by the correction factor. This factor is given by the formula:

$$\text{Correction factor} = \sqrt{\frac{N-n}{N-1}}$$

where N = population size, and n = sample size. Hence, with our example of a sample of size $n = 3$, drawn from a population of size $N = 5$, the correction factor $= \sqrt{0.5} = 0.707$. We would then apply this correction, by multiplying the standard error (calculated as $s \div \sqrt{n}$) by 0.707.

 ### RS - Ends

In our example of sampling from a very small population, we have seen the effect of sample size on the precision of an estimate. Do not forget, though, that in practice, we take only one sample. We do not know whether we have selected a sample with a mean close to the population mean or far away. We do know, however, that the larger the sample, the more likely it is that we obtain a sample mean close to the population mean.

Now let's look at a more realistic example, with a large population. Let's say we are interested in finding out about the weight of people living in a small town with a population of 10 000. It is not practical, or necessary, to measure everyone, so we are going to take a random sample of 200 (sampling fraction of 2 per cent), and find the sample mean weight, termed $\bar{x}_1$ (pronounced 'x bar'). The mean that we are estimating is, of course, the population mean, termed μ (pronounced 'mew'), and it is important to remember that our survey of 200 people will not tell us what this population mean weight actually is; it will only estimate the population mean with the sample mean ($\bar{x}_1$). The following diagram summarises what we are doing:

POPULATION (N = 10, 000)

This *population* has a mean weight, termed μ. Let us say it is 70 kg, but of course we will never actually know this because we are not going to measure the weights of all 10,000 people.

For practical reasons, we take a *simple random sample* (of n = 200 people in this example)

SAMPLE ($n = 200$)

The mean of this sample is termed $\bar{x}_1$ and let's say that the value turns out to be 69.7 kg. As you can see, it is not exactly the same as the value of μ, although very close. Now, if we have taken a *representative sample* (it was *random*, so it should be, so long as there is no *selection bias*), then the only factor preventing our sample mean from being identical to the population mean is chance (we will also ignore the possibility that the scales are not accurate). This is *sampling error*, and occurs because it is extremely unlikely that the 200 people selected will have weights with a mean of exactly 70 kg, even though they were randomly selected from a population with a mean weight of 70 kg.

Imagine now that we started all over again, and took another sample of $n = 200$, and calculated the mean of that group. Let's call this $\bar{x}_2$, as it is the second sample. By chance, $\bar{x}_2$ will be a bit different from $\bar{x}_1$ and from μ. Let's say that the mean in this second sample comes out at 71.9 kg. If we repeated this exercise many times, we would end up with many estimates of the population mean μ, which we can term $\bar{x}_1, \bar{x}_2, \bar{x}_3$, and so on.

There are many, many possible samples of size 200 which could be chosen from a population of 10 000 – millions of them. If we prepare a histogram of the sampling distribution of all the possible sample means ($\bar{x}_1, \bar{x}_2, \bar{x}_3$, and so on), the intervals are very narrow and the histogram has a smooth shape. The *sampling distribution of the sample mean* is shown in 4.4.1.

The distribution in Figure 4.4.1 is the *normal distribution* that we introduced in Section 2.4.3 of Chapter 2. The mean of the sampling distribution is 70 kg, the population mean weight, and the standard deviation of the sampling distribution (which we now know as the *standard error* of the mean) depends on the population standard deviation, which we label σ (pronounced 'sigma'), and the sample size, $n = 200$. For different sample sizes we obtain different sampling distributions, all with the same mean (70 kg) but with different standard errors (Figure 4.4.2).

The sampling distributions have the same basic shape (a normal distribution), but are more and more closely centred on the population mean as sample size increases. What is surprising, though, is that if the sample size is large enough (at least 30), the sampling distribution of the mean always has a normal distribution, no matter what the shape of the population distribution (this is

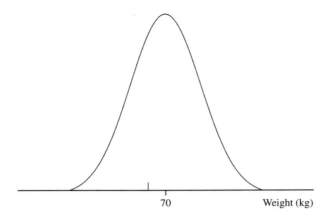

70　　　　　　　　　Weight (kg)

Figure 4.4.1 The sampling distribution of the sample
mean from a population with mean weight 70 kg

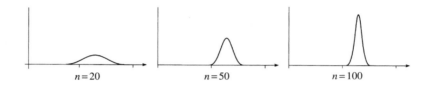

$n = 20$　　　　　　　$n = 50$　　　　　　　$n = 100$

Figure 4.4.2 Sampling distributions of the sample mean for different sample sizes

known as the Central Limit Theorem). This rather convenient phenomenon is illustrated below.
Figure 4.4.3 shows a rough picture of the population distribution of women's weekly earnings in
the UK in 1994.

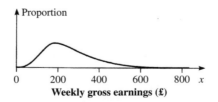

Figure 4.4.3 Weekly gross earnings of all women in the UK in 1994

Although the population distribution is clearly right skewed, look at the sampling distributions of
the mean for various sample sizes (Figure 4.4.4, below).

As the sample size increases, the sampling distribution becomes more and more bell-shaped and
symmetric (normal). It also becomes more peaked and compressed – the standard error decreases.

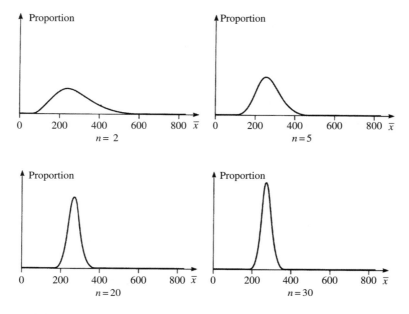

Figure 4.4.4   Sampling distributions of the sample mean from a skewed population

As a rough guide, if the sample size is larger than 30, the sampling distribution of the sample mean can be assumed to have a normal distribution whatever the shape of the population distribution. This is important, because we often do not know the shape of the population distribution.

Summary: sampling distributions and standard error of the sample mean

1. We label the population mean μ and the population standard deviation σ. We do not usually know these values, and estimate them from a sample of size n.

2. There are many different samples of size n which could be chosen. Each sample has a particular mean $\bar{x}$ and standard deviation s. In practice, only one sample will be chosen.

3. The distribution of all the possible sample means is called the sampling distribution of the sample mean.

4. The standard deviation of the sampling distribution is called the standard error of the sample mean. It is a measure of how precisely a sample mean estimates the population mean.

5. The standard error depends on the population standard deviation (σ) and on the sample size n: standard error $= \sigma/\sqrt{n}$.

(Continued)

6. Where the sampling fraction is greater than (about) 10 per cent, adjustment to the standard error can be made by the finite population correction factor.

7. The sampling distribution of the sample mean is always normal for sample sizes larger than about 30, whatever the shape of the population distribution.

8. If the population distribution is normal, the sampling distribution of the sample mean is normal even for small samples ($n \leq 30$).

4.4.3 The normal distribution

Although we refer to the normal distribution, there are many different normal distributions – in fact an infinite number. They all have the same symmetric bell shape and are centred on the mean, but with different means and standard deviations. The normal distribution is defined by a formula, so it is possible to calculate the proportion of the population between any two values. For any population with a normal distribution, about 68 per cent of the values lie within one standard deviation of the mean ($\mu \pm 1\sigma$), about 95 per cent lie within two standard deviations of the mean ($\mu \pm 2\sigma$), and almost the whole of the distribution (99.7 per cent) lies within three standard deviations ($\mu \pm 3\sigma$) (Figure 4.4.5). In fact, exactly $\mu \pm 1.96$ standard deviations include 95 per cent of the values, and this explains where the figure 1.96 comes from in earlier sections.

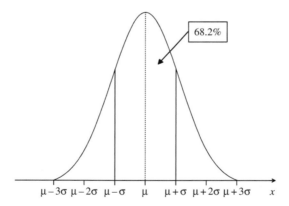

Figure 4.4.5 The normal distribution: 68.2 per cent of all values lie between $\mu - \sigma$ and $\mu + \sigma$ (see text)

Summary: the normal distribution

• A normal distribution is bell-shaped, and symmetric about its mean value.

• A normal distribution is defined by its mean and standard deviation.

- About 68 per cent of the values lie within ($\mu \pm 1\sigma$), about 95 per cent lie within ($\mu \pm 2\sigma$), and almost the whole of the distribution (99.7 per cent) lies within ($\mu \pm 3\sigma$).

- Exactly 95 per cent of the values lie within ($\mu \pm 1.96\sigma$).

4.4.4   Confidence interval (CI) for the sample mean

Our discussion of sampling error has been built around the theoretical position of taking repeated samples of the same size from a given population. In reality, of course, we do not take repeated samples: in the weight example, we have one estimate derived from 200 people, and we have to make do with that. We do not know whether we had a lucky day and this single estimate has a value very close to the population mean (say, 69.7 kg, only 0.3 kg out), or a bad day and we got the value 71.9 kg (1.9 kg out), or worse. What we can do, however, is to calculate a range of values, centred on our sample mean, which we are fairly confident includes the true population mean. This is called a **confidence interval (CI)**, and is much more informative than just quoting the sample mean. It is common to calculate a **95 per cent CI for the population mean**. With such an interval, 'we are 95 per cent confident that the specified range includes the population mean'. We have seen that approximately 95 per cent of a normal distribution falls within two standard deviations of the mean, and exactly 95 per cent falls within 1.96 standard deviations of the mean. Since the distribution of sample means is normal with mean μ and standard deviation $\sigma/\sqrt{n}$ (the standard error), there is a 95 per cent chance that we choose a sample whose mean lies in the interval $\mu - 1.96\sigma/\sqrt{n}$ to $\mu + 1.96\sigma/\sqrt{n}$. This is illustrated in Figure 4.4.6.

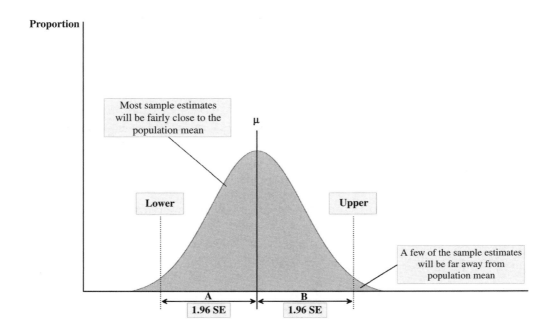

Figure 4.4.6   The sampling distribution of the sample mean

The range covered by the arrows A and B between the upper and lower dotted lines, is ±1.96 standard errors from the true population mean, and includes 95% of possible sample means.

 ### Self-Assessment Exercise 4.4.1

1. On Figure 4.4.6, mark a value $\bar{x}_1$ between the upper and lower dotted lines. Is it true that the range $\bar{x}_1 \pm 1.96$ standard errors includes the value μ (that is, the population mean that we want to know)?

2. What percentage of sample means lie in the area between the dotted lines?

3. Mark a value $\bar{x}_2$ either to the left of the lower line or to the right of the upper line. What percentage of values lie outside these lines?

4. Is the value of μ included in the range $\bar{x}_2 \pm 1.96$ standard errors? What is the implication of your answer to this?

Answer in Section 4.8

To summarise, in order to calculate this CI, we first need the sample mean $\bar{x}$ of a random sample, the sample size n, and the population standard deviation σ. We know the first two after collecting information about the members of the sample, but we do not know the standard deviation of the population. However, provided the sample is reasonably large (again, more than about 30), we can use the sample standard deviation s to estimate the population standard deviation σ. A 95 per cent CI for the population mean μ is therefore shown as follows:

---

95 per cent CI for a population mean

$$(\bar{x} - 1.96s / \sqrt{n}, \ \bar{x} + 1.96s / \sqrt{n}) \text{ or } \bar{x} \pm 1.96 \text{ SE}$$

where SE stands for 'estimated standard error of the sample mean': that is, the standard error with σ replaced by s. The CI is stated to the same accuracy (number of decimal places) as the sample mean.

For our weight example, suppose our sample of 200 people has a mean weight of 69.7 kg and standard deviation of 15 kg. Then a 95 per cent CI for the mean weight of the population (10 000 people) is

$$69.7 \pm 1.96 \times 15 / \sqrt{200} = (67.6, \ 71.8)$$

Hence, we are 95 per cent confident that the mean weight of the population lies between 67.6 and 71.8 kg. In this example, the CI does include the population mean (70 kg), but of course we would not actually know this. Although 95 per cent of all the possible random samples of size 200 will result in a CI that includes the population mean, 5 per cent will not. Put another way, we do not know for certain whether or not the CI for our sample has captured the population mean, but we are 95 per cent sure it has.

 ## Self-Assessment Exercise 4.4.2

The following summary statistics for the lifetime number of partners for women aged 16–44 years were obtained from the NATSAL 2000 study.

Number of lifetime partners for women aged 16–44 years	
Mean	6.5
Median	4
Standard deviation	9.7
Sample size (weighted)	5390

Using these summary statistics, find a 95 per cent CI for the mean number of lifetime partners for all women aged 16–44 years.

Answer in Section 4.8

Summary: CI for the population mean

- A CI (for a mean) is a range of values which is likely to include the population mean.

- A 95 per cent CI for the population mean is $\bar{x} \pm 1.96$ SE where SE $= s/\sqrt{n}$. This formula requires the sample to be large ($n > 30$) and random.

- 95 per cent of such CIs will include the population mean.

- For any particular sample, we do not know for sure whether or not the 95 per cent CI includes the population mean. There is a 5 per cent chance that it does not.

4.4.5 Estimating sample size

The 95 per cent CI allows us to quantify the precision of a population estimate measured in a sample. Being able to quantify the precision of a sample estimate in this way also means that it is possible to calculate the *sample size* required to estimate a population value to a desired level of accuracy. Now that we have calculated the 95 per cent CI for the sample mean, it is a relatively simple step to work out the sample size needed to estimate the sample mean with a precision that we can specify.

4.4.6 Sample size for estimating a population mean

We have seen that, for a large ($n > 30$) random sample there is a 95 per cent chance that the sample mean lies in the interval $\mu - 1.96\sigma/\sqrt{n}$ to $\mu + 1.96\sigma/\sqrt{n}$ (for small samples ($n < 30$) we need to use the t-distribution, which is introduced in Chapter 5). As sample size n increases, the standard error $\sigma/\sqrt{n}$ decreases, and the sample mean is a more precise estimate of the population mean. In order to determine the sample size needed, we first specify the error range we will allow, termed ε (epsilon). If we want to be 95 per cent certain of achieving the specified error, drawing on the formula for a 95 per cent confidence interval, we set the error (ε) to $1.96\sigma/\sqrt{n}$. The sample size required is therefore as follows:

Sample size (n) for estimating a population mean to within $\pm\varepsilon$

$$n = \frac{1.96^2\sigma^2}{\varepsilon^2}$$

The derivation of this formula from that for the 95 per cent CI is quite simple, and is shown in the reference section below.

RS - Reference section on statistical methods

We start with the expression for the 95 per cent CI, which is $\pm 1.96\sigma/\sqrt{n} = \varepsilon$ (note that the full range of the 95 per cent CI is $\pm\varepsilon$). In order to 'extract' the sample size, which is n, we square the whole expression:

$$\frac{1.96^2\sigma^2}{n} = \varepsilon^2 \quad \dots \text{which is equivalent to} \dots \quad n = \frac{1.96^2\sigma^2}{\varepsilon^2}$$

RS - ends

To calculate the sample size, we need to estimate σ, the population standard deviation – which we do not know. We have to substitute an estimate of σ from data already available, expert opinion or previous experience, or carry out a pilot study to obtain a rough estimate. Fortunately, this estimate need not be very precise in order to calculate the approximate size of sample required. An example and exercise will now show how all this works in practice.

Example

In a study of the effects of smoking on birthweight, it was required to estimate the mean birthweight of baby girls to within $\pm 100\,\text{g}$. Previous studies have shown that the birthweights of baby girls have a standard deviation of about $520\,\text{g}$. The required sample size is therefore

$$n = \frac{1.96^2 \times 520^2}{100^2} = 103.88.$$

So, a sample of 104 baby girls is required.

A calculated sample size should be used only as a guide, and we would not generally use the exact number calculated. Thus, for this example, we would be cautious and decide on, say, 120.

We would then need to allow for parents of some of the selected babies refusing to participate in the study. If we expected a 20 per cent refusal rate, we would need to select a sample of $120 \times 100/80 = 150$ babies.

 Self-Assessment Exercise 4.4.3

1. Using data from the example (above) on birthweight of baby girls, calculate the sample size required to estimate the mean to $\pm 50\,g$.

2. What sample size is required to estimate the mean birthweight to $\pm 25\,g$? What do you notice happens to the sample size when the error is halved?

Answers in Section 4.8

4.4.7   Standard error and 95 per cent CI for a population proportion

We will now look at how these concepts and methods for standard error, 95 per cent CIs, and sample size for precision of an estimate, apply to proportions. In fact, although the formulae differ, the principles are the same.

Suppose now that we want to estimate the proportion P of a population with some characteristic, such as a disease; that is, we want to estimate the disease prevalence in the population. The estimate of P is the proportion of the sample with the characteristic. If there are n individuals in the sample, and r of them have the characteristic, the estimate is conventionally written as $p = r/n$. When we are referring to the sample proportion, we use lower case for proportion (p) and upper case for the population proportion (P). To calculate the 95 per cent CI for a sample proportion, we first need the standard error, which is derived as follows:

> The *standard error of a sample proportion* is
>
> $$\sqrt{\frac{P(1-P)}{n}}$$

If we have a large sample (more than 30), the sampling distribution of the sample proportion is approximately normal, and a 95 per cent CI for the population proportion P is derived as follows:

> **95 per cent CI for a population proportion**
>
> $$p \pm 1.96\ \text{SE}$$
>
> where SE is the estimated standard error of p, which is
>
> $$\sqrt{p(1-p)/n}$$

Self-Assessment Exercise 4.4.4

The following summary statistics for the percentage of men cohabiting were taken from the NATSAL 2000 study.

Percentage of men cohabiting	
Percentage	16.5%
Sample size (weighted)	5679

Calculate the 95 per cent CI for the percentage of men cohabiting.

Answer in Section 4.8

4.4.8 Sample size to estimate a population proportion

To find the sample size required to estimate the population proportion to within a specified precision, we follow the same reasoning as we used for the mean, but use the standard error of a proportion. In order to estimate a population proportion P to within a specified level of error $\pm\varepsilon$, we require:

$$1.96\sqrt{\frac{P(1-P)}{n}} = \varepsilon$$

and the required sample size is as follows (this formula is derived in the same way as for the mean, by squaring the expression and extracting the sample size term, n – see Reference Section in Section 4.4.6):

> **Sample size for estimating a population proportion to within**
>
> $$\pm\varepsilon$$
>
> $$n = \frac{1.96^2 P(1-P)}{\varepsilon^2}$$

An important point to note when calculating the standard error, is that the quantity of interest, P, may be expressed as a proportion (as we have done so far), as a percentage (rate per 100), or a rate per 1000, and so on. The standard errors of the sample estimates are then as follows:

P	*Standard error of* p
As a proportion	$\sqrt{P(1-P)/n}$
Per 100 (as a percentage)	$\sqrt{P(100-P)/n}$
Per 1000	$\sqrt{P(1000-P)/n}$

Moreover, be careful to ensure that the error term (ε) is in the same units. As with calculating sample size for the mean, we generally do not have the population value P, but we can use and estimate from a sample; that is, p

Example

Suppose we want to estimate the percentage of smokers in some population to within ± 4 per cent of the true value. If the population percentage is 30 per cent, the required sample size is

$$n = \frac{1.96^2 \times 30 \times 70}{4^2} = 504.21$$

A sample of 505 people is required. Note we have used the formula for percentages (rather than proportion), and that the units for the percentage smoking and the error are the same (per cent).

 ## Self-Assessment Exercise 4.4.5

1. If the true prevalence of a specific but uncommon sexual behaviour is estimated to be 1 per cent, what sample size is required to estimate it to within ± 0.2 per cent?

2. If we have a sample of size 500, to what precision can the prevalence of this behaviour be estimated?

Answers in Section 4.8

Assumptions

The sample size calculations presented are based on certain assumptions:

1. The sample is selected by simple random sampling.

2. The sample size is large ($n > 30$).

3. The sampling fraction is less than 10 per cent (see Section 4.4.2 for explanation of the sampling fraction).

It is important to remember that the calculations shown here are based on simple random sampling. Stratification will increase precision compared with a simple random sample of the same size, so a smaller sample can be selected. Cluster sampling will reduce precision compared with a simple random sample of the same size, so a larger sample will be needed. We will not look further here at methods for these adjustments to sample size. In general, it is recommended that advice on sample size calculation be sought from a statistician. If the calculation results in a very small sample, assumption (2) above does not hold, and alternative methods must be used to calculate sample size. If the calculation results in a large sample size relative to the population size (large sampling fraction), assumption (3) does not hold, and a modification of the calculation is required.

Summary: sample size calculations for precision of sample estimates

1. To estimate a population mean to within $\pm\varepsilon$ of the true value with a 95 per cent CI, we need a sample of size of

$$n = \frac{1.96^2\sigma^2}{\varepsilon^2}.$$

2. To estimate a population proportion to within $\pm\varepsilon$ of the true value with a 95 per cent CI, we need a sample of size of

$$n = \frac{1.96^2 P(1-P)}{\varepsilon^2}.$$

4.5 Response

4.5.1 Determining the response rate

Having selected a representative sample, we now have to think about who actually ends up being studied. As we have seen, there are in fact two groups of people who, although selected for the sample, do not contribute to the study:

- People who cannot be contacted, because, for instance, they have moved on from the selected address.

- People who are spoken to, or receive a postal questionnaire, but who decline to take part in the study.

The percentage of the selected sample that does take part in the study is called the ***response rate***. Note that response can be calculated in two different ways. The ***overall response rate*** usually excludes people who could not be contacted. Although it is important to achieve a high response rate, the most important question is whether those who do not take part, the ***non-responders***, are different from those who do, the ***responders***. If the non-responders differ substantially from the responders, especially with respect to some of the factors under study, then this will result in ***non-response bias***. We will now return to the NATSAL 2000 study: please now read the following excerpt from the results section of paper A:

Results

From the 40,523 addresses visited, 16,998 households were identified with an eligible resident aged 16–44 years. At 1425 (3·5%) addresses, eligibility was not known as no contact was achieved (after a minimum of four attempts) or all information was refused. Interviews were completed with 11,161 respondents of whom 4762 were men and 6399 were women. The unadjusted response rate was 63·1%. Response rates were lower in London, and an adjustment taking account of the over-sampling of London, gave a response rate of 65·4%. Response rates were calculated excluding those who did not speak English, were sick or away from home (545 selected residents), and after estimating the likely proportion of ineligibles in the 1425 households, where there was no information about residents.

Self-Assessment Exercise 4.5.1

What was the response rate in the NATSAL 2000 study?

Answer in Section 4.8

4.5.2 Assessing whether the sample is representative

It is very important to find out whether the sample is representative of the population, or, more realistically (since no sample is perfect!), how representative it is. In order to do this, we need to find some way of comparing the sample with the population, and the key to this is finding some characteristic(s) about which there is information available from both the sample and the population. This can usually be done, although it is often not as simple as it may appear at first sight. Among other things, we have to be sure that a given characteristic has been measured in the same way in both the sample and in the data source we are using for the population. For the NATSAL 2000 study, the team compared estimates for key socio-demographic characteristics with (i) mid-1999 population estimates (based on the most recent census, adjusted for births, deaths and migration, etc.) and (ii) data on marital status, social class and percentages of households with and without children from the 1998 Health Survey for England (Table 4.5.1).

Table 4.5.1 Comparison of key demographic characteristics from NATSAL 2000 study with mid-1999 population (age and region) and 1998 Health Survey of England (marital status and social class)

Characteristics	NATSAL 2000 sample after final weighting		Population estimates	
	Men	**Women**	**Men**	**Women**
Age	%	%	%	%
16–19	12.1	12.0	12.2	12.0
20–24	14.6	14.4	14.5	14.4
25–29	17.6	17.4	17.6	17.4
30–34	20.0	19.9	19.8	19.8
35–39	19.3	19.4	19.4	19.5
40–44	16.5	16.9	16.4	16.9
Percentage of sample	**50.9**	**49.1**	**51.0**	**49.0**
Government office region	%	%	%	%
North East	4.4	4.5	4.3	4.4
North West	11.7	11.7	11.7	11.7
Yorkshire and Humberside	8.8	8.6	8.7	8.6
East Midlands	7.1	7.1	7.1	7.1
West Midlands	9.1	9.0	9.0	9.0
South West	7.9	7.8	7.8	7.8
Eastern	9.1	9.2	9.2	9.2

Table 4.5.1   (Continued)

Characteristics	NATSAL 2000 sample after final weighting		Population estimates	
	Men	Women	Men	Women
Inner London	5.9	6.0	6.1	6.1
Outer London	8.5	8.3	8.5	8.3
South East	14.0	13.9	13.9	13.9
Wales	4.6	4.7	4.8	4.8
Scotland	8.9	9.1	8.9	9.2
Marital status	%	%	%	%
Single	39.3	29.9	38.8	31.3
Married	39.8	44.2	42.4	45.7
Separated	1.6	2.8	1.9	3.1
Divorced	2.8	4.6	2.6	5.5
Widowed	0.1	0.3	0.1	0.5
Cohabiting	16.5	18.2	14.1	13.8
Social class	%	%	%	%
Professional	7.5	3.3	6.2	2.7
Managerial and technical	29.2	27.2	26.2	22.8
Skilled non-manual	13.3	38.0	14.5	38.5
Skilled manual	30.5	8.4	30.0	7.6
Partly skilled manual	14.7	18.3	17.1	22.4
Unskilled manual	4.9	4.7	6.0	6.1

 Self-Assessment Exercise 4.5.2

1. Compare the breakdown of the sample by (a) age, and (b) government office region with that obtained from the mid-1999 estimates.

2. Now compare the breakdown of the sample by (a) marital status, and (b) social class with that obtained from the Health Survey of England, and comment on what you find.

Answers in Section 4.8

4.5.3   Maximising the response rate

Achieving a good response rate is therefore important for keeping *response bias* to a minimum. Research teams have some control over the response to any given study, and the following table summarises some of the ways of improving this.

- For a postal survey, include a covering letter signed by a respected person.
- Explain the reason(s) for the study, conveying the relevance to the target audience.

- If possible, arrange for the age, gender and ethnicity (including language spoken) of interviewers to be appropriate to the audience and subject matter.

- Contact subjects in advance to inform them that a study is planned and they may/will be contacted shortly to ask whether they would be prepared to take part (more practical and relevant in, for example, studies of health service users).

- Reminders are routinely used and are an acceptable technique. These can be sent up to two (rarely three) times after the initial contact, at roughly 1–2-week intervals. It is also acceptable to telephone courteously, and to make a personal visit in certain circumstances.

- Always respect the individual's right not to take part, and ensure that procedures agreed with an ethical committee are not exceeded.

 Self-Assessment Exercise 4.5.3

Draft a (brief) covering letter which could be used to accompany a postal questionnaire for a research project on asthma among men and women aged 20–59 that you are carrying out in collaboration with a general practice.

See Section 4.8 for a specimen letter

We have now seen how a sample is drawn and contacted, and how to maximise and then assess the response rate. We are now ready to think about asking these people questions, taking measurements, etc., to collect the data that we are interested in.

Summary

- It is important to determine the response rate in surveys.

- While achieving a high response is obviously desirable, the most important issue is to minimise non-response bias.

- Non-response bias can be assessed by comparing the characteristics (e.g. age, social class, marital status) of responders with the same characteristics among non-responders, so long as such information is available for non-responders.

- Non-response bias can also be assessed by comparing the sample of responders with independent sources of information about the population the sample has been designed to represent.

- There are a number of practical steps that can be followed to increase the response in any given situation.

- The right of individuals not to take part in research must always be respected.

4.6 Measurement

4.6.1 Introduction: the importance of good measurement

In the planning of the original NATSAL 1990 study, the research team recognised that

> Sexual behaviour is regarded as intensely personal by most people: reported accounts of behaviour have to be relied on, there are few possibilities for objective verification, and disclosure may include acts which are socially disapproved of, if not illegal. The twin issues of veracity (truthfulness) and recall particularly exercise those who have doubts about the validity of sexual behaviour surveys. (Wellings, K. et al. (paper B))

These comments illustrate well the measurement problems faced by the NATSAL team. Although especially pertinent to a study of sexual behaviour, the issues they mention of truthfulness, recall, the opportunity for objective verification, and so on, are principles that apply to the measurement of much more mundane behaviours such as smoking and drinking, for example. Furthermore, while we will be concentrating here on good measurement in relation to aspects of knowledge and human behaviour, these principles apply to measurement in general, including other characteristics of human populations (such as height, blood pressure, and presence or absence of a given disease), as well as characteristics of the environment (such as air pollution and quality of housing). Measurement issues relating to some of these other characteristics will be explored later in this chapter, and in other chapters.

There are a number of factors to consider in the design of their survey that can improve the accuracy of measurement. Paper B from the NATSAL 1990 study includes a good discussion of these issues in respect of the assessment of behaviour, and suggests that the following are important in ensuring accurate measurement

> A non-judgmental approach.
>
> Thorough development work, leading to the choice of meaningful language in the wording of questionnaires.
>
> Careful consideration of when to use various data-collection methods, including interviews, self-completion booklets, computer-assisted methods, the more private methods being used for the most sensitive information.
>
> Use of precise definitions.
>
> Recognition of the problems that people face in accurate recall, and the inclusion of devices to help people remember as accurately as possible.

4.6.2 Interview or self-completed questionnaire?

You will have seen that in NATSAL, the team used both interviews and self-completed question-naires. Self-completed questionnaires can be completed either in the form of a booklet, as was done in NATSAL 1990, or, as in NATSAL 2000, by computer-assisted self-interview (CASI). So, in any given situation, how do we decide which to use, and which will give the best results? As in much of research, the decision is a trade-off between the best scientific method for obtaining the information required, and practical considerations of cost and time. The principal advantages and disadvantages of interviews and self-completed questionnaires are as follows:

Interview or self-completed questionnaire?

Method	Advantages	Disadvantages
Interview	• The interviewer can ensure questions are understood. • Can explore issues in more depth. • Can use more *'open'* questions (discussed in Section 4.6.3 below).	• Greater cost and time. • Need to train interviewer. • The interviewer may influence the person's answers; this is called *interviewer bias*.
Self-completed questionnaire	• Quicker and cheaper in booklet format, as many can be mailed or distributed at the same time. • Avoids *interviewer bias*. • Self-completion, including CASI, allows respondents to record privately their responses to sensitive issues, and directly on to a computer.	• Research team may be unaware that respondent has misunderstood a question. • If, when questionnaires are checked, it is found that some questions have not been answered, it may not be possible to go back to the respondent. • Need to rely more on *'closed'* questions (see Section 4.6.3 below). • The questionnaire must not be long or complex.

4.6.3 Principles of good questionnaire design

Good questionnaire design is achieved through a combination of borrowing other people's ideas (especially their good, proven ideas), your own innovation, and paying attention to the 'rules' of good practice. We will look briefly at some of these rules, but if you are involved in questionnaire design, you may also wish to look at specialist references on the topic (for example, Bradburn *et al.*, 2004).

Question type: open and closed questions

One of the principal distinctions in question type is the extent to which these are *open* or *closed*. A closed question is one in which we specify in advance all of the 'allowable' answers to which the respondents' comments have to conform. This is done to ensure consistency in the range of answers that are given, and for ease of analysis, as each response can be given a predetermined code number. Here is an example of a closed question to respondents who are known to be unemployed:

Why are you unemployed?	Tick one box.
(1) I was made redundant.	☐
(2) I am unable to work for health reasons.	☐
(3) I cannot find a job.	☐
(4) I do not wish to work.	☐

This rigid channelling of answers into predetermined categories may be convenient for coding and data handling, but it does not encourage respondents to tell us much of interest, and by the same token provides very little to go on if we want to understand more about the real reasons for their response. If we wish to capture more of this information content of the response, we can ask respondents to answer in their own words. This is called an open question, and here is the same example expressed in an open way:

Please explain in the space below, why you are unemployed.
- -
- -

As noted in the summary table above, self-completed questionnaires generally require questions which are more closed in nature, but that does not mean that open questions cannot be used. Note also that questions can lie anywhere on a spectrum from fully closed to fully open, and the two approaches can be combined: for instance, we could add to the closed question example (above) a additional line such as 'Please write in the space below any further information about the reason(s) why you are not employed.'

Length of the questionnaire

Acceptable questionnaire length depends on the audience, and how specific and relevant the subject matter is to their experience. In general, though, it is important to make the questionnaire as short as possible, so avoid including anything that is not really needed. As a rough guide, an interview should not exceed 20–30 minutes (but longer interviews are certainly possible and not uncommon), and a self-completion questionnaire should not exceed about 10–12 pages. The acceptability of the questionnaire length should be assessed as part of *pretesting* and *piloting*, which are described in more detail in Section 4.6.4.

General layout

This is most critical for self-completion questionnaires, although it is also important that an interview schedule be well laid out for the interviewer to follow. In self-completion questionnaires (particularly), it is important to:

- avoid crowding the questions and text;

- have a clear and logical flow;

- avoid breaking parts of questions over pages.

Ordering of questions

This will to a great extent be determined by the range of subject matter under study. However, there are some useful guidelines on question order:

- It is wise to avoid placing the most sensitive questions in the early part of a questionnaire.

- Use ordering creatively. For example, in the NATSAL study design, respondents were asked about first sexual experience before later experiences, to help them to trigger recall of experiences that are less easily remembered.

- A variation on the above example is known as *funnelling*, whereby questions are constructed to go from the general to the specific, and thereby focus (funnel) the respondent's attention on the detailed information that is really important.

Phrasing and structure of questions

The way questions are phrased and structured is critical, especially when dealing with sensitive material. In the NATSAL study, for example, great care was taken to find the best language to use. The way in which the question is structured can also help. Suppose we wish to ask people how much alcohol they drink, and are especially interested in people who drink heavily. Since this is medically and (to some extent) socially disapproved of, it is helpful to phrase the question in such a way that the respondent senses that the study is not a part of this disapproval.

In the following example (for spirits; similar questions would be given for other types of alcoholic drink), the categories of consumption have been designed to cover the full range of consumption from none to extremely heavy, in such a way that a relatively heavy drinker does not appear to be giving the most extreme response (the very heaviest drinkers would, but that is unavoidable). Thus, since the recommended limit for all alcohol consumption is 3–4 units a day for men and 2–3 for women (a unit is 8 g of alcohol), moderate and heavy drinkers (say, males drinking 5–6 or 7–9 units per day) are still in the upper-middle categories of response, and not at the extreme:

On average, how many units of spirits do you drink each day (one unit is equivalent to a single measure of whisky, gin, etc.)?

Please tick one box only.

None	☐	5–6 units	☐
1 unit	☐	7–9 units	☐
2 units	☐	10–14 units	☐
3–4 units	☐	15 or more units	☐

There is more to good phrasing of questions, however, than not offending people over the wording of embarrassing subjects. Whatever the subject matter, sensitive or mundane, it is vital to avoid ambiguities in the wording which can confuse, annoy, convey different things to different people, and so on. Here are two questions with problems of this type.

 Self-Assessment Exercise 4.6.1

See whether you can (a) spot some problems with these questions, and (b) try rewording to avoid the problem(s). (Note: these are just examples – you may well find other problems!)

1. How important is it to you to take exercise and eat healthy food?
                              Tick one.
     Very important   ☐
     Fairly important   ☐
     A bit important   ☐
     Not at all important   ☐

2. These days, more and more people are turning to alternative medicine such as homoeopathy. How effective do you think homoeopathic medicines are?

Answers in Section 4.8

Skip questions

The use of skip questions is part of the ordering and flow of a questionnaire, but we will consider this under its own heading because it requires some further emphasis, especially for self-completion questionnaires. A skip question is used when we want to direct respondents past questions which are not relevant to them. In the example of alcohol consumption, it is pointless to expect lifelong non-drinkers to plough through detailed questions on their spirit, beer and wine-drinking histories. So, having established that they are lifelong non-drinkers, it is necessary to design the questionnaire in such a way as to direct them to the next section without anything being missed. This requires clear layout, numbered questions, and simple, clear instructions about which question to go to. Arrows and boxing off the parts to be skipped can also be useful, although complicated, fussy layout should be avoided.

4.6.4 Development of a questionnaire

The process for developing, *pretesting* and *piloting* an interview or self-completion questionnaire is summarised in Figure 4.6.1. While it is important not to cut corners in the development of a measurement instrument, there is no point reinventing perfectly good ones.

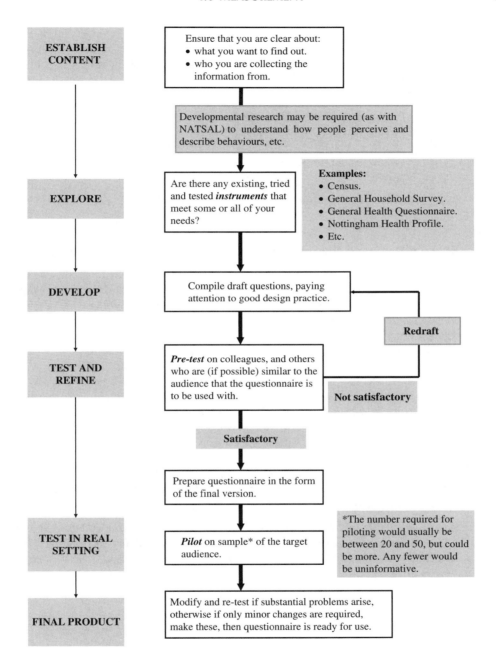

Figure 4.6.1 Summary of process for questionnaire development

---

Summary on questionnaire design

- Interviews and self-administered questionnaires each have their advantages and disadvantages, and one method will often be better suited to a given situation and research purpose than the other.

- Principles of good questionnaire design should be employed. Preparing a questionnaire is a process requiring research, development and testing. If other languages are needed, ensure that colloquial terms are known, and have the questionnaire back-translated (by a third party) to ensure meaning has not been changed.

- There is no need to reinvent questionnaires when there are already well-used, tested instruments that meet your requirements – see, for example, Bowling and Ebrahim (2005).

4.6.5   Checking how well the interviews and questionnaires have worked

We have seen how, in the NATSAL studies, the research team designed what they believed would be a representative sampling method, and then, having obtained the sample, they checked their sample against a range of information sources. We will now examine how the team assessed the success of their measurement techniques; that is, the interviews and self-completion questionnaires.

At first sight, it may seem that the team would have a problem with this. How else can one 'measure' sexual behaviours and knowledge other than by asking people questions? They have, if you like, already used the best available method. All is not lost, however, as there are a number of ways in which the success of the measurement methods can be assessed. We shall also be returning to this concept of comparison with an objective 'gold standard', in exploring how we can quantify the quality of measurement in Section 4.6.6 of this chapter, and in Chapter 10 when we discuss screening tests. These checks were described in considerable detail for the NATSAL 1990 study, so we will look first at that. These checks can be divided into two categories:

- Comparisons of some characteristics measured in the study with independent sources of information about the same characteristics, derived from routine data or other surveys. This is known as checking ***external consistency***.

- Comparisons made within the study data, of information on the same issue collected in different ways. Thus, information on a certain topic might be obtained initially in the interview, and for a second time by self-completion booklet (or CASI in NATSAL 2000). This is known as checking ***internal consistency***.

Comparison with independent, external data sources

Since one of the main reasons for doing the original NATSAL study was the lack of existing information about sexual attitudes and behaviours in a representative sample of the British population, the team was obviously not going to find an adequate alternative source against which to compare the most important data on sexual behaviours. The study did, however, include some less specific – but nevertheless quite relevant – items that could be compared, including reported therapeutic abortions. Comparison of rates of reported abortions with routinely available national abortion statistics provided one means of checking external consistency. Table 4.6.1 shows data used for this comparison in the 1990 study.

Table 4.6.1 Rates of abortions in the last year per 1000 women reported from the NATSAL 1990 study and from national figures derived from records of abortions for the same year

Age (years)	Great Britain: rates per 1000 women, 1990	NATSAL 1990 study (women aged 16–44)	
		Rate per 1000 women	95% CI
16–19	25.2	23.5	14.5–35.0
20–24	27.1	21.4	14.1–31.5
25–29	18.1	14.5	8.9–22.0
30–34	12.0	8.9	4.8–6.2
35–39	7.5	6.1	2.3–12.0
40–44	2.7	4.0	1.3–9.5
Total	15.3	12.7	10.2–15.5

Source: Reproduced from Wadsworth (1993).

 Self-Assessment Exercise 4.6.2

1. Describe the rates reported in NATSAL 1990 in comparison with the national data.

2. What do you conclude about the accuracy with which this sensitive topic has been recorded in NATSAL 1990?

3. What are the implications for measurement of other sensitive information in the NATSAL study?

Answers in Section 4.8

This comparison may seem rather inadequate in a number of ways. It is not the most important information that is being checked, and comparisons are made with data collected and/or measured in different ways. No comparison was available for men. These points are all fair criticism, but it is often the best that can be done, and better than making no checks at all. Furthermore, these external comparisons are only one of a number of ways in which the adequacy of data collection has been checked in the study. This leads to the second approach used to check consistency.

Checking internal consistency

The NATSAL 1990 study reported that:

> A further measure of validity of the data is that of internal consistency between responses to different questions. For example, respondents were asked to give some information about homosexual experience during the face-to-face interview, using show cards which allowed respondents to select from a choice of written responses by using an identifying letter only, and again in more detail in the self-completion booklet. This device deliberately provided more than one opportunity for disclosure. (Wadsworth, 1993)

A large number of internal consistency checks were included; in fact, a total of 185. The following table summarises the percentages of men and women with no inconsistencies, one or two, and three or more:

Number of inconsistencies	Men	Women
None .	78.6%	82.4%
One or two	19.2%	16.2%
Three or more	2.2%	1.4%

It was found that people were more likely to report censured behaviour in the self-completion booklet, suggesting that the responses in the booklet were closer to the truth. It does not prove it, of course, since the 'truth' is not available. Note that internal checks such as these can be built into an interview, or a self-completion questionnaire, and it is not necessary to have one method (interview) to check the other (self-completion). If, on the other hand, both data-collection methods are required to meet the study aims, as was the case with NATSAL on account of the sensitive information required, then it makes sense to make comparisons between them.

Summary

- A variety of methods are available for assessing the accuracy of measurement techniques.

- It is important to anticipate how these checks might be made at the design stage, particularly with internal consistency, since these comparisons cannot be made unless the necessary questions are built in to the interviews and/or self-completion questionnaires.

4.6.6 Assessing measurement quality

We have seen from this review of NATSAL that the ***instruments*** used to collect information can result in measurement error in a number of ways. Applying the principles of good design, backed up by developmental research and testing, should result in instruments that keep error to a minimum. Nevertheless, it is important to be able to assess (measure) how well these instruments perform, over time, in different settings, or with different groups of people, and so on. The two key components of this performance are ***validity*** and ***repeatability***.

Validity

Validity is in essence a measure of accuracy of a test or instrument, and is defined as follows:

Validity is the capacity of a test, instrument or question to give a true result.

An instrument is said to be valid after it has been satisfactorily tested, repeatedly, in the populations for which it was designed. Different forms of validity are commonly described, and examples of these are presented in Table 4.6.2 in relation to questionnaire design in the assessment of back pain.

We will describe the statistical measurement of validity (including sensitivity, specificity and predictive value) in the context of screening tests, in Chapter 10.

Table 4.6.2 Definitions of validity and examples in respect of a questionnaire designed to measure disability (restriction of activities of daily living) associated with back pain

Validity type	Description	Example
Face	The subjective assessment of the presentation and relevance of the questionnaire: do the questions appear to be relevant, reasonable, unambiguous and clear?	During questionnaire development, a focus group is held, including five patients with back pain (including both acute and chronic symptoms). The group is used to ensure face validity, ensuring it is easily comprehensible and unambiguous to potential respondents.
Content	Also theoretical, but more systematic than face validity. It refers to judgements (usually made by a panel) about how well the content of the instrument appears logically to examine and comprehensively include, in a balanced way, the full scope of the characteristic or domain it is intended to measure.	For content validity, another focus group is held, including a physiotherapist, a rheumatologist and an occupational therapist with an interest in back pain together with additional patients. They ensure that the questionnaire measures the full spectrum of disabilities that might be related to back pain, and, specifically, that it includes disability items from the such domains as physical, psychological/emotional and self-care.
Criterion	This relates to agreement between the measure and another measure, which is accepted as valid (referred to as the 'gold standard'). This is often not possible as there are no gold standards for topics such as quality of life, so proxy measures are used instead. Criterion validity is usually divided into two types: concurrent and predictive validity: • Concurrent: the independent corroboration that the instrument is measuring what it is designed to. • Predictive: is the instrument able to predict future changes in key variables in expected directions?	Questions relating to a restricted range of movement are assessed for criterion validity as follows: 50 patients with acute and chronic back pain are given the questionnaires to complete. Each then receives a physical examination to measure the range of back movement, using a standardised technique. The level of disability assessed by questionnaire is then compared with the measurements from the physical examination to assess *concurrent* criterion validity. Six weeks later, the patients repeat the questionnaire and physical examination. To assess the *predictive* criterion validity, the change in patients' disability between the original questionnaire score and that 6 weeks later is compared to the change in range of back movement.

Table 4.6.2   (Continued)

Validity type	Description	Example
Construct	This is the extent to which the instrument tests the hypothesis or theory it is measuring. There are two parts to construct validity • Convergent construct validity requires that the measure (construct) should be related to similar variables. • Discriminant construct validity requires that the measure (construct) should not be related to dissimilar variables.	A disability score is calculated by combining 25 self-reported disability items for the 50 patients with back pain. These scores are then compared to self-rated severity of low back pain, an item that has also been included in the questionnaire and is measured on a 10-point scale; 1 = minimal pain, 10 = very severe pain. The correlation between these measures of disability and pain severity, which we would expect to be related, allows assessment of *convergent* construct validity. *Discriminant* construct validity would be assessed by comparing the disability score with a variable we would not expect to be related.

Repeatability

This describes the degree to which a measurement made on one occasion agrees with the same measurement made on a subsequent occasion. Synonymous terms are *reproducibility* and *reliability*. We have all probably experienced the frustration of making a measurement – for instance, on a piece of wood we plan to saw – and then gone back to check it, only to get a slightly different result and then wonder which one is right? In this situation, we can be fairly sure that it is our carelessness that has caused the error, but in health research the situation is rather more complex. The following example will help to illustrate why this is so. The table shows the mean systolic and diastolic blood pressures of a group of 50 middle-aged men who were screened in a well-man clinic in a general practice, and then followed up on two further occasions. The blood pressures were taken by a variety of different staff in the practice (doctors and practice nurses).

	Mean systolic (mmHg)	Mean diastolic (mmHg)
Screening	162	85
First follow-up	157	82
Second follow-up	152	78

So, why are the mean values different on the three occasions? There are a number of possible explanations for this:

- Chance: We must consider chance variations, but this is unlikely to be due to the pattern of a progressive decrease in both systolic and diastolic. We could calculate the 95 per cent CIs around these mean values to see whether the changes are within the range of random variation. The 95 per cent CIs in fact show that chance is very unlikely to be the explanation.

- Real Change: The men's blood pressures are actually lower because they are getting used to the procedure and the staff: this is a real change in the men's measured blood pressures, but one related to the measurement setting.

- Artefact or Bias: The screening and follow-up blood pressures were taken by different staff, and their technique of blood-pressure measurement could have varied. This type of inconsistency between people making measurements is known as **observer variation**. This may occur **within the observer** (for instance, the same doctor uses a different technique on two occasions), or **between observers** (for instance, the doctor uses a different technique from the nurse). Observer variation is a potentially important source of **bias**.

- Artefact or Bias: The sphygmomanometers (blood pressure-measuring equipment) used were in need of maintenance and **calibration**, and some were leaking at the time of the follow-up measurements and consequently gave lower readings. This is another potential source of bias.

Example from NATSAL

We will now look at some of the changes between the 1990 and 2000 NATSAL studies, and consider whether differences are likely to be the result of chance or artefact, or are real.

 Self-Assessment Exercise 4.6.3

1. Use the following table to compare findings in 1990 and 2000 (with 95 per cent CIs), for the behaviours listed.

Behaviour among men	NATSAL 1990		NATSAL 2000	
	(%)	95% CI	(%)	95% CI
Ever had homosexual partners (all areas)	3.6	3.1–4.2	5.4	4.8–6.1
Injected non-prescribed drugs, last 5 years (all areas)	1.3	1.0–1.7	1.3	1.0–1.7
Condom use on all occasions in last 4 weeks (all areas)	18.3	17.1–19.7	24.4	22.8–26.1

2. Drawing on your learning so far on sources of error and the interpretation of differences, make brief notes on the possible explanations for 1990 and 2000 findings.

Answers in Section 4.8

When you have checked your answer, please read the following section from the discussion section of paper A, in which the authors discuss the possible reasons behind the issue of increased reporting of sexual behaviours in greater detail.

Discussion

While interpreting the changes in reported behaviours over time, we have considered whether the results are due entirely to changes in behaviour, or may in part result from changes in methodology or in respondents' willingness to report socially censured behaviours. Natsal 1990 and 2000 achieved similar response rates, 66·8% and 65·4% respectively, and, where questions were repeated, used identical question wording.[2]

Methodological improvements in survey research between 1990 and 2000 have led to improved data quality.[13] We used computer-assisted interviewing techniques in Natsal 2000 rather than the pen-and-paper questionnaire used in Natsal 1990. In a randomised comparison of CASI with pen-and-paper self completion, we showed that CASI resulted in lower rates of question non-response and greater internal consistency of responses, and we found no consistent evidence of an increased willingness to report sensitive behaviours.[13] Turner and colleagues[24] have noted increased willingness to report injecting drug use and other sensitive behaviours using audio-CASI in a sample of male adolescents in the USA, but the generalisability of this result to other demographic groups is uncertain. Despite the general increase in reporting sexual activity, we found no consistent increase in the rate of reporting recent injecting drug use, which is evidence against a generalised increase in willingness to report.

Elsewhere,[25] we have examined the evidence for change in reporting between surveys, by comparing a limited number of behaviours occurring before the time of Natsal 1990 among the age cohorts eligible for both surveys (those born between 1956 and 1974). Where there were differences, these were in the direction of greater reporting of sensitive behaviours and in particular, homosexual experience before age 20 years, in Natsal 2000. These differences perhaps arise from greater willingness to report socially censured behaviours, and thus, more accurate reporting. This conclusion is consistent with an analysis of attitudes from the two surveys, which shows greater tolerance in Natsal 2000 to male and female homosexuality and to casual partnerships.[25] However, changing attitudes may also alter behaviour, and the increased liberalisation of attitudes since 1990 is consistent with the direction of observed changes in behaviour.

4.6.7 Overview of sources of error

The following table summarises the main sources of error we have looked at so far in epidemiological research. We will return to this classification in later sections as we explore some of these sources of error in more detail, and look at ways to overcome them. For now, it is important to note that there are two principal types of error in this table:

- *Systematic error* or *bias*, which falsely alters the level of a measurement.

- Chance, or *random error*, which causes the sample estimate to be less precise.

This is a very important distinction, as we can deal with the two problems in quite different ways. Thus, one of the main ways to reduce random error is by increasing the number of subjects or measurements: this is why sample size estimation is such an important aspect of study design. On the other hand, bias must be avoided (or at least kept to a minimum) by representative sampling and the use of valid (accurate) measurement instruments.

Table 4.6.3   Summary of sources of error in surveys

Source	Type of error	Comment
Sampling	Sampling error	Random imprecision arising from the process of sampling from a population, and quantified by the standard error (if the sampling is random).
	Selection bias	Non-random systematic error, arising from a non-representative sampling method, or non-response bias.
Measurement – instrument	Inaccuracy (poor validity)	Systematic error (bias) in measurement due to inadequate design of the measurement 'instrument', or poorly calibrated or maintained equipment.
	Poor repeatability (unreliability)	This may be due to variable performance in different situations, or with different subjects (which may be mostly random), or may be a systematic drift over time which is bias (and in effect a change in accuracy).
Measurement – observer	Between observer	A systematic difference (bias) between measurements obtained by different observers, arising from the way they carry out the measurements, their training, etc.
	Within observer	Measurements by the same observer vary between subjects and over time, due to inconsistencies in technique, etc. This is mainly random variation, but may also drift over time in the same way as described for instruments.

 Self-Assessment Exercise 4.6.4

A study of nutrition was carried out among 1000 women attending an antenatal clinic. Women were allocated randomly to see one of two dietitians (A and B), who asked them about their diet during the pregnancy in a standard interview questionnaire. The estimated iron intake based on this questionnaire for the women seeing dietitian A was 25 per cent lower than that for dietitian B. Discuss which of the following could explain the observed difference:

a) A real difference in iron intake?

b) Between-observer bias?

c) Instrument unreliability?

Answers in Section 4.8

Self-Assessment Exercise 4.6.5

The diagram illustrates four targets in a firing range, each of which has been shot with 10 bullets. For each target (a–d), describe the validity (accuracy) and reliability (repeatability).

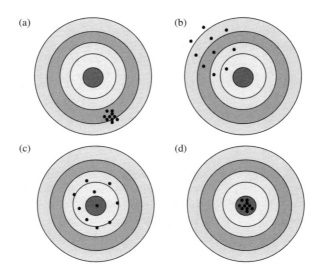

Answers in Section 4.8

Summary on measurement quality

- The validity of a measurement instrument describes how accurately it measures the true situation.

- The validity of measurement should be checked where possible: both internal consistency checks and external comparisons offer opportunities to do this. Some forward planning is often required to make these checks possible.

- Repeatability describes how consistently the instrument functions on different occasions.

- Error in measurement falls into two broad categories: random and systematic (bias), and may arise from sampling, measurement instruments, and from the 'observers' who carry out the measurements.

4.7 Data types and presentation

4.7.1 Introduction

A survey such as NATSAL generally results in a vast amount of data. In their raw state, the data tell us little. We need to *summarise* the data to make sense of the information they contain, and we need to present this information in an appropriate way. We need to *analyse* the data to get answers to our questions and make *inferences* about the population. The ways in which data are summarised, presented and analysed depend on the type of data. In Chapter 2 we looked in some detail at presenting and summarising *continuous* data. In the NATSAL study, we meet other types of data which require different methods, which are discussed here.

4.7.2 Types of data

Quantities which vary from person to person, such as age, sex and weight, are called *variables*. Measured values of these variables are *data*. For example, weight is a variable. The actual weights of five people (say, 62.5, 68.4, 57.3, 64.0 and 76.8 kg) are data. Values may be measured on one of the following four measurement scales:

Type	Description
Categorical (nominal)	A nominal scale has separate, named (hence 'nominal') classes or categories into which individuals may be classified. The classes have no numerical relationship with one another; for example, sex (male, female) or classification of disease.
Ordered or ranked categorical (ordinal)	An ordinal scale has ordered categories, such as mild, moderate or severe pain. Numbers may be used to label the categories, such as $1 =$ mild, $2 =$ moderate, $3 =$ severe, and so on, but this is only a ranking: the difference between 1 and 2 does not necessarily mean the same as the difference between 2 and 3.
Interval	An interval scale is so called because the distance, or interval, between two measurements on the scale has meaning. For example, $20\,°C$ is 30 degrees more than $-10\,°C$, and the difference is the same as that between $60\,°C$ and $30\,°C$.
Ratio	On a ratio scale, both the distance and ratio between two measurements are defined: 1 kg (1000 g) is 500 g more than 500 g and also twice the weight. An additional property is that the value zero means just that, whereas with an interval scale such as degrees Celsius, $0\,°C$ does not mean 'no thermal energy'.

Interval measurements can be further classified into *continuous* or *discrete*. Continuous measurements can take any value within a range, the only restriction being the accuracy of the measuring instrument. Discrete measurements can take only whole-number values - a household may contain one, two, three or more people, but not two and a half people. Note that interval measurements are also ordered. Discrete interval data may be treated as ordered categories or continuous, depending on the number of discrete values and how they are distributed (we will return to this).

As there are a number of interchangeable terms for data types, from now on we shall refer to *categorical; ordered categorical, discrete* (interval) and *continuous* (interval, ratio) data. We shall now look at some of the variables measured in the NATSAL 2000 study, which include:

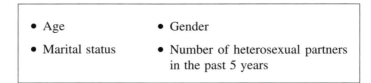

- Age
- Marital status
- Gender
- Number of heterosexual partners in the past 5 years

 Self-Assessment Exercise 4.7.1

For each of the variables above, think about how each one is likely to have been measured and so classify them into categorical (including whether or not ordered) or continuous variables (type of scale, and whether or not discrete).

Answers in Section 4.8

4.7.3 Displaying and summarising the data

We generally start by describing the number of study participants and their basic characteristics, such as age, sex, ethnicity and so on. We will now look at how this is done for categorical variables.

Categorical data

Often, many of the data collected in surveys are categorical, such as sex (male, female), behaviours such as smoking (never, ex-smoker, current smoker), or a disease classification (present or absent). Data on one categorical variable can be summarised by the number of individuals in each category. This is the *frequency distribution*, and it is simpler to construct for a categorical variable than for a continuous variable (Chapter 2, Section 2.4.2) because we do not have to decide how to divide the range of the data into intervals. Table 4.7.1 shows the frequency distribution of marital status of participants in the NATSAL 2000 study taken from Table 1 of paper A.

Table 4.7.1 Frequency distribution of marital status in the NATSAL 2000 study

Marital status	Number
Single	3873
Cohabiting	1931
Married	4687
Separated/widowed/divorced	670
Total	11161

It is easier to compare the relative numbers in each category by percentages or proportions of the total number. These are the *relative frequencies* introduced in Section 2.4.4 of Chapter 2. They are particularly useful for comparing two distributions, as when we compared marital status of the NATSAL sample with the Health Survey for England.

Table 4.7.2 Relative frequency distribution of marital status in the NATSAL 2000 sample

Marital status	Number	Percentage
Single	3873	34.7
Cohabiting	1931	17.3
Married	4687	42.0
Separated/widowed/divorced	670	6.0
Total	11161	100.0

The frequency and relative frequency distributions can be displayed in a *bar chart* or a *pie chart*.

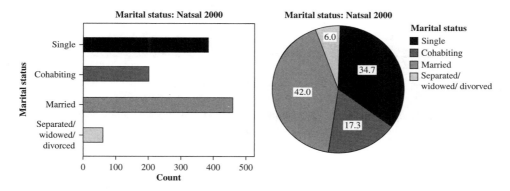

Figure 4.7.1 Data on marital status from NATSAL 2000 presented as (a) bar chart of frequency distribution and (b) pie chart of relative frequency distribution

Note that there are spaces between the bars of the bar chart. A histogram does not have spaces between intervals, because they are parts of a continuous scale. In the pie chart, the angle of each sector is proportional to the frequency (or relative frequency). The *modal category* of the distribution may sometimes be stated. This is simply the category with the highest frequency/relative frequency. The modal category of marital status in NATSAL 2000 is 'married'.

Discrete data

Discrete data are tabulated in exactly the same way as categorical data (Table 4.7.3). The frequency distribution shows the frequency of each separate value.

The frequency distribution can be displayed as a *line chart* or a bar chart (Figure 4.7.2).

Table 4.7.3 Hypothetical frequency distribution of number of children in 62 families

Number of children	Frequency
0	17
1	8
2	21
3	13
4	2
5	1
Total	62

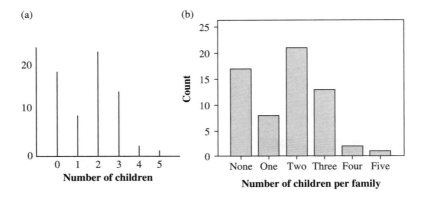

Figure 4.7.2 (a) Line chart and (b) bar chart of the frequency distribution of number of children in a sample of families

If there are many different values in the data, they may be grouped. This is not generally into equal sized groups, but in such a way that the most frequently occurring values are shown individually, and the less common values grouped. For example, the number of heterosexual partners in the past 5 years is grouped in Table 2 of paper A as follows (Table 4.7.4):

Table 4.7.4 Relative frequency distribution of number of heterosexual partners in the past 5 years of men in the NATSAL 2000 sample

Number of partners	Percentage
None	9.0
1	42.4
2	12.1
3–4	15.1
5–9	12.9
10+	8.4
Total (base = 5522)	100.0

Table 4.7.5 Methods for presenting and summarising data

Type of data	Presenting the data	Summarising the data
Categorical (including ordered)	Frequency/relative frequency table Bar chart Pie chart	Percentages Modal category
Discrete	Frequency/relative frequency table Bar chart Line chart	Mean and standard deviation (symmetric distribution) Median and interquartile range (skewed distribution)
Continuous	Frequency/relative frequency table* Histogram Box and whisker plot**	Mean and standard deviation (symmetric distribution) Median and interquartile range (skewed distribution)

* For continuous data, a frequency/relative frequency table would be obtained by dividing the data into subgroups.
** Box and whisker plots are illustrated and explained in Chapter 11, Section 11.3.5.

The location and spread of discrete data may be summarised by the mean and standard deviation or the median and interquartile range, depending on whether the distribution is approximately symmetric or is skewed. The same criteria apply as for continuous data (Chapter 2, Section 2.4.3).

Table 4.7.5 provides an overview of methods recommended for presenting and summarising the main types of data.

4.8 Answers to self-assessment exercises

Section 4.1

Exercise 4.1.1

Reasons for carrying out the NATSAL 2000 study

(a) General background reasons

- Changes in public attitudes to sexual matters accompanied by a decline in HIV education and increased attention to school sex education.

- Indications that sexual behaviour may have changed over time.

- Need for new population estimates of some aspects of sexual behaviour due to advances in understanding of transmission of sexually transmitted disease.

(b) Immediate needs

Updated estimates of the distribution of different sexual behaviours are required to assess changes in reported sexual behaviour over time.

Section 4.2

Exercise 4.2.1 Probability

1. The probability that a smoker is chosen is

$$\frac{\text{Number of smokers in population}}{\text{Total population}} = \frac{25000}{100\,000} = 0.25$$

2. The probability the person has had IHD is

$$\frac{875 + 750}{100\,000} = 0.01625$$

3. The probability that the person chosen is a smoker who has suffered IHD is

$$\frac{875}{100\,000} = 0.00875$$

Exercise 4.2.2 Quota sampling

1. A quota of 70 women aged 20–24 is required (28 per cent of 250).

2. If they were to do this, it would of course badly under-represent people in employment, and the sample would be very biased.

3. It is not very easy to find a quota of, say, 75 males aged 15–19 who are representative of everyone in that age group. Contrast this with a random sampling method in which a name and address is specified, and the research team has to keep trying (within limits!) until the specified person is contacted and can be offered the opportunity to take part in the study. Nevertheless, in expert hands, quota sampling can be very effective, and can be made more representative by

breaking the quotas down into more subgroups (for instance, men, aged 20–24, in employment; men, aged 20–24, unemployed; etc.), so that a more representative structure is imposed on the sampling and quota-finding process.

Exercise 4.2.3 Weighting

1. The overall percentage of people in the sample reporting the behaviour of interest is $1080/10\ 900 = 9.9$ per cent.

2. This is incorrect because it does not allow for the fact that, for example, people from inner London have (a) a much higher prevalence of the behaviour, and (b) are three times more likely to be in the sample.

3. $900/3 = 300$ people.

4. $225/3 = 75$ people.

5. The weighted answer would be $(630 + 100 + 75) \div (9000 + 500 + 300) = 8.2$ per cent. This is considerably different from the unweighted answer to question 1 of 9.9 per cent.

Exercise 4.2.4 Sampling methods

1. *Cardiovascular disease*

   Simple random sampling would be appropriate. Cluster sampling would probably not be necessary or appropriate in an area such as a district. It did form part of the NATSAL sampling method, with wards as clusters, but this was in part due to the very large area that needed to be covered and visited by interviewers (locations across the whole country). Quota sampling would be a poor method unless relatively simple information was required quickly. It would be a very inappropriate way to approach people if a physical examination and blood tests were required. A convenience sample would be inappropriate, and very unlikely to yield a representative sample.

2. *People aged over 75 in residential homes*

   Simple random sampling would be difficult given that the residents are spread very unevenly in the population, but a cluster sample would be appropriate, as the homes are in effect clusters. We could select the homes randomly, and then sample people randomly within homes, or survey all residents in the selected homes, depending on the sample size required. A snowball sample is inappropriate and unnecessary, as it is not difficult to identify and contact the subjects, so that a more satisfactory random sampling technique is quite possible. Quota sampling would also be inappropriate and unnecessary, for the same reasons.

3. *Drug users*

   A cluster sample would be inappropriate as the women will be living in many different situations, and not in any identifiable clusters. A snowball sample may be a good approach, depending on whether the available networks and contacts could yield a sample with this hard-to-reach group. Simple random sampling is unlikely to work as it would be hard to identify people, and contacting the women via a standard sampling frame (e.g. addresses) will probably be ineffective. Quota sampling would be inappropriate because we have no basis for working out quotas.

Section 4.3

Exercise 4.3.1 Sampling frames

Here are some examples of sampling frames (not including the postcode address files used in NATSAL):

Sampling frame	Advantages	Disadvantages
Electoral register	• updated each year.	• restricted to people of voting age (18+). • addresses, but no personal details. • losses due to non-registration and mobility.
GP lists	• considerable amount of information on individuals available (subject to permission).	• loss due to inaccurate addresses and non-registration may be serious; e.g. younger people in urban areas. • list may also be inflated by people who have actually moved away but not yet been removed from the list.
School registers	• all children required to attend school, so almost complete and updated. • age and sex information available subject to permission.	• may be difficult to include independent (private) schools.
Employee registers	• should be complete. • personal information available subject to permission. • good for studying employment-related issues.	• not representative for population survey purposes, as excludes the unemployed, long-term sick, etc.

In the NATSAL study, the team also needed to choose from various options, and, on balance, the postcode sectors and address files were judged best to meet their needs.

Section 4.4

Exercise 4.4.1 Sampling distribution

1. Yes, in this case the range ± 1.96 SE does include μ, as the sampling distribution is centred on the population mean.

2. 95 per cent of sample means.

3. 5 per cent of sample means.

4. No, it is not included. This shows that there is a 5 per cent (1 in 20) chance that the 95 per cent CI around a given sample estimate will not include the true population mean.

Exercise 4.4.2 CI for a mean

For the mean number of lifetime partners for women aged 16–44 years in the NATSAL 2000, we have

$$\bar{x} = 6.5$$

$$s = 9.7$$

$$n = 5390$$

So the 95 per cent CI $= \bar{x} \pm 1.96$ SE $= 6.5 \pm 1.96 \times 9.7 \big/ \sqrt{5390} = (6.24, 6.76)$.

Note that the CI for the mean number of lifetime partners for women is narrower than the one for men: the estimate is more precise. This is because, although the sample size is similar, the standard deviation is smaller, resulting in a smaller SE.

Exercise 4.4.3 Sample size for estimating a mean

1. $n = 1.96^2 \times 520^2 \big/ 50^2 = 415.5$, so the required sample size should be around 420 (not allowing for refusals).

2. If the precision is doubled (ε halved), the sample size is multiplied by 4, so the sample size required is $4 \times 415.5 = 1662$. A common mistake in calculating sample size is to think ε is the required width of the entire 95 per cent CI, when it is in fact *half* the width as the error range is specified as $\pm\varepsilon$.

Exercise 4.4.4 CI for a proportion/percentage

The sample percentage is 16.5 per cent, and the sample size 5679

$$\text{SE} = \sqrt{\frac{0.165(1 - 0.165)}{5679}} = 0.0049255.$$

95% CI $= 0.165 \pm (1.96 \times 0.0049255) = (0.155, 0.175)$, or in percentages (15.5–17.5 per cent). As with the mean, because the sample size is large, the 95 per cent CI is very narrow. We interpret this as we are 95 per cent certain that the percentage of men aged 16–44 in Britain who are cohabiting is between 15.5 per cent and 17.5 per cent.

Exercise 4.4.5 Sample size for estimating a proportion

a) The sample size formula for estimating a proportion using percentages is $n = 1.96^2 P(1 - P) \big/ \varepsilon^2$. Substituting $P = 1\%$ and $\varepsilon = 0.2\%$, the required sample size is $1.96^2 \times 1 \times 99/0.2^2 = 9508$. If the prevalence was expressed as a proportion, we would use the formula $n = 1.96^2\, P(1 - P)/\varepsilon^2$ with P $= 0.01$ and $\varepsilon = 0.002$.

b) If we have a sample of only 500 people, $\varepsilon = 1.96\sqrt{[P(100 - P)/n]} = 1.96\sqrt{[1 \times 99/500]} = 0.87$.

That is, using a 95 per cent CI, we have a 95 per cent chance of obtaining an estimate of the prevalence to within ± 0.87 per cent of the true value. This is large relative to 1 per cent: we cannot obtain a very precise estimate from a sample of 500. This emphasises why the sample size for the NATSAL 2000 study had to be large. Some subgroups were considerably smaller, however, so these estimates (drug use, for example) have not been measured with the same precision.

Section 4.5

Exercise 4.5.1 NATSAL response rate

A total of 16 998 households were identified with an eligible resident. Of these, at 1425 (3.5 per cent of all addresses), no contact was achieved. Interviews were completed on 11 161 respondents. The unadjusted response is 63.1 per cent, adjusted 65.4 per cent (allowing for over-sampling and a lower response rate in London, and excluding those who were sick, did not speak English, and were expected to be ineligible from the 1425 where no contact was made). So, is a response of 65.4 per cent adequate? It is not particularly good, but perhaps not bad given the subject matter of the survey. However, the critical question is whether the non-responders differed substantively from the responders, and we will look at that question next.

Exercise 4.5.2 Representativeness of sample

1. The percentages for men and women, for age and region match the population data very closely, and the research team comments that 'the NATSAL II (2000) sample closely reflects the general population'.

2. Percentages for marital status are quite similar, with the largest difference being for cohabiting (women), suggesting that cohabiting couples are over-represented relative to some of the other categories. For social class, in both men and women, there is a tendency for higher social classes to be over-represented compared to lower social classes. But which of the two samples, NATSAL II (2000) or Health Survey of England, is most representative of the true situation in the country? The research team does comment on these differences, but notes 'these [differences] were thought too small to warrant additional weighting'.

Exercise 4.5.3 Specimen invitation letter

The Health Centre
Yellow Brick Rd
Liverpool LXX 9XX
Tel: 0111-111-1111

Dr A. Brown
25 January 2007
Dear *Mr Patterson*

I am writing to ask for your assistance in a study we are carrying out jointly with the University of Liverpool, on the treatment of chest problems such as asthma and bronchitis. The purpose of the study is to help the practice develop and improve the service we can offer our patients.

I would be grateful if you would complete the enclosed questionnaire, and return it in the postage-paid reply envelope provided.

All information will be treated confidentially. If you have any questions about the study, please contact Ms Jenny Smith of the Department of Public Health at the University on 0222-222-2222, who will be pleased to assist you.

Yours sincerely
Anthony Brown
Dr A. Brown

There are of course many ways to phrase such a letter, but here are the key features of good practice incorporated in this one:

- It is from a respected person known to the subject. The fact that the person is known should help, but be aware that it can be inhibiting if (for example) the study is about quality of services and the respondent is reluctant to criticise the GP's service in case this affected the way the respondent is treated in the future.

- The letter has a personal touch, with handwritten name and signature.

- The reason for the study and its relevance are explained.

- A postage-paid reply envelope is provided.

- Confidentiality is explained.

- There is a contact name for assistance, and note that this person is not at the practice. This may be of help provided the respondent has been made aware of why people other than the practice staff are involved.

- The letter is short and clear.

Section 4.6

Exercise 4.6.1 Question phrasing

1. The problem here is that the initial question contains two important but quite different ideas, namely exercise and healthy eating. The respondent may well feel differently about the two, and hence cannot answer the question meaningfully. This is called a ***double-barrelled question***, and the most obvious solution is to ask two separate questions.

2. In this question, the opening statement implies growing interest, acceptability and approval of homoeopathy. This could well convey to the respondent that an approving answer is the correct one, or at least expected, and is therefore a ***leading question*** (it is not neutral, and leads respondents towards one type of answer). A more neutral way of setting the context might be to start by asking respondents whether or not they had used homoeopathic medicines.

Exercise 4.6.2 Comparison of abortion rates in NATSAL and Great Britain

1. All the age-specific rates are lower in the NATSAL sample, with the exception of the 40–44-year age group. Although the 95 per cent CIs are wide (and all include the national rates), the fact that almost all age groups are lower for NATSAL suggests that these differences are systematic rather than due to chance (sampling error).

2. On the face of it, there seems to have been under-reporting of abortions in the NATSAL study. The authors comment, however, that '[national] abortion statistics may include a slight excess of temporary residents using UK addresses and women having more than one abortion in a year'. Hence, the difference may in part be due to artefact.

3. It is difficult to say with any certainty what might be going on with other sensitive information, particularly for men for whom no external comparisons were made. Overall, we may conclude that although there is some evidence of under-reporting where comparative information was available (therapeutic abortions), this was not substantial and may in any case be largely due to artefact.

Exercise 4.6.3

Question 1

- Ever had homosexual partners (all areas): an increase from 3.6 per cent to 5.4 per cent, with non-overlapping 95 per cent CIs.

- Injected non-prescribed drugs, last 5 years (all areas): no change (1.3 per cent).

- Condom use on all occasions in last 4 weeks (all): an increase from 18.3 per cent to 24.4 per cent with non-overlapping 95 per cent CIs.

Question 2

Ever had homosexual partners (all areas)	• Chance: 95 per cent CIs exclude this.*
	• Artefact: could improved methods (CASI), etc., have improved reporting? Could changes in social acceptance of homosexual behaviour have encouraged a higher level of disclosure?
	• Real: if not due to greater willingness to report and not due to chance, we can conclude this is a real increase.
Injected non-prescribed drugs, last 5 years (all areas)	• Chance: 95 per cent CIs are small, but there are no differences.
	• Artefact: probably not relevant, as there was no change (although, of course, this does not mean there is no effect of artefact occurring).
	• Real: if real, interesting that no change reported. This could be taken as evidence that there has not been a generally greater willingness to disclose sensitive information between 1990 and 2000 either due to use of CASI and/or changed social acceptance (although it is, of course, possible that there may have been different trends in social acceptance of injecting drug use and homosexual behaviour).
Condom use on all occasions in last 4 weeks (all)	• Chance: 95 per cent CIs exclude this.*
	• Artefact: similar considerations as above; an added factor may be that respondents in 2000 wished to appear more responsible in their answers than was the case in 1990.
	• Real: if real, this is quite a large increase. Is this in line with expectations of increased condom use?

*95 per cent CI excludes chance, by convention, although. as we have seen. there is still a 5 per cent chance that the population value lies outside the CI of the sample estimate.

Exercise 4.6.4 Nutrition study

a) A 25 per cent mean difference is very unlikely to be real, given the random allocation and the relatively large numbers (about 500 for each nurse).

b) Bias arising from *between-observer variation* is the most likely explanation. When obtaining the dietary information from the women, dietitian A tends, on average, to obtain results on iron intake 25 per cent lower than dietitian B. Of course, this does not tell us which one is nearer the truth (most valid). The solution to this problem is to ensure standardised training for both dietitians.

c) **Instrument unreliability** is unlikely, as both dietitians are using the same standard questionnaire, and even if there is a lot of variation in how it works from subject to subject, this type of variation is mainly random in nature and will not produce such marked systematic differences (bias) between observers.

Exercise 4.6.5 Targets

a) Validity is very poor (shots are a long way from the bullseye, which in this analogy is the 'truth', or measurement we are seeking to make), but the repeatability is very good. This pattern might be caused by poorly adjusted (calibrated) sights on a rifle that was otherwise in very good condition, and which was being shot with very consistent technique.

b) Poor validity and poor repeatability.

c) Good validity, but poor repeatability: we can see that, on average, these 10 shots are on target, but there is scatter. This scatter is more or less random, and could, for example, be caused by poor shooting technique or a worn barrel. Thus, in measurement analogy terms, we can see this result as an accurate estimate, but one with an excessive amount of random imprecision.

d) The desired result: high validity and high repeatability.

Section 4.7

Exercise 4.7.1

Age
A bit more difficult than it looks. Age can take any value of between 16 and 44 (in this study), so it is a **continuous** variable, even though it may be measured only to an accuracy of whole years. However, for the purposes of analysis, age is often presented in groups as an **ordered categorical** variable (16–24, 25–34, etc.). It is most likely that age either was recorded as age last birthday or was calculated from the respondent's date of birth and the interview date, and then grouped into categories for the purpose of presentation.

Gender
This is a **categorical** variable, with possible values being male and female.

Marital status
There are a number of categories, but these are not ordered in any way, so this is simply a **categorical** variable.

Number of heterosexual partners in the last 5 years
Again, as with age, we do not know how this variable was measured. It is likely that the actual number of partners was recorded, in which case it is (or can be treated as) continuous. The number of partners must, however, be a whole number (including 0), so this is a **discrete** variable. Unlike age (even in years), the number of partners for any given study respondent cannot take a value between whole numbers, such as 3.6, although it is meaningful to present such values as group averages.

5

Cohort studies

Introduction and learning objectives

Survey methods have provided us with a way of studying population groups of our own choice and better-quality information on issues that may not be available from routine data sources. These methods have also allowed us to examine associations in greater detail, but are not able to provide particularly strong evidence about factors that cause disease.

In the next two chapters of this book, we will study two research designs that offer marked advantages over the descriptive methods examined so far. These are called *cohort* and *case-control* studies. We will look at cohort studies first because the design, analysis and interpretation of case-control studies is more complex. However, many of the design issues that occur in this chapter are also relevant to case-control study design. You may find it useful to refer to table 2.7.1 which was introduced at the end of Chapter 2 to refresh your memory of the concepts we introduced at that stage. In particular you should focus on how the cohort study ideas fit into the overall framework of studies so far.

The defining feature of the cohort study is the follow-up of subjects over time. Obtaining sufficient information from a cohort to enable reliable estimation (for example, of disease incidence, or mortality) generally requires a large sample, a long follow-up period, or both. A cohort study may also be referred to as a longitudinal study, a prospective study, an incidence study, or a follow-up study.

Learning objectives

By the end of Chapter 5, you should be able to do the following:

- Describe the purpose and structure of the cohort study design, within an overall framework of epidemiological study designs.
- Give examples of the uses of cohort studies, including examples from your own field.

(*Continued*)

Quantitative Methods for Health Research   Nigel Bruce, Daniel Pope and Debbi Stanistreet
© 2008 John Wiley & Sons, Ltd

- Describe the strengths and weaknesses of cohort studies.

- Describe the various types of bias that can arise with cohort studies, including measurement and observer error, and how these can be minimised.

- Define relative risk, and how this is derived from a cohort study.

- Explain the use of, carry out, and interpret the appropriate hypothesis test for categorical data (chi-squared test).

- Explain the use of, carry out, and interpret the appropriate hypothesis test for continuous data (Student's t-test).

- Describe the information required to carry out a sample size calculation for a cohort study, including the concept of power.

- Define confounding, with examples.

- Describe the criteria used to assess whether an association is causal (the Bradford Hill guidelines), with examples.

- Explain the uses of, and interpret, simple linear regression.

- Describe the uses of, and principles underlying, multiple linear regression.

- Describe how adjustment for confounding by regression methods helps meet the Bradford Hill guidelines, with examples.

The cohort study that we will look at investigates the association between physical activity and risk of cancer in middle-aged men (paper A). This study was part of a much broader programme, the British Regional Heart Study (BRHS), designed primarily to investigate cardiovascular disease (CVD) in Great Britain.

We will also refer to the original BRHS publications where necessary to provide more details of the methods used (papers B and C).

Resource papers

(A) Wannamethee, S. G., Shaper, A. G. and Walker, M. (2001). Physical activity and risk of cancer in middle-aged men. *Br J Cancer* **85**, 1311–1316.

(B) Shaper, A. G., Pocock, S. J., Walker M. *et al.* (1985). Risk factors for ischaemic heart disease: the prospective phase of the British Regional Heart Study. *J Epidemiol Community Health* **39**, 197–209.

(C) Walker, M. and Shaper, A. G. (1984). Follow up of subjects in prospective studies based in general practice. *J R Coll Gen Pract* **34**, 365–370.

5.1 Why do a cohort study?

5.1.1 Objectives of the study

We will begin our examination of cohort studies by finding out exactly why the team chose this design to investigate their research question. Please now read the summary and introduction section of paper A, which are given below:

Summary

A prospective study was carried out to examine the relationship between physical activity and incidence of cancers in 7588 men aged 40–59 years with full data on physical activity and without cancer at screening. Physical activity at screening was classified as none/occasional, light, moderate, moderately-vigorous or vigorous. Cancer incidence data were obtained from death certificates, the national Cancer Registration Scheme and self-reporting on follow-up questionnaires of doctor-diagnosed cancer. Cancer (excluding skin cancers) developed in 969 men during mean follow-up of 18.8 years. After adjustment for age, smoking, body mass index, alcohol intake and social class, the risk of total cancers was significantly reduced only in men reporting moderately-vigorous or vigorous activity; no benefit was seen at lesser levels. Sporting activity was essential to achieve significant benefit and was associated with a significant dose-response reduction in risk of prostate cancer and upper digestive and stomach cancer. Sporting (vigorous) activity was associated with a significant increase in bladder cancer. No association was seen with colorectal cancer. Non-sporting recreational activity showed no association with cancer. Physical activity in middle-aged men is associated with reduced risk of total cancers, prostate cancer, upper digestive and stomach cancer. Moderately-vigorous or vigorous levels involving sporting activities are required to achieve such benefit.

Introduction

There is increasing evidence that physical activity is associated with altered risk of total cancers and certain specific types of cancer, especially colon and prostate (Lee, 1995; Oliveria and Christos, 1997; Gerhardsson, 1997; McTiernan et al, 1998; Moore et al, 1998; Shephard and Shek, 1998). In particular, the evidence strongly supports the role of physical activity in reducing risk of colon cancer (Lee, 1995; Oliveria and Christos, 1997; Gerhardsson, 1997; McTiernan et al, 1998; Moore et al, 1998; Shephard and Shek, 1998; Giovannucci et al, 1995; Slattery et al, 1997); the findings relating to prostate cancer have been inconsistent (Albanes et al, 1989; Thune and Lund, 1994; Oliveria and Lee, 1997; Hartman et al, 1998; Giovannucci et al, 1998; Liu et al, 2000). A few prospective studies have suggested an inverse relationship with lung cancer (Lee and Paffenbarger, 1994; Thune and Lund, 1997; Lee et al, 1999). Data on physical activity and other types of cancer are limited and the amount and type of physical activity required to confer protection remains unclear for many of the cancers. There is some indication that a high level of activity (vigorous) is required to achieve benefit for prostate cancer (Giovannucci et al, 1998). The inconsistent findings between studies for the various cancer types may relate to the different levels of activity in the populations studied. This raises the question of how much activity is required to achieve benefit and in particular, whether light to moderate physical activities have any effect on diminishing risk. This paper examines the relationship between physical activity and the incidence of total cancers and some site-specific cancers and assesses the type and amount of activity required to achieve benefit in a prospective study of middle-aged men.

Self-Assessment Exercise 5.1.1

1. Make a list of all the research issues and the aim of the study noted in this passage.

2. Which of these do you think could be addressed adequately by descriptive and survey methods, and which might require a more sophisticated research design (such as is offered by a cohort study)?

Note: in working through this exercise, do not be concerned that we have not yet studied cohort designs. Use your knowledge of descriptive epidemiology and surveys to identify what could be done reasonably effectively with these methods, and what may require a more sophisticated approach.

Answers in Section 5.10

5.1.2 Study structure

Before looking at various aspects of the methods in detail, we will consider the overall structure of a cohort study. This will help to tie in what we have identified about the research issues and aim of the study with the research design chosen to address them. Figure 5.1.1 summarises the structure of a cohort study with a 5-year follow-up period.

5.2 Obtaining the sample

5.2.1 Introduction

We have seen that the first stage in this study design is to obtain a sample of people to study. You will recall from Chapter 4, Section 4.2.2, that a sample is taken to provide a representative group of subjects, and that this group must be large enough to allow conclusive results. We will not examine the statistical methods for determining sample size in a cohort study until Section 5.6, but will look at how the sample was chosen, and identify what population the sample was designed to represent.

Please now read the section below taken from paper A entitled 'Subject and Methods'.

Subjects and Methods

The British Regional Heart Study (BRHS) is a prospective study of cardiovascular disease comprising 7735 men aged 40–59 years selected from the age-sex registers of one group general practice in each of 24 towns in England, Wales and Scotland initially examined in 1978–80. The criteria for selecting the town, the general practice and the subjects as well as the methods of data collection, have been reported (Shaper et al, 1981). Research nurses administered a standard questionnaire that included questions on smoking habits, alcohol intake, physical activity and medical history. Height and weight were measured and body mass index (BMI) defined as height/weight^2. The classification of smoking

---

habits, alcohol intake, social class and physical activity have been reported (Shaper et al, 1988, 1991). The men were classified according to their current smoking status: never smoked, ex-cigarette smokers and current smokers at four levels (1–19, 20, 21–39 and ≥40 cigarettes/day).

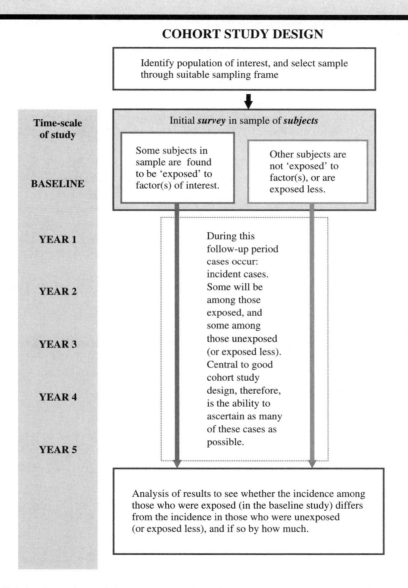

COHORT STUDY DESIGN

Figure 5.1.1 Overview of the structure of a cohort study with a 5-year follow-up period

The following excerpt from paper C provides more detail about how the towns and subjects were selected.

In brief 24 towns were primarily selected from those with populations of 50,000–100,000 (1971 census). They were chosen to represent the full range of cardiovascular mortality and water hardness, and towns in all the major standard regions were included. One general practice in each town was selected after consultation with the District Medical Officer who listed practices apparently fulfilling the required criteria. These included a patient list greater than 7500, an interested group of doctors and a social class distribution in the practice that reflected the social class distribution of the men of that town. All practices on the shortlist were visited and the most suitable group selected. If there was no up-to-date age-sex register, one was established for the practice. From each age-sex register, about 420 men aged 40–59 years were selected at random to produce five-year age groups of equal size. The list of names was reviewed by the doctors in the practice, who were asked to exclude those whom they considered could not participate because of severe mental or physical disability. Close scrutiny of the returned annotated lists reduced the exclusions to approximately 6–10 names per practice.

The remaining subjects were invited to take part in the study by a letter signed by their general practitioner. A response rate of 78 per cent was achieved, and 7735 men – approximately 320 men per town – were examined over a period of two and a half years at the rate of one town per month. The 22 per cent of non-responders comprised men who;

1. Did not reply to the invitation and one reminder, but as far as was known lived at the address supplied by the practice.

2. Were not available to attend the examination in the two-week period offered because of work commitments.

3. Refused without reason.

The sampling procedure was designed to provide a representative sample, but women were not included.

 Self-Assessment Exercise 5.2.1

1. What population was this study designed to investigate?

2. Why do you think the research team restricted their investigation to men?

3. What sampling frame was used?

4. From the information given in the two excerpts you have just read, including the reported response rate and exclusions, how representative do you think the sample was of the defined population?

Answers in Section 5.10

5.2.2   Sample size

A total of 7735 men were included in the study. This may seem like a very large number, but in fact it is not particularly large for a cohort study. We have to bear in mind that in this type of study, it is necessary to wait for cases of disease to occur in the original sample (Figure 5.1.1), and unless the sample is large, it would be necessary to wait a very long time for enough cases to occur – even with a condition as common as cancer. In the BRHS, the size of the sample would have been calculated to provide adequate numbers of cases within a reasonably manageable follow-up period (although as noted the study was designed originally to study CVD rather than cancer outcomes).

Summary: sampling

- Sampling involves obtaining the most representative group possible. The sample also needs to be of sufficient size to meet the objectives, but not too large as to be impractical, and too costly for the budget available. Sometimes a pragmatic balance between these various demands needs to be struck.

- No sampling method is perfect.

- For the BRHS, sampling through general practice had the advantage of preparing the system that was to be used for the follow-up. This will be studied in Section 5.4.

5.3   Measurement

5.3.1   Importance of good measurement

One of the other very important issues we identified in Chapter 4, Section 4.6, was the importance of good measurement, and avoiding the bias that can arise with poor questionnaire design and inconsistent administration of interviews, for example. A wide range of measurements were made in the BRHS, and considerable care was taken to avoid bias during the survey and follow-up periods.

5.3.2   Identifying and avoiding measurement error

From reading the subjects and methods section of paper A, you will have noted that a number of characteristics of interest were measured. Some data were collected by means of a nurse-administered questionnaire and some by physical examination. When designing the study, the authors would have needed to give considerable thought to ensuring that each of the different variables was measured accurately (precisely) to reduce random error and bias. This is more difficult to do than might initially appear to be the case. For example, let's consider the measurement of blood pressure, a routine measurement taken in many epidemiological studies.

5.3.3   The measurement of blood pressure

Most, if not all, of us have had our blood pressure measured, and no doubt it seems a straightforward procedure. If you break down the various components of blood pressure measurement, you can appreciate that it is actually rather complex, and subject to all kinds of error. Indeed, a lot of error does arise in blood pressure measurement in clinical as well as in research settings.

 Self-Assessment Exercise 5.3.1

1. Think about how blood pressure is measured, and make a list of the equipment used and activities that go on during this procedure.

2. Against each item in your list, write down all the sources of error that you think could arise during the process of measurement.

3. Against each source of error you have identified, suggest ways in which the error could be minimised.

Answers in Section 5.10

This exercise emphasises how complex and open to error an apparently simple measurement procedure can be. This example has identified issues that will apply to a greater or lesser extent to any type of measurement in research, or clinical practice. In general terms, these sources of measurement error, their nature, and the means of addressing them can be summarised as in Table 5.3.1.

Table 5.3.1 Types of measurement error and bias

Type of error	Nature	Comment
Observer error	Systematic differences between observers.	Systematic observer error (bias) can best be avoided by careful standardisation of techniques through training, and checking performance. For some measures (as we have seen with blood pressure), special measurement equipment may help.
	Variation within observers, e.g. from day to day, which is mainly random.	An individual observer's performance will vary from day to day. Since there is usually no consistent pattern with this type of error, it is mostly random and just adds 'noise' to the data, effectively increasing the standard error. We will return to this issue.
*Instrument error	Systematic differences between instruments.	These systematic differences may result from design factors, faults, poor maintenance, etc. If possible, these differences should be detected and removed or reduced.
	Variation in how the instrument performs from day to day. May be random.	This applies principally to reliability of equipment, since for questionnaires this variation arises from the observer (interviewer). Equipment unreliability may be random, but watch out for systematic effects developing over time (drift). Random variation will increase the standard error (as with the within- observer error), but systematic 'drift' over time will result in bias.

*The term instrument refers to the tool used to make a measurement, and can include a machine, self-administered questionnaire, interview schedule, etc.

In fact, for the BRHS, even these precautions could not overcome the problem. The research team felt that the residual *observer bias* they were able to detect was large enough to warrant 'adjustment' of all the blood pressure data before they were used in the analysis of the cohort study. We will look at what is meant by adjustment in Section 5.8.

In the physical activity and cancer study, the researchers developed an instrument to measure levels of physical activity among participants. A total physical activity score was calculated for each participant based on frequency and intensity of physical activity reported, and a physical activity index with six levels (an ordered categorical variable) was created which ranged from 'inactive' to 'vigorous exercise'. Such measurement of physical activity is open to error (including bias) in a number of ways. The researchers therefore compared the use of the index, using heart rate and 'forced expiratory volume' (a measure of lung function) measurements as a means of validation.

5.3.4 Case definition

The set of criteria used to determine what is, and what is not, a case of cancer is known as *case definition*. Identifying cases is known as *case finding*. Overall, this process is termed *case ascertainment*. Please now read the following section from paper A, entitled 'Ascertainment of cancer cases':

Ascertainment of cancer cases
Cancer cases up to December 1997 were ascertained by means of: (1) death certificates with malignant neoplasms identified as the underlying cause of the death (ICD140–209); (2) Cancer registry: subjects with cancer identified by record linkage between the BRHS cohort and the National Health Service Central Register (NHSCR); and (3) postal questionnaires to surviving members in 1992, 1996 and in 1998. In each survey the men were asked whether a doctor had ever diagnosed cancer and if so, the site and year of diagnosis. Smoking related cancers were regarded as cancers of the lip, tongue, oral cavity and larynx (ICD codes 140, 141, 143–149), oesophagus (ICD 150), pancreas (ICD157), respiratory tract (ICD 160–163), bladder (ICD 188) and kidney (ICD 189).

 Self-Assessment Exercise 5.3.2

How effective do you think case ascertainment would have been in this study? If you are unsure of the process of death certification and generation of mortality statistics, refer back to Chapter 2, Section 2.1.

Answers in Section 5.10

This exercise shows the care that needs to be taken in defining and finding cases. In working through these questions, you will have seen that for the cancer study, information was required from a number of sources: the official death registration system, the cancer registration system, and direct contact with study participants (by questionnaire).

In the next section, we will look further at the methods used in cohort studies for following up participants and finding cases, while meeting the criteria demanded by the case definition. It is fine having precise and comprehensive case definitions, but if the follow-up system can only find 50 per cent of the people who have developed the outcomes (e.g. cancer), the results may be very misleading. In other words, good case finding is as important as good case definition in minimising the possibility of bias.

Summary: measurement

- Good measurement is vital, as poor measurement can lead to bias and/or an unnecessary increase in random error.

- Measurement error can arise from a variety of sources, including the instrument (equipment, questionnaire, etc.), and the observer (the person making the measurements).

- Measurement error can be reduced in a number of ways, including:

  - observer training and calibration against standards

  - clear, unambiguous case definition

  - careful design and testing of questionnaires

  - good maintenance and regular calibration of equipment

  - special measurement equipment.

- These precautions should reduce measurement error, but will rarely remove it altogether.

5.4 Follow-up

5.4.1 Nature of the task

Think about the problem for a moment. The research team has identified and studied a group of almost 8000 men, living in 24 towns throughout the country. These men responded to an invitation to come into a survey centre in their town, and then went home and got on with their lives. Somehow or other the team had to follow up these men over the next 15–20 years, to identify those who went on to develop some form of cancer. The men were all registered with a GP at the time of the baseline survey, but of course some would move to other parts of the country and change GP, and a few would emigrate. A cohort study depends very much on the ability to carry out such a demanding logistic exercise, and this is why these studies are complex, time-consuming and expensive. The BRHS provides a good illustration of the complexities of the follow-up procedure in cohort studies, and of how these can be successfully addressed.

The aim of good *case ascertainment* is to ensure that the process of finding cases, whether deaths, illness episodes, or people with a characteristic, is as complete as possible. In a number of countries (including the UK), there are systems that make tracing deaths relatively straightforward. We will begin by looking at the follow-up of deaths (mortality), and then move on to the more difficult task of finding the non-fatal cases (morbidity).

5.4.2 Deaths (mortality)

The system used for tracing deaths among the study sample relies on the records held by the National Health Service (NHS) Central Register. Following certification, every death is notified to the NHS register, so this provides a convenient and very complete means of finding out about the deaths, and obtaining information on the cause of death. When carrying out a study it is possible to flag individuals who have been recruited to the study so that if a death occurs among one of the study participants, the research team would be notified.

5.4.3 Non-fatal cases (morbidity)

Finding the non-fatal cases is not so simple. Fortunately, in the cancer study, the researchers were able to utilise a national database of cancer morbidity, the Cancer Registry. Even so, the team also used questionnaires to contact participants and find out whether any cases had 'slipped through the net' of cancer registration.

For many diseases, there is no central register in the same way as for deaths or non-fatal cancer, so the only way to find these events is to pick them up through the general practices and hospitals concerned, and by asking the subjects themselves. For example, in the original arm of the BRHS, the researchers needed to identify all non-fatal ischaemic heart disease. In that study, co-ordinators were identified from each of the group practices with responsibility for mailing and updating morbidity reports, notifying the study centre of all deaths and address changes, and reviewing the medical records at set intervals to ensure that no cases had been missed. Even a common occurrence such as change of address requires a well-organised system to prevent study subjects from being lost to follow-up. The method used by the BRHS team relied on the systems used for administration of general practice, and the transfer of records when a person leaves one practice and later registers at another one. This system is described in paper C, and is worth reviewing as it clearly demonstrates the attention to detail required to achieve effective follow-up in cohort studies.

5.4.4 Assessment of changes during follow-up period

We saw that the cohort study began by selecting a sample, and then carrying out a survey to measure all of the social, lifestyle, health and other baseline characteristics of interest. This survey provides information on levels of *exposure* to risk and possible protective factors that will be used in the analysis, such as whether a person exercises and how much. A man reporting that he exercises moderately at the time of the baseline survey, however, may not continue to exercise at the same rate during the follow-up period. Indeed, he might give up the day after the survey, or, conversely, he may exercise more over the ensuing years. If the research team has no further contact with the study subjects after the initial survey, or there are no records providing valid and representative information on subsequent changes in risk factors, then it has to be assumed that the information obtained at baseline applies for the entire period of follow-up.

Random changes in risk factors over the follow-up period would simply increase random (misclassification) error in the analysis, resulting in less *precision* but not necessarily *bias*. However, bias will arise if a defined group in the sample, such as men in higher socio-economic groups, are more likely to increase the amount that they exercise during the follow-up period than other men. If the research team does not know this, it will lead to bias in the results, especially with respect to any analysis involving socio-economic factors. This is because the apparent benefits in this group will be artificially increased. This is illustrated in the example in Figure 5.4.1.

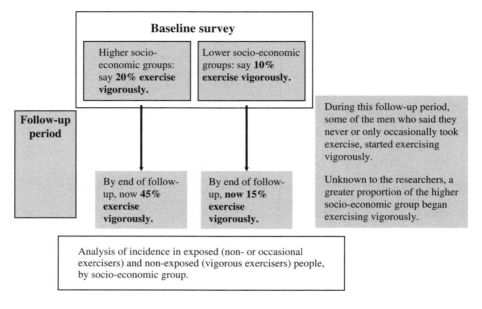

Figure 5.4.1 Hypothetical scenario in cohort study with socio-economically related changes in exercise behaviour

In this scenario (Figure 5.4.1), the association between exercise and cancer is being studied. Exercise level and frequency are measured at the baseline survey, and a lower prevalence of vigorous exercise is found among subjects in lower socio-economic groups. However, during the follow-up, a greater proportion of 'none or occasional exercisers' in the higher socio-economic group begin to exercise vigorously. Whereas, at baseline, lower socio-economic groups were half as likely to exercise vigorously (20 per cent versus 10 per cent), by the end of the study they were three times less likely to be vigorous exercisers (45 per cent versus 15 per cent). If the researchers do not know about this, bias will occur in analysis of socio-economic group and the impact of exercise on cancer. In this example, the benefit will be overestimated in the higher socio-economic group, as the observed reduction in cancer risk will be associated with a lower prevalence of vigorous exercise than is actually the case.

 Self-Assessment Exercise 5.4.1

1. What further exposure information was collected during the follow-up period of the physical activity and risk of cancer study (paper A)?

2. What might be the impact on the results if during the follow-up period, those who exercised more vigorously had been more likely to give up smoking?

Answers in Section 5.10

Summary: follow-up

- The follow-up (including case ascertainment) is the most critical and demanding part of a cohort study.

- Generally, follow-up for mortality is more straightforward than for morbidity, especially where there are systems available such as the flagging of records at the NHS Central Register.

- The percentage of the sample lost to follow-up should be kept to an absolute minimum.

- Changes in the level of exposure to key risk factors, after the initial survey and during the follow-up period, are a potentially important source of random error and/or bias. One or more interim assessments, such as the 5-year questionnaire in the BRHS, are time-consuming but may be of considerable value.

5.5 Basic presentation and analysis of results

5.5.1 Initial presentation of findings

We have completed the follow-up component of the study, and can now look at the findings of the baseline survey to see how these are related to subsequent deaths and non-fatal cases that occurred. Referring back to Figure 5.1.1, which summarises the cohort study design, we see that analysis involves calculating how the *incidence* varies by level of *exposure* to a *risk factor*. This exposure level will be expressed in different ways, according to the type of data:

- As the presence or absence of the risk factor (e.g. whether or not there is a family history of a specific cancer), which are dichotomous categorical variables.

- As categories (which may be ordered), such as never, ex-, or current smoker.

- As an actual numerical value, such as body mass index and age, which are continous variables.

Incidence of study outcome (cancer)

Table 5.5.1, reproduced (Table 2 from paper A) below, shows, in column 4, the incidence rates of cancer for each of the different categories of physical activity. You will recall that in order to calculate the incidence, we need a *numerator* (number of cases), a *denominator* (number of people at risk), and a *time period*. In this study, the authors have calculated *incidence density*, expressed as a rate per 1000 person years (p-y).

The final columns show adjusted relative risks (and 95 per cent CIs). We will look at relative risk in Section 5.5.2, and consider confounding and the methods used for adjustment in Sections 5.7–5.9.

Table 5.5.1 Physical activity and age-adjusted cancer rates/1000 person-years and adjusted relative risks for all cancers (excluding skin cancer) in 7,588 middle-aged British men

Physical activity	No.	Cases	Rates /1000 p-y	Relative risks (95% CI)	
				A	B
None/Occ	3017	424	8.4	1.00	1.00
Light	1749	234	7.8	0.93 (0.79, 1.09)	0.95 (0.80, 1.11)
Moderate	1196	163	8.1	0.95 (0.80, 1.14)	1.04 (0.86, 1.24)
Moderate-vigorous	1113	101	5.8	0.68 (0.54, 0.84)	0.78 (0.62, 0.97)
Vigorous	513	47	5.7	0.65 (0.44, 0.88)	0.76 (0.56, 1.04)
Test for linear trend				P < 0.0001	P = 0.02

A = age-adjusted
B = adjusted for age, cigarette smoking, BMI, alcohol intake and social class
Source: Reproduced with permission from Wannamethee *et al., 2001.*

  Self-Assessment Exercise 5.5.1

Use the incidence density rates from Table 5.5.1 (Table 2 from paper A) (column 4) to answer the following questions:

1. What is the incidence in the 'none/occasional' group?

2. What is the incidence in the 'vigorous' group?

3. How much lower is the incidence in the 'vigorous' group than in the 'none/occasional' group? What does this tell you?

Answers in Section 5.10

5.5.2 Relative risk

The concept of relative risk

We will now look at how we define, and calculate, the risk of disease associated with a given factor such as smoking, cholesterol, or physical activity. First, here are some everyday examples of risk:

> 'I have smoked 20 cigarettes a day for the last 20 years. What are the chances of my getting lung cancer compared to my friend who never smoked?'
>
> 'If I wear a helmet when I go cycling, how much does this reduce my chance of a serious head injury if I am knocked off my bike in traffic?'

Relative risk describes how the risk of a disease varies according to the level of exposure to a risk factor, such as smoking relative to not smoking, or wearing a cycle helmet relative to not wearing one at the time of an accident.

This idea is the same as that introduced in Exercise 5.5.1 when we looked at the way in which the incidence of cancer varied among those who took no exercise or only occasional exercise compared to those who exercised vigorously. Indeed, it is the comparison of *incidence rates*, which provides us with the measure known as *relative risk (RR)*:

$$\text{Relative risk} = \frac{\text{Incidence of disease in } \textbf{\textit{exposed}} \text{ group}}{\text{Incidence of disease in } \textbf{\textit{unexposed}} \text{ group}}$$

Often, relative risk is calculated as a comparison of rates in more exposed and less exposed, rather than the absolutes of exposed and unexposed. Returning to our data in Exercise 5.5.1, the relative risk for those who exercised vigorously compared with those who took no or only occasional exercise was the ratio of the two incidence rates, which we calculate as $5.7 \div 8.4 = 0.68$, or 68 per cent. A relative risk of 1 would mean that the risk of cancer among the two groups was the same. A relative risk of less than 1 implies the exposure has a protective effect in relation to the outcome. In other words, the relative risk of cancer among vigorous exercisers is 32 per cent less or 0.68 times the risk of those who take no or only occasional exercise.

You will see that the relative risks quoted in Table 5.5.1 (Table 2 reproduced from paper A) are slightly different from what you calculated in Exercise 5.5.1. This is because these have been adjusted for the confounding factors listed at the bottom of the table, using regression methods. These methods will be introduced in Sections 5.8 and 5.9 of this chapter.

In another arm of the BRHS, researchers were interested in the relative risk of heart disease among smokers compared to non-smokers, data for which are shown in Table 5.5.2.

Table 5.5.2 Incidence of ischaemic heart disease (IHD) among non-smokers, ex-smokers and current smokers, after an average of 4.2 years of follow-up

Cigarette smoking	Cases	Total men	Per cent	Rate/1000/year
Never	18	1819	0.99	2.36
Ex-smoker	76	2715	2.80	6.66
Current	108	3185	3.39	8.07

Source: Reproduced with permission from Shaper *et al.*, 1985 (paper B).

 Self-Assessment Exercise 5.5.2

1. Calculate the relative risks of ischaemic heart disease (IHD) for (a) smokers and (b) ex-smokers compared to never smokers.

2. Given that we have taken the never smokers as the ***reference group***, have a go at interpreting the values of relative risk you have just calculated for the ex-smokers, and the value for the current smokers.

3. One explanation for smokers having a higher incidence of IHD than never smokers is that smoking causes IHD. Can you think of any other explanations for this finding?

Answers in Section 5.10

> ### Summary: relative risk
>
> - With relative risk, we can express the risk of an outcome (e.g. IHD) for men with a level of a risk factor (e.g. current smoker), relative to men with another level (e.g. never smoked).
>
> - We can place a value on this risk; that is, we can quantify the risk.
>
> - If an exposure category has a relative risk greater than 1, it means that the people in that category have a higher risk of the outcome than the people in the reference category.
>
> - If the relative risk is less than 1, the people in that exposure category have a lower risk of the outcome than the reference category.
>
> - If the relative risk is 1, the people in that exposure category have the same risk as the people in the reference category.

 Self-Assessment Exercise 5.5.3

Look again at Table 5.5.1 (Table 2 reproduced from paper A) (Section 5.1.1).

1. What group was taken as the ***reference group*** for calculating relative risk?

2. Why was this an appropriate reference group?

Answers in Section 5.10

5.5.3 Hypothesis test for categorical data: the chi-squared test

Real association or a chance finding?

It appears from the cancer study that exercise is associated with a decreased risk of cancer. From exercise 5.5.2, we found that the relative risk for 'none or occasional exercisers' compared with those who exercise vigorously was found to be 0.68 (without adjustment for confounding factors). This is lower than 1.00, the relative risk if the risk of cancer is the same for both groups. In fact, the risk of cancer among vigorous exercisers is 32 per cent less than the risk of cancer among people who take no or only occasional exercise.

But does the observed association in this sample of men mean that cancer and exercise are associated in the population of all middle-aged British men? If we studied another sample from the population, we would probably obtain a different value for the relative risk. Any possible sample will provide an estimate of the relative risk in the population, and the estimate will vary from sample to sample: this is the **sampling distribution** we introduced in Chapter 4, but now applied to sample estimates of relative risk.

We need an objective way of deciding whether the association between cancer and exercise that we have observed in this particular sample is evidence of a real association in the population of middle-aged British men. This is the process of **inference** that was referred to in Chapter 1. This objective assessment of the evidence provided by the sample is called an **hypothesis test**. We shall now develop the idea of **hypothesis testing** and carry out a test to investigate whether cancer incidence and level of physical activity are statistically 'significantly' associated – that is, the association we observe in this study sample is very unlikely to be the result of chance arising from sampling error.

Contingency tables

We shall consider the risk of cancer for those who never or occasionally exercise and those who exercise vigorously, as you have already done in previous exercises. The relevant data from Table 5.5.1 (Table 2 from paper A) are given in Table 5.5.3.

Table 5.5.3   Exercise and cancer

Exercise category	Cancer				Total
	Cases		**Other men**		
	No.	%	**No.**	%	
None/occasional	424		2593		3017
Vigorous	47		466		513
Total					

 Self-Assessment Exercise 5.5.4

1. Table 5.5.3 is defined by the two variables, *cancer* and *exercise*. What values can each of these two variables take? Are they categorical, ordered categorical, discrete or continuous variables?

2. Insert the percentage of 'none/occasional' exercisers who became cases and the percentage who did not become cases in Table 5.5.3.

3. Do the same for vigorous exercisers and for everyone in the sample (the *Total* row).

4. Interpret the findings.

Answers in Section 5.10

Table 5.5.3 is defined by two categorical variables, also called **factors**, and each of the four possible combinations of the variables is called a **cell**. The figure in each cell is a frequency, or count. A cross-tabulation of frequencies such as this is called a **contingency table**.

Hypothesising about the population

We want to use these data to answer the question, 'Is there an association between exercise and cancer in middle-aged British men?' It is more complex to measure how strongly associated these two factors are, but what we can do is analyse the sample data to see whether an assumption of no association between exercise and cancer is reasonable. If this assumption turns out to be unreasonable on the basis of the information we have from the sample, we will conclude that there is evidence of an (inverse) association between exercise and cancer for middle-aged British men. Assumptions about populations are called *hypotheses*, and so this analysis is an *hypothesis test*.

The assumption of no association is called the ***null hypothesis***, abbreviated to H_0, and the alternative, that there is an association, is called the ***alternative hypothesis***, H_1. These must be stated precisely, so that we know exactly what we can conclude after we have tested the null hypothesis. The hypotheses we are interested in may be written:

> H_0: There is no association between exercise and cancer for middle-aged British men, and any observed association has arisen by chance (RR $= 1$).
>
> H_1: There is an association between exercise and cancer for middle-aged British men (RR $\neq 1$).

The symbol $\neq$ means 'not equal to'. The hypotheses must clearly state (i) the variables between which there may be an association, and (ii) the population about which we are hypothesising.

 ### Self-Assessment Exercise 5.5.5

For H_0 and H_1 as given above,

1. State the (outcome and exposure) variables we are investigating,

2. State the population about which we are hypothesising.

Answers in Section 5.10

If the null hypothesis is unreasonable – that is, the data are not in agreement with such an assumption – we reject the null hypothesis in favour of the alternative hypothesis. We then say there is evidence that exercise and cancer are associated for middle-aged British men.

We can assess the strength of evidence against the H_0 provided by the data because we can work out how likely the observed frequencies are to have arisen if there is no association. The measurement of 'how likely' is known as probability. The usual convention is that if the probability of the observed frequencies arising, assuming no association, is less than 0.05 (5 per cent, or 1 in 20), then it is sufficiently unlikely that H_0 is true. Therefore, there is an association.

Testing the null hypothesis

We shall now work through the hypothesis test using the data in Table 5.5.3, and then summarise the procedure. In most circumstances, hypothesis tests are done with a computer, but it will aid understanding of the purpose and process of hypothesis testing to see how the most commonly used tests are calculated.

The first step is to find the frequencies we would expect if the null hypothesis (no association) were true. These are calculated for each of the four cells by multiplying together the totals of the row and column the cell is in and dividing by the total number in the sample.

$$\text{expected frequency} = \frac{\text{row total} \times \text{column total}}{\text{total sample size}}$$

For example, taking the top, left-hand cell (cases who take non/occasional exercise), if there really is no association between exercise and cancer, then of the sample of 3530 men we would expect 402.55 men to be cases of cancer in that cell. The calculation of this expected number is shown below:

$$\text{expected frequency} = \frac{\text{row total} \times \text{column total}}{\text{total sample size}} = \frac{3017 \times 471}{3530} = 402.55$$

Of course, it is not possible to have 402.55 cases. By the 'expected' frequency, we mean that, if we were to observe lots of different samples of 3530 men, then the average number of men in each sample who took none/occasional exercise and were cases would be 402.55 if there is no association between exercise and cancer. This calculation of expected frequency is based on the fact that if there is no association between exercise and cancer, we would expect the same proportions of none/occasional exercisers and vigorous exercisers to develop cancer.

 Self-Assessment Exercise 5.5.6

Calculate the expected frequency for each of the four cells of Table 5.5.3 and complete the following table:

Table 5.5.4   Exercise and cancer: expected frequencies

	Cancer		
Exercise category	Cases	Other men	Total
None/occasional	402.55		
Vigorous			
Total			

Answers in Section 5.10

Note that the expected frequencies add up to the same totals as the observed frequencies. This is always true (apart from small rounding errors), so this can be used to check whether the expected frequencies are correct. We now need to calculate the differences between the observed and expected frequencies in each cell. These are called the **residuals**. For cases of cancer who took none/occasional exercise (top left cell), the residual is

$$424 - 402.55 = 21.45$$

The residual is always calculated this way round; that is, the observed frequency minus the expected frequency.

 Self-Assessment Exercise 5.5.7

Complete the table of residuals, below:

Table 5.5.5 Exercise and cancer: residuals

Exercise category	Cancer		Total
	Cases	Other men	
None/occasional	21.45		
Vigorous			
Total			

Answers in Section 5.10

The row and column totals of the residuals should always be zero – apart from small rounding errors. The sign $(+/-)$ of a residual shows whether the observed frequency is larger or smaller than expected, and the size of the residual shows how large the difference is. We now combine these residuals to obtain an overall measure of the difference between what we have observed and what we expect under the null hypothesis of no association. The measure we use is the sum of the squared residuals each divided by the corresponding expected frequency:

$$\sum \frac{(\text{observed frequency} - \text{expected frequency})^2}{\text{expected frequency}} = \sum \frac{\text{residual}^2}{\text{expected frequency}}$$

This expression is generally written as:

$$\sum \frac{(O - E)^2}{E}$$

and is called the ***chi-squared statistic*** (*chi* is pronounced 'ky'). Thus, in our example, for cases of cancer who took none/occasional exercise, the first value contributing to the chi-squared statistic is:

$$\frac{(21.45)^2}{402.55} = 1.14$$

It is convenient to put these values in another table, called the chi-squared table, which is illustrated after the following brief reference section on the chi-squared statistic.

RS - Reference section on statistical methods

This statistic is called the chi-squared statistic because it can be proved that all the possible values it can have form a distribution with a particular shape, called the chi-squared distribution. This is often abbreviated to the χ^2 distribution, using the Greek letter *chi*. This is a theoretical distribution, like the normal distribution, and the shape of the distribution can be described by a known formula.

RS - ends

In this final exercise on the chi-squared hypothesis test, we will calculate the statistic, and then interpret the result.

Self-Assessment Exercise 5.5.8

Complete the chi-squared table (Table 5.6) and calculate the value of the chi-squared statistic.

Table 5.5.6 Cancer and exercise: chi-squared table

	Cancer		
Exercise category	**Cases**	**Other men**	**Total**
None/occasional	1.14		
Vigorous			
Total			

Answers in Section 5.10

The value of the chi-squared statistic for these data is thus 9.08. This is a measure of how the observed frequencies differ from the frequencies we would expect to occur if the null hypothesis, that there is no association between cancer and exercise, were true.

If the observed and expected frequencies are similar (that is, the data are consistent with the null hypothesis), then the differences 'observed frequency–expected frequency' will be small, and the value of the chi-squared statistic will be small. Conversely, if the observed frequencies are very different from the expected frequencies, either smaller or larger (that is, the data are not consistent with the null hypothesis), then the value of the chi-squared statistic will be large. So a large value is evidence against the null hypothesis.

If the value is large enough, it is *very unlikely* that we could have obtained the observed frequencies if H_0 is true, and we reject H_0 and conclude that cancer and exercise are associated. We will now look at how we decide whether the chi-squared statistic is 'large enough' to reject the null hypothesis.

p-values, degrees of freedom and the test result

To decide whether the chi-squared value is 'large enough' and the observed frequencies 'unlikely' to be consistent with H_0, we use computer software or printed tables to find the probability of obtaining such a value, or a larger one, when H_0 is true. This probability is called the ***p-value***. As already noted, we generally consider a probability of less than 0.05 to be small enough for the observed data to be so unlikely that H_0 must be untrue.

If we are looking our p-value up on a chi-square table, we first need to calculate ***degrees of freedom***. The chi-squared distribution can have different shapes, depending on the size (how many rows and columns) of the contingency table. The quantity which defines the size of a contingency table is called the degrees of freedom (df), and each value of degrees of freedom defines a different chi-squared distribution. The degrees of freedom are calculated by multiplying together the number of rows minus one and the number of columns minus one:

'Degrees of freedom' of a contingency table

If a contingency table has r rows and c columns, the degrees of freedom are

$$df = (r-1)(c-1)$$

Such a table is called an $r \times c$ contingency table.

In our case, we have only two rows ('None/occasional' and 'Vigorous' exercise) and two columns ('Cancer case' and 'Other'), so the degrees of freedom are $(2-1)(2-1) = 1$. We then look up our p-value on a table of critical values of the chi-squared statistic under one degree of freedom.

The level of probability below which we consider the sample provides evidence to reject the null hypothesis is called the ***significance level*** of the test. It is usually written as a percentage. So if we choose a probability of 0.05, we say the hypothesis test is carried out at the 5 per cent significance level. If the null hypothesis is rejected, we may say that H_0 is rejected at the 5 per cent significance level, or that the value of the chi-squared statistic obtained is significant at the 5 per cent level. An alternative name for a hypothesis test is a ***test of significance***. By 'significant', we mean a difference that cannot reasonably be explained by chance alone.

The required significance level should always be decided before carrying out an hypothesis test. The value of 5 per cent is very commonly used, but is arbitrary. In different situations, we may require either more evidence (a lower significance level, e.g. 1 per cent) or less evidence (a higher significance level, e.g. 10 per cent, although this is uncommon) in order to reject the null hypothesis.

The critical value of the chi-squared statistic associated with a 0.05 probability with one degree of freedom (df = 1) is 3.84. Our chi-squared statistic was 9.08, and there is a probability of only 0.003 (three in a thousand) of obtaining a chi-square value as large as this on one degree of freedom, or a larger value, if H_0 is true. This is a probability much smaller than 0.05. If the null hypothesis of no association between exercise and cancer were true, it is very, very unlikely that we would observe the frequencies in Table 5.5.3 (but it is not quite impossible – the p-value is greater than 0!). The null hypothesis is therefore unreasonable, and we reject it. We conclude that there is evidence to suggest that exercise and cancer are associated in middle-aged British men.

If we had calculated a chi-squared statistic which was smaller than 3.84, then we would not reject the null hypothesis at the 5 per cent significance level. However, we would not accept the null hypothesis either, and conclude that there is no association between exercise and cancer. This is because we can never know whether the null hypothesis is true unless we observe everyone in the population. On the basis of the information we have from the sample, we do not have enough evidence to reject H_0, but we cannot say it is true. We therefore say that we do not reject H_0 at the 5 per cent significance level and conclude that there is insufficient evidence of an association, or that it is possible that there is no association (possible but not certain).

We have talked in terms of the sample providing 'evidence' against the null hypothesis, and hypothesis testing is often explained by analogy with a criminal trial. The accused is found guilty only if there is sufficient evidence of guilt ('beyond reasonable doubt'). In the case of failing to reject the null hypothesis, we can think of a person being found 'not guilty' through lack of evidence. The person may in fact be guilty – being found 'not guilty' does not mean they are innocent!

Test assumptions and summary

The chi-squared test is used to determine whether or not, on the basis of information in a random sample, there is evidence of an association between two categorical variables in the population from which the sample is drawn. Use of the test is subject to a set of assumptions, which are summarised below.

Summary: the chi-squared test

1. The chi-squared test is based on statistical theory which requires certain assumptions to be fulfilled for the test to be valid. These assumptions are:

   (a) The two variables must be categorical.

   (b) The groups defined by the variables must be independent. This means a person can be in only one group – for example, a person takes 'none/occasional exercise' or takes 'vigorous exercise' – but cannot be in both categories.

   (c) The sample must be large. The usual rule for determining whether the sample is large enough is that 80 per cent of the expected frequencies must be greater than 5 and all the expected frequencies must be greater than 1.

2. It does not matter which variable defines the rows of the contingency table, and which defines the columns.

(Continued)

3. The hypotheses and conclusions are about the population from which the sample is taken.

4. The null hypothesis may be stated in several different forms. The following are equivalent:

   • There is no association between exercise and cancer.

   • Exercise and cancer are independent.

   • The probability of a person who takes vigorous exercise becoming a cancer case is the same as the probability of someone who never exercises becoming a cancer case.

   • The relative risk of cancer for people who exercise vigorously compared with those who never exercise is 1.

5. The chi-squared test can be applied to any size of contingency table. The calculation is exactly the same, just more time-consuming. With larger tables, it is more likely that the conditions for a large sample are not fulfilled (1 (c) above). If there are too many small expected frequencies, variable categories (that is, rows and/or columns) can be combined to ensure the conditions are satisfied.

6. It is usually sufficient to calculate expected frequencies and chi-squared values to two decimal places.

Interpreting the chi-squared test

The chi-squared test uses sample information to determine whether or not there is evidence of an association between two categorical variables in the population. However, we cannot conclude from the test the direction of any association: the test result (Section 5.5.3) does not tell us whether men who exercise are more or less likely to develop cancer than those who never or only occasionally exercise, but only that there is evidence of an association. Nor does the chi-squared test tell us how strongly the variables are related: the chi-squared statistic is not a measure of the strength of an association.

If we conclude from the test that there is evidence of an association between the variables, then we need to return to the observed frequencies and percentages to describe how they are related. In Exercise 5.5.4 we found that the percentage of none/occasional exercisers who developed cancer was larger than the percentage of vigorous exercisers who became cases. Now with the result of the chi-squared test, we can say that this is evidence of a higher risk of cancer for none/occasional exercisers in the population of middle-aged British men compared to men who regularly exercise vigorously.

We could quantify the difference in risk by the difference between these percentages, and give a range of likely values of this difference in the population by calculating a CI for the difference. This is how the results of an analysis of a 2×2 contingency table are usually summarised. However, in the particular case of a cohort study, the primary aim is usually to estimate the relative risk, and it is appropriate to summarise the results in terms of relative risk rather than percentages. The relative risk is a measure of the strength of association.

Summary: categorical data and hypothesis testing

- A contingency table is a table of frequencies, defined by two categorical variables.

- An hypothesis is a statement about the population of interest.

- We use an hypothesis test to decide whether the information we have from a sample is in agreement with an hypothesis about the population.

- A chi-squared test is used to test the null hypothesis of no association between two factors of interest defining a contingency table.

- The probability of obtaining the observed test result (or a more extreme one) is the p-value of the test.

- If the p-value is small (e.g. less than 0.05), we reject the null hypothesis.

- The value below which the p-value must be in order to reject H_0 is the significance level of the test.

- A chi-squared test does not tell us the strength or direction of any association between factors.

We will now look at hypothesis testing for continuous data. It will be reassuring to know that the underlying principles are essentially the same as those we have introduced for categorical data – although we have to use a different type of test. This test, which you will probably have come across in its most familiar form, the *t-test*, is based on the ideas we covered in Chapter 4, Section 4.4, on the standard error of sample means.

5.5.4 Hypothesis tests for continuous data: the *z*-test and the *t*-test

We have seen that we can use the chi-squared test to investigate relationships between categorical variables such as exercise (none or occasional, light, moderate, etc.) and cancer (case, non-case). However, if we wish to investigate whether continuous variables are associated with cancer we need to employ a different method. Continuous variables were investigated in the physical activity and cancer study, such as age and body mass, but the values of these variables were not reported in this paper. We will therefore refer to the original BRHS report on heart disease to provide an example of carrying out an hypothesis test on continuous data (paper B).

During the study a number of potential risk factors for ischaemic heart disease (IHD) were investigated, including cholesterol levels, blood pressure, smoking and body mass index. As reported in paper B, after a mean follow-up of 4.2 years, 202 cases of IHD had been identified. In this section we shall examine whether there was a statistically significant difference in systolic blood pressure among men who experienced IHD and men who did not.

Table 5.5.7 is reproduced from Table 3 of paper B and shows the mean SBP for cases (of IHD) to be 155.4 mmHg and for non-cases to be 144.9 mmHg. The table also gives a '*t*-value' – this is the result of the hypothesis test, a *t*-test. There is a substantial difference between the two means – in this group of men, systolic blood pressure was, on average, 10.5 mmHg higher among men who suffered from IHD. Can we infer that this is evidence of an association between high systolic blood pressure and IHD in all middle-aged British men?

Table 5.5.7   Means of risk factors in cases and other men (continuous variables) (paper B)

	Cases ($n = 202$)	Other men ($n = 7533$)	t-value
Age (years)	52.8	50.2	7.1
Systolic blood pressure (mmHg)	155.4	144.9	6.1
Diastolic blood pressure (mmHg)	87.9	82.1	5.1
Body mass index (kg/m^2)	26.44	25.46	4.1
Total cholesterol (mmol/l)	6.78	6.29	6.0
Triglyceride* (mmol/l)	2.10	1.73	4.1
HDL-C (mmol/l)	1.08	1.15	−3.5

* Geometric mean used (the geometric mean will be explained in more detail later in the book).
Source: Reproduced with permission from Shaper *et al.*, 1985.

Comparing the means of large samples: the two-sample *z*-test

We will see shortly that the *t*-test is used for both large and small samples, and when a hypothesis test for comparing means is carried out using computer software the *t*-test is most commonly calculated. For large samples such as the BRHS, however, we can use the two-sample *z-test*, although (as we will demonstrate) the conclusion is almost identical to that produced by the *t*-test. Again, to aid understanding of the process and (as shown below) to link this to our discussion of sampling distributions and the standard error in Chapter 4, we will first calculate the *z*-test.

The basic principle of hypothesis tests for continuous data is the same as for the chi-squared test. We formulate hypotheses and calculate a test statistic. We use this to determine the likelihood of observing these sample means if the null hypothesis were true. If it is very unlikely, we reject the null hypothesis.

Stating the hypotheses

The question of interest is, 'In middle-aged British men, does average systolic blood pressure differ significantly between those who become IHD cases and those who do not?' The null hypothesis may be stated as follows:

H_0: there is no difference, on average, between the systolic blood pressure of middle-aged British men who become IHD cases and the systolic blood pressure of middle-aged British men who do not become IHD cases.

This can be written more concisely by symbols. We use μ_1 to denote the mean systolic blood pressure in the population of middle-aged British men suffering IHD, and μ_2 to denote the mean systolic blood pressure in the population of middle-aged British men who do not suffer IHD. The hypotheses are then

$$H_0 : \mu_1 = \mu_2$$
$$H_1 : \mu_1 \neq \mu_2$$

Testing the null hypothesis

We have evidence of a real difference (that is, the null hypothesis is unlikely to be true) if the difference between the sample means is 'large enough'. Labelling the sample means $\bar{x}_1 = 155.4$ and $\bar{x}_2 = 144.9$ the observed difference is $\bar{x}_1 - \bar{x}_2 = 10.5$ mmHg. Whether this is 'large' depends on how much this difference can vary from sample to sample; that is, the **precision** of this estimate of the difference between means. This precision is measured by the *standard error of the difference between means*, described below.

The standard error (SE) of the difference between means

The estimated standard error of $(\bar{x}_1 - \bar{x}_2)$ for use with the z-test is

$$\text{SE} = \sqrt{\frac{s_1^2}{n_1} + \frac{s_2^2}{n_2}}$$

where s_1 and s_2 are the standard deviations of the sample of systolic blood pressures of cases and the sample of systolic blood pressures of non-cases respectively.

Moving now to the hypothesis test, the test statistic is called z. It is the difference between the sample means relative to the standard error of the difference between the means:

$$z = \frac{\bar{x}_1 - \bar{x}_2}{SE}$$

In order to calculate the standard error of the difference between means, we require an estimate of the standard deviations, which we obtain from the sample. Paper B does not report the sample standard deviations of systolic blood pressure, so in order to illustrate the z-test we shall use some plausible values. Suppose that the standard deviation of the sample of men with IHD is $s_1 = 26.1\,\text{mmHg}$, and of the sample of men without IHD is $s_2 = 24.1\,\text{mmHg}$. We have:

	Cases	Non-cases
$\bar{x}$	155.4	144.9
s	26.1	24.1
n	202	7533

The estimated standard error of the difference in means is:

$$\sqrt{\frac{26.1^2}{202} + \frac{24.1^2}{7533}} = 1.8573$$

and the value of the z-statistic is

$$\frac{155.4 - 144.9}{1.8573} = 5.653$$

Obtaining the p-value for the test

You will normally carry out hypothesis testing on a computer which will produce the relevant p-value. In order to find the p-value associated with the value of z that we have calculated, we have to look up the critical value of z in a table of the normal distribution. It is useful for you to know that these tables exist (as they also do for the chi-squared distribution), and examples are illustrated in Chapter 11. The critical value for the z-statistic at the 0.05 probability level is 1.96. For our z-statistic of 5.653, the relevant p-value from the table is $p < 0.001$. This is the probability that this value of the z-statistic could have arisen by chance.

Interpreting the result of the test

This p-value is small, very small in fact, as it indicates a probability of less than 1 in 1000. If we adopt the convention of rejecting the null hypothesis if the p-value is less than 0.05 (1 in 20), then we reject H_0 and conclude that there is a significant difference between the mean systolic blood pressure of men who suffer IHD and those who do not suffer IHD. We have then rejected the null hypothesis at the 5 per cent significance level.

Summary: the two-sample z-test

This is used to test the null hypothesis that the means of two populations are equal. To use the z-test:

- The data must be continuous.

- The samples must be random.

- The samples must be independent (i.e., a person cannot be in both samples).

- The samples must be large (each exceed about 30 in number).

1. State the hypotheses

$$H_0 : \ \mu_1 = \mu_2, \quad H_1 : \ \mu_1 \neq \mu_2$$

   defining μ_1 and μ_2, the population means.

2. Decide on the significance level. Call this α. (Typically $\alpha = 0.05$).

3. If calculating the z-statistic, use the formula:

$$z = \frac{\bar{x}_1 - \bar{x}_2}{SE}$$

   where $SE = \sqrt{\dfrac{s_1^2}{n_1} + \dfrac{s_2^2}{n_2}}$,

   $\bar{x}_1$ and $\bar{x}_2$ are the sample means, and s_1 and s_2 are the sample standard deviations.

4. If calculated, compare the value of z with the normal distribution and determine the p-value.

5. If $p < \alpha$, reject the null hypothesis. Otherwise do not reject H_0.

(If $z < -1.96$ or $z > +1.96$, H_0 is rejected at the 5 per cent significance level).
   State the conclusion and interpret the result.

Comparing the means of smaller samples: the two-sample t-test

So far, in the z-test, we have assumed that the samples from which we wish to make inferences about the population are large. Smaller samples (by which we mean less than 30 values) still give us information about the population, but we need different techniques to make these inferences. If we want to use small samples to investigate whether population means differ, we should use a *two-sample t-test*, provided we can reasonably assume that (i) the two samples are from populations with (roughly) normal distributions, and (ii) the two populations have the same (or at least similar) standard deviations. If these assumptions are not reasonable, we can use a 'non-parametric' test: these tests are covered in Chapter 11.

Calculating the *t*-test

We calculate a test statistic, called *t*, in very much the same way as we did in the *z*-test,

$$t = \frac{\bar{x}_1 - \bar{x}_2}{SE}$$

However, the standard error of the difference between means (SE in formula) differs from that used for the *z*-test, as explained in the reference section below.

 RS - Reference section on statistical methods

The standard error for difference between means (*t-test*)

Since for the *t*-test we are assuming that the populations have the same (or at least similar) standard deviations, we use information from both samples to estimate this common standard deviation. The estimate is called the ***pooled standard deviation***, s_p, and its square, the estimated variance, is

$$s_p^2 = \frac{(n_1 - 1)s_1^2 + (n_2 - 1)s_2^2}{n_1 + n_2 - 2}$$

The estimated standard error of the difference between means is

$$SE = \sqrt{\frac{s_p^2}{n_1} + \frac{s_p^2}{n_2}}.$$

 RS - ends

To calculate the *t*-test result for our example, we can start with the difference between the means – which is the same as for the *z*-test (10.5 mmHg). The standard error, using the formula stated above, is 1.722, and the *t*-statistic is 6.097. We are now ready to determine the p-value, but, to do so, we have to know the degrees of freedom. As with the chi-squared distribution, there are different *t* distributions, each defined by a number of degrees of freedom. For the *t*-statistic, the degrees of freedom are the total number in both samples minus 2:

$$\text{df (degrees of freedom)} = n_1 + n_2 - 2 = 7733$$

The probability of obtaining a value of the *t*-statistic of 6.1 on 7733 degrees of freedom (or a value more extreme) is <0.001, the same result that we obtained using the *z*-test.

Use of the *t*-test or *z*-test?

We saw that the results of using *t*-test and *z*-test were in effect identical with the large sample in the BRHS, so how should these two tests be used? A *t*-test applies whenever the populations can be considered to have normal distributions, whatever the sample size. So it is never wrong to use the t-test in this situation. However, it would be wrong to use the z-test for small samples, that is, smaller than the (arbitrary) cut-off of 30 suggested as a guide in most situations. As noted, computer software generally calculates only a t-statistic, so this is most commonly quoted in journals. The z-statistic is easier to calculate without a computer. The t-test, like the chi-squared test, is subject to a number of assumptions, which are listed below as part of a summary of the procedure.

Summary: the two-sample t-test

This is used to test the null hypothesis that the means of two populations are equal, when the samples are small. To use the t-test:

- The data must be continuous.

- The samples must be random.

- The samples must be independent (i.e. a person cannot be in both samples).

- The samples must be from populations with normal distributions.

- The populations must have the same (or similar) standard deviations. A rule of thumb is that if the larger of the sample standard deviations divided by the smaller of the sample standard deviations is < 2, then we can assume sufficiently similar population standard deviations.

1. State the hypotheses
$$H_0 : \ \mu_1 = \mu_2 \ H_1 : \ \mu_1 \neq \mu_2$$
   defining μ_1 and μ_2, the population means.

2. Decide on the significance level. Call this α (typically $\alpha = 0.05$).

3. Calculate the square of the pooled standard deviation
$$s_p^2 = \frac{(n_1 - 1)s_1^2 + (n_2 - 1)s_2^2}{n_1 + n_2 - 2}$$
   where s_1 and s_2 are the sample standard deviations.

4. Calculate the t-statistic,
$$t = \frac{\bar{x}_1 - \bar{x}_2}{SE} \quad \text{where } SE = \sqrt{\frac{s_p^2}{n_1} + \frac{s_p^2}{n_2}},$$
   and $\bar{x}_1$ and $\bar{x}_2$ are the sample means.

5. Compare the value of t with the t-distribution on $n_1 + n_2 - 2$ degrees of freedom and determine the p-value.

6. If $p < \alpha$, reject the null hypothesis. Otherwise do not reject H_0.

7. State the conclusion and interpret the result.

5.6 How large should a cohort study be?

5.6.1 Perils of inadequate sample size

In Chapter 4, we discussed the importance of sample size for precision of estimates of means and proportions, and looked at the information needed to calculate these sample sizes. Sample size is just as important when designing an analytic study or trial, but we need to introduce additional components when comparing values (e.g. means, rates) if we are to avoid making what are termed type I and type II errors, which are explained in Table 5.6.1 in the context of a cohort study.

Table 5.6.1   Type I and type II errors

Type I error	In a cohort study, the effect of exposure to (for example) smoking, is being studied. For our example, let's say smoking does not in reality affect the risk of the disease. By chance, however, the study shows a relative risk of 1.25 (25 per cent increase in risk). We would be making a ***type I error*** if we were to conclude that smoking really does increase the risk of the disease.
	We reach a conclusion by carrying out an hypothesis test (e.g. a chi-squared test). A type I error occurs if we reject the null hypothesis when it is in fact true (that is, there is no increased risk, as in this example). The chance, or probability of a type I error is called the ***significance level*** of the test and is usually denoted by α, and as we have seen in Section 5.5, we typically choose a significance level of 5 per cent; thus, the probability of a type I error occurring is 5 per cent or 0.05. Let's say the result of the hypothesis test is p = 0.086, and as a result we do not reject the null hypothesis. The hypothesis test, set at the 0.05 level, has helped us to avoid making a type I error.
Type II error	In another situation, let's say the exposure (smoking) really does increase the risk of the disease, and the true relative risk is 1.25 (25 per cent increase in risk). A ***type II error*** occurs if this genuine increase in risk is not recognised as being real. The probability of a type II error is denoted by β. This will happen if the study is too small, relative to the amount of sampling error; let's say that when the hypothesis test is applied the result is p = 0.086 (non-significant) and, consequently we do not reject the null hypothesis.
	A study must therefore be designed to be large enough to be fairly certain of avoiding this mistake. This is described as ensuring that the study has enough statistical ***power***. The power is the probability that we reject the null hypothesis (conclude there is evidence of an association) when it is in fact false (there really is an association); in other words, we arrive at the right conclusion. Since the probability of the type II error is β, the power of the study – which is the probability of avoiding this error – is $1 - \beta$. Typically, we may choose a power of 80 per cent or 90 per cent, so β, the probability of a type II error occurring, is then 20 per cent or 10 per cent respectively.

Avoiding these errors is clearly very important. We will now look at the method for calculating sample size for a cohort study.

5.6.2 Sample size for a cohort study

There are a variety of approaches to calculating the sample size required for a cohort study. One relatively easy-to-use method that will help us to understand the information needed, and the process is provided by the StatCalc programme in Epi Info (a useful data-analysis programme that is free to use, and available from the Centers for Disease Control: http://www.cdc.gov). The information required to calculate sample size using StatCalc is as follows:

Sample size parameters for a cohort study

- The level of significance of the hypothesis test (α) – typically set at 0.05.

- The power ($1 - \beta$) – typically around 80 per cent.

- The expected frequency of the disease in the unexposed group (the proportion of subjects getting the disease over the projected follow-up period) – for example, 1 per cent (this would be equivalent to an incidence of 10 in 1000 per year for a 1-year study).

- Ratio of the number of unexposed to the number exposed – this is in effect the prevalence of exposure – for example, 50 per cent, a 1:1 ratio.

- The relative risk that is to be detected – for example, 2.0.

The choice of levels of the parameters to be used to calculate a sample size (for example, the relative risk you wish to detect) should ideally be based on previous experience using information from the published literature of studies investigating similar topics. In reality, however, it is not always possible to obtain such information, especially if the research topic is new, and values will have to be estimated. We will see how changes in parameters entered into a sample size calculation affect the required sample size (for example, increasing numbers are required as the required relative risk decreases) in Section 5.6.3.

It is strongly recommended that you always seek statistical advice about this crucial aspect of study design. It is, however, valuable for you to be able to understand the type of information that is required as it will be you (the researcher) rather than the statistical consultant who will need to make the decisions about what is important.

5.6.3   Example of output from Epi Info (StatCalc)

The information in Table 5.6.2 shows the values for the parameters of the sample size calculation we listed above entered into Epi Info (StatCalc).

Table 5.6.2   Information for sample size in a cohort study using Epi Info (statCalc)

Information needed for sample size calculation	Values for this example
Probability that if two samples differ this reflects a true difference in the two populations (confidence level or $1 - \alpha$)	95.00% (equivalent to the α. value of 0.05)
Probability that if two populations differ, the two samples will show a 'significant' difference (power or $1 - \beta$)	80.00%
Ratio (number of exposed: Number of unexposed):	1:1
Expected frequency of disease in unexposed group	1%
Please fill in the closest value to be detected for one of the following:	
• Risk ratio (RR) or relative risk – closest to 1.00	2.00
• % disease among exposed – closest to % for unexposed	(Automatic when RR completed)

The output from the sample size calculation using StatCalc in Epi Info is shown in Table 5.6.3.

Table 5.6.3 Output from sample size calculation for a cohort study using Epi Info

```
C:\Documents and Settings\All Users\Start Menu\Programs\Epi Info\StatCalc.lnk    - ⊟ ×
  EpiInfo Version 6                Statcalc                  November 1993
      Unmatched Cohort and Cross-Sectional Studies (Exposed and Nonexposed)
              Sample Sizes for 1.00 % Disease in Unexposed Group
                                Disease    Risk    Odds        Sample Size
Conf.     Power    Unex:Exp   in Exposed   Ratio   Ratio    Unexp.   Exposed    Total
95.00 %   80.00 %    1:1        2.00 %     2.00    2.02      2,514    2,514     5,028

90.00 %     "         "      ╷─────────────────────╴@       2,021    2,021     4,042
95.00 %     "         "      │ Change values for   │        2,514    2,514     5,028
99.00 %     "         "      │ inputs as desired,  │        3,647    3,647     7,294
99.90 %     "         "      │ then press F4 to     │       5,242    5,242    10,484
95.00 %   80.00 %     "      │ recalculate.        │        2,514    2,514     5,028
   "      90.00 %     "      E─────────────────────╯        3,300    3,300     6,600
   "      95.00 %     "                                     4,034    4,034     8,068
   "      99.00 %     "                                     5,622    5,622    11,244
   "      80.00 %    4:1                                    5,780    1,445     7,225
   "        "        3:1                                    4,695    1,565     6,260
   "        "        2:1                                    3,610    1,805     5,415
   "        "        1:2                                    1,957    3,914     5,871
   "        "        1:3                                    1,768    5,305     7,073
   "        "        1:4                                    1,673    6,691     8,364

   F1-Help                         F5-Print      F6-Open File      F10-Done
```

Conf.: confidence – this is $1 - \alpha$, the level of the hypothesis test. Power: this is $1 - \beta$, the power.

From this table (the first row), it can be seen that a total of around 5000 subjects are required for an α level of 0.05, power of 80 per cent, 1 per cent disease incidence in the unexposed, 1:1 ratio of unexposed to exposed, and a relative risk to be detected of 2.00.

We can also see how the required sample size becomes larger when (i) the required significance level (Conf.) is increased (e.g. from 95 per cent to 99 per cent), (ii) the required power is increased (e.g. from 80 per cent to 90 per cent), and (iii) the prevalence of the exposure becomes more common (e.g. from 50 per cent (1:1) to 80 per cent (4:1)) or becomes less common (e.g. from 50 per cent (1:1) to 20 per cent (1:4)).

By varying the required relative risk for the calculation, we can also see that the smaller the risk is to be detected, the larger the required sample size (Table 5.6.4 below).

Table 5.6.4 Example from Epi Info (StatCalc) of how the sample size for a cohort study changes with the value of the relative risk

Unmatched cohort and cross-sectional studies (exposed and non-exposed) Sample sizes for 1.00% disease in unexposed group

Conf	Power	Unex:Exp	Disease in Exp	Risk ratio	Odds ratio	Sample size		
						Unexp	Exposed	Total
95.00%	80%	1:1	2.00%	2.00	2.02	2, 514	2, 514	5, 028
95.00%	80%	1:1	3.00%	3.00	3.06	865	865	1, 730
95.00%	80%	1:1	1.50%	1.50	1.51	8, 145	8, 145	16, 290

As with sample size for precision of estimates, we should make allowance for the expected initial response rate. Additionally, because cohort studies involve follow-up, it is important to make allowance for losses to follow-up that can arise from losing contact with study subjects (e.g. migration), refusals to continue in the study, and deaths from causes that may not be relevant to the study. As a result, the eventual required sample size will always be larger than that obtained from the statistical calculation.

5.7 Confounding

5.7.1 Introduction

Determining whether an association is causal is a very important issue in the interpretation of research evidence. Our ability to make judgements about causation depends on the type and extent of the evidence, and there are a number of pointers that can help us reach a conclusion. These are commonly referred to as the Bradford–Hill guidelines, and are shown in Table 5.7.1.

Table 5.7.1 Bradford Hill guidelines with explanations and examples

Criterion	Explanation and example of application
Exposure preceding the onset of the disease	If a factor is causing a disease, it stands to reason that the exposure to that factor must have occurred before the disease process began. Also, the exposure must be shown to have occurred long enough before the onset of disease to allow for the *latency period*, this being the time it takes for the exposure to lead to overt disease in a human. An example is the relationship between radiation exposure and leukaemia: it takes several years after exposure to radiation before leukaemia appears. An important advantage of the prospective study design (cohort studies) is that clear information is usually available on the time sequence of exposure and disease onset.
Strength of association	The stronger an association, the more likely it is to be causal. A good example is the association between smoking and lung cancer, for which the relative risk has generally been found to be at least 10. This effect is so strong that it is extremely unlikely to be anything other than causal. It is important to distinguish between the strength of the association (as estimated by a relative risk), and the p-value that arises from an hypothesis test used to examine that association. Thus, a very large study could well identify a very modest relative risk of something like 1.05 with a p-value of <0.001: this is a highly statistically significant finding of a very weak association.
Independence of confounding	It is important to be able to demonstrate that the association is not explained by confounding factors. Matching in case-control studies and randomisation in trials are used to avoid confounding, while multiple-regression techniques are used in the analysis to adjust associations for confounding. Even with modern statistical methods, however, some humility is still required in the face of confounding with observational study designs: there may well be confounding factors that have not been considered, or not measured adequately enough to adjust for.

Consistency across populations with differing exposure	If a factor is causal, it would be expected that populations with a high level of exposure would have higher incidence of the disease in question than populations with lower levels of exposure. For instance, if high serum cholesterol really is an important cause of IHD, then populations such as Japan with low levels should have correspondingly low IHD incidence rates, as is indeed the case. If on the other hand, Japan had high IHD incidence, or we found populations with high cholesterol levels and low IHD incidence, we would have to question whether cholesterol really is causal.
Consistent evidence from studies in different settings	We would expect that a genuine causal association would show up in studies of different types, and in different populations. Of course, some causal effects may be dependent on, or modified by, genetic or other factors associated with ethnic group, but a degree of consistency across studies in different settings can nonetheless be expected.
Dose – response relationship	If an association is causal, we would expect that the greater the exposure (dose), the greater is the effect on the outcome (response). If, for example, heavy lifetime smokers had a similar risk of lung cancer as, or lower risk than, light smokers, or people who smoked for only a few years, we would have to question whether smoking could cause lung cancer. Although there may be threshold effects for some exposures (for example, above a certain level there is no further increase in risk), it is usual to find evidence of a dose-response relationship across most of the range of exposure encountered.
Biologically plausible	It would be unwise to suggest that an association is causal if it does not make any sense given what we know of the biological mechanisms involved. Equally, if it is plausible, that would strengthen our view of causality. For example, if we have observed an association between bladder cancer and a certain carcinogenic (cancer-causing) substance, and we know this substance is excreted in the urine, it would be reasonable to use this biological evidence to strengthen our case for this being a causal association. On the other hand, if the toxin is handled by the liver and converted to metabolites with no known carcinogenic effect, we may be more cautious in assuming causation. Alternatively, we may not know enough about the biological mechanisms involved to exclude the possibility of causation.
Evidence from animal studies	Animal experimentation creates a good deal of controversy, not only from the animal welfare point of view, but also because of the relevance of animal models to humans. If an effect is seen in rats or monkeys, how do we know it applies to humans? And just because an effect is not seen in animals, does this mean that it cannot occur in humans? Despite these uncertainties, experience has shown that animal evidence can be relevant, and where it exists should be taken into account.
Removal of the exposure reduces risk	Perhaps the most powerful evidence of causation comes from experiments that measure the effect of reducing exposure to the suspected causal factor. In the 'ideal' form (from a scientific point of view), the randomised, controlled trial has the capacity to study the effect of changing the level of exposure, in a comparison where only the factor of interest differs between the groups being studied.

We will review these guidelines again in later chapters when looking at the results from other study designs. By then, we will have encountered most of these guidelines in one form or another, and it will be a matter of bringing them together to see how they help in making judgements about causation.

One of the most important of the Bradford Hill guidelines that we have already begun to think about is that the association should be independent of *confounding*. This is a suitable point to look at what confounding means, and to begin thinking about how to deal with it.

5.7.2   What is a confounding factor?

The conditions necessary for a factor to confound an association are as follows: for a factor (X) to *confound* an association between a *potential cause* (A) and the *outcome* (B), it must:

- be associated with the potential cause (A)

- be a risk factor for the outcome (B)

- not be in the causal pathway for the effect of (A) on (B).

In order to illustrate this more clearly, we will return to the example of smoking and heart disease. We are interested in the question of whether smoking is *causally* associated with IHD, and whether that association is being *confounded* by other factors.

The factors that it is suggested may confound the smoking–IHD association, must themselves be *associated* with smoking. Compared to non-smokers, people who smoke would therefore have to take less exercise, have higher blood cholesterol, etc. This is true, certainly among some population groups.

In order for factors such as exercise and blood cholesterol to confound the smoking–IHD association, the factors must themselves be capable of causing the outcome. Thus, lack of exercise and high cholesterol would need to be risk factors for IHD, and we also know this to be the case.

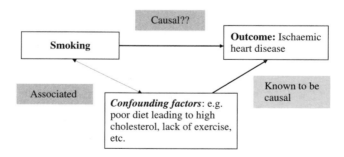

It has been stated that confounders should not be on the causal pathway, and an example may help explain why this is important. Smoking in pregnancy causes low birthweight. It is generally believed that this occurs mainly because smoking leads to increased levels of carbon monoxide (CO) in the blood. The CO combines with haemoglobin (Hb), the substance in red blood cells that transports oxygen, to produce carboxyhaemoglobin (COHb). COHb is not so good at delivering oxygen to the tissues and organs of the body, including to the placenta, so the fetus receives less and its growth is restricted. Let us now consider this in our model of confounding through the following two diagrams, the first (A) a model of confounding, and the second (B) showing how CO fits into the causal pathway.

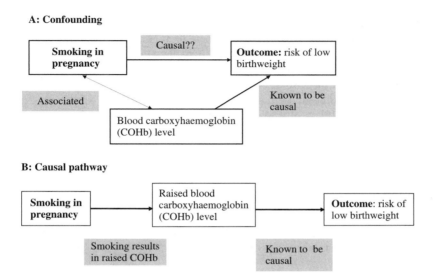

A: Confounding

B: Causal pathway

The question then is, does COHb act as a confounding factor in the association between smoking in pregnancy and low birthweight? Raised COHb is associated with smoking, and does cause low birthweight, but it is *not* confounding the association because it is one of the main mechanisms by which smoking has this effect on birth weight. It is in the ***causal pathway***. This is an important conclusion because if we were to 'allow' (adjust) for the effect COHb, we would as a consequence remove the effect of smoking as well. We would then erroneously conclude that smoking is not the problem.

5.7.3 Does smoking cause heart disease?

It is now accepted that smoking does indeed cause a wide range of diseases, including IHD. In our discussion of confounding of the smoking–IHD association, we suggested that factors such as cholesterol and lack of exercise might be confounders. So are they? Well, in some population groups, they certainly could partly confound an association between smoking and heart disease, but they would never explain that association completely. That is to say, even after taking into account the effects of these confounding factors, smoking still has a strong independent association with IHD, which we believe to be causal.

We can summarise this conclusion as follows. The observed association between smoking and IHD is mainly due to the fact that smoking causes IHD. In some situations, it is also partly due to the fact that smokers have other characteristics (such as taking less exercise or eating less healthily) which add to their risk of IHD. In these situations, the observed association between smoking and IHD is partly confounded by other lifestyle factors. When we allow for these other lifestyle factors in the analysis, the independent effect of smoking is still clearly apparent.

5.7.4 Confounding in the physical activity and cancer study

The authors of paper A were also concerned about the possibility of confounding in their study. There was a possibility that some factors associated with the amount of physical activity an individual takes might also be associated with cancer, such as age, cigarette smoking, body mass index, alcohol intake and social class. In order to adjust for these potential confounders, it was necessary to collect data on these for each individual in the study. So how did the authors then carry out this all-important analysis to demonstrate the independent effect of physical activity on the risk of cancer? This was done by using a method of analysis called **regression**, which we will introduce in the next section of this chapter. The following exercise will help to consolidate your understanding of the concept of confounding, and the differing extents to which confounding can operate. This will be useful background for when we look at regression methods in Section 5.8.

 Self-Assessment Exercise 5.7.1

Based on the information given in the following diagrams, which of the following three models of association between factor A and outcome B, could be confounded by factor X?

Model 1: Could heavy alcohol consumption confound an association observed between cigarette smoking and high blood pressure?

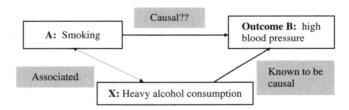

Model 2: Could cigarette smoking confound an association between radon gas exposure and lung cancer? (Radon gas is a naturally occurring product of uranium in the ground, especially in areas of the country with granite: it collects in the house and leads to human exposure.)

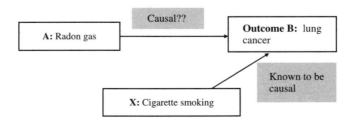

Model 3: Could poverty confound an association between damp housing and respiratory illness?

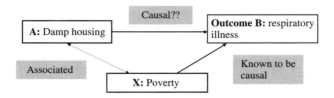

Answers in Section 5.10

5.7.5 Methods for dealing with confounding

There are a number of other aspects of study design and analysis that we need to cover before going into this more thoroughly, but it is worth considering in general terms how we set about dealing with confounding. There are essentially two approaches:

- We can design the study in a way that minimises the effect of confounding factors. We will return to this when we look at matching in case-control studies (Chapter 6), and randomisation in intervention trials (Chapter 7).

- We can use statistical methods for adjusting for the effects of confounding. The main methods of doing this are *standardisation* (which we looked at in Chapter 3 when we adjusted for the effects of differing age structures in two populations) and *multivariate analysis* by regression techniques, which will be introduced in Section 5.9 of this chapter.

Summary: confounding – main messages

- There are often complex interrelationships between variables being studied.

- These interrelationships can result in confounding, if the potential confounder is associated with the possible cause, is itself a risk factor for the outcome, and is not in the causal pathway.

- Confounding is often partial; that is to say, it partly explains an association between a risk factor and an outcome.

- The potential for confounding must be recognised in planning research, assessed, and, if necessary, allowed (adjusted) for before meaningful conclusions can be arrived at.

- Confounding can be minimised at the study design stage by matching or randomisation (we will look at these techniques in Chapters 6 and 7), and/or adjusted for in the analysis by standardisation or multivariate regression analysis.

5.8 Simple linear regression

5.8.1 Approaches to describing associations

In Chapter 2 we started looking at relationships between two continuous variables (such as birthweight and gestational age), each measured on the same individuals. You will recall that:

- Two continuous variables each observed for the same individuals can be displayed on a *scatterplot*.

- We describe any relationship between the variables in terms of its *form, strength* and *direction*.

- The *correlation coefficient* is an objective numerical measure which summarises the strength and direction of *linear association* between the variables.

We will now look at what is generally the next stage in investigating such relationships: that is, to describe how one variable (the *outcome* or *dependent* variable) depends on the other variable (the *explanatory* or *independent* variable). For example, in the case of birthweight and gestational age (an association we studied with correlation), having observed that there is an approximately linear relationship between the variables, we may wish to describe how birthweight *depends* on gestational age. Note that it does not make sense to consider how gestational age depends on birthweight.

Birthweight is the dependent (or y) variable. Gestational age is the independent (or x) variable. As noted above, a dependent variable may also be called an *outcome variable*. Also, an independent variable may also be called an *explanatory variable*, because it explains, to some extent, how the outcome varies. The simplest description of a relationship between two continuous variables is a straight line. A straight line is defined by an *intercept* (where the line crosses the y axis) and a slope (the *gradient*):

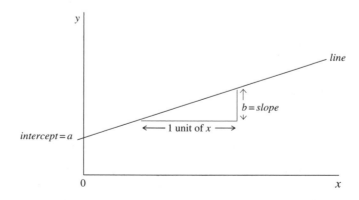

Figure 5.8.1　Components for the equation of a straight line

The intercept is the value of y when x is zero, and the slope is the amount y increases for each unit increase in x. Thus, the equation for the line is:

y (outcome variable) $= a$ (intercept) $+ b$ (slope) x (explanatory variable)

Returning to our example of birthweight and gestational age, we saw that there was a fairly strong, positive, linear relationship between the two variables, Figure 5.8.2:

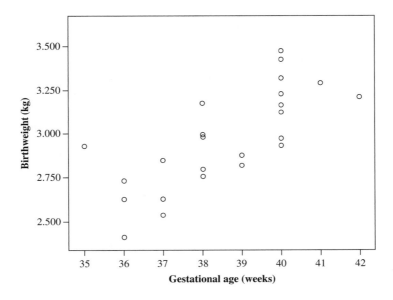

Figure 5.8.2 Birthweight and gestational age of babies

Clearly, a straight line cannot exactly describe this relationship, as few of the values could lie on such a line. However, a line which is close to the data values summarises the relationship. It tells us by how much birthweight increases, on average, for an increase of 1 week in gestational age. The statistical method of estimating the relationship between variables is called *regression*. When we describe the relationship between one outcome variable and one explanatory variable by a straight line, it is called *simple linear regression*.

5.8.2 Finding the best fit for a straight line

How do we decide which is the straight line that best summarises the relationship? That is, what do we mean by a line which is 'close' to the data? There are various ways of defining closeness. The most common definition involves the differences between the observed y-values and a straight line. That is, the vertical deviations from the line (Figure 5.8.3).

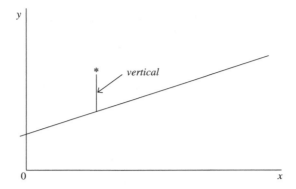

Figure 5.8.3 Difference between observed y-value and a straight line

We choose the line which results in the smallest possible value when all the deviations are squared and added together. This method of choosing the 'best' line to describe the relationship is called *least squares regression*. The statistical basis for this calculation is beyond the scope of this book, and the parameters summarising the *line of best fit* are given by all statistical software. The least squares regression line summarising the relationship between birthweight (y) and gestational age (x) is calculated as $y = -1.4850 + 0.1155x$.

Plotting the line [$y = -1.4850 + 0.1155x$], on the scatterplot shows us how much the data vary about the line (Figure 5.8.4).

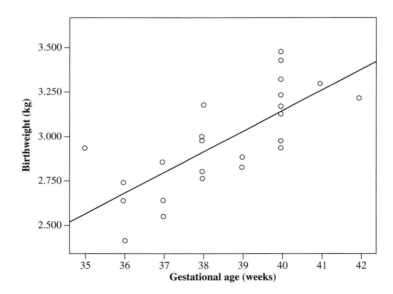

Figure 5.8.4 The regression of birthweight on gestational age

The following exercise involves using the regression equation to calculate some values of birthweight and see whether they fit the line.

Self-Assessment Exercise 5.8.1

1. Use the regression equation to calculate the value of birthweight (in kgs) for 37 weeks, and for 41.5 weeks.

2. Do your answers lie on the line in Figure 5.8.4?

3. Do you think it would be reasonable to use this line to calculate the birthweight of a baby of 28 weeks' gestation?

Answers in Section 5.10

5.8.3 Interpreting the regression line

The equation we have calculated is a summary of the relationship. It does not tell us the actual birthweight of a baby born at a particular gestational age. We know that birthweight varies for any particular gestational age, because gestational age is only one of several factors associated with birthweight.

The equation shows us the average birthweight of babies of a particular gestational age. It also shows us how birthweight changes with gestational age over the range of 35–42 weeks: for each extra week of gestational age, birthweight increases by 0.1155 kg (about 120 g) on average.

Note that the intercept (that is, where the line crosses the y-axis, which is for a gestational age of 0 weeks) is negative (-1.4850), implying a negative birthweight for a gestational age of 0 weeks. Of course, this does not make any sense, and clearly somewhere between 35 weeks' gestation and conception the relationship we have described with this regression equation changes. It is therefore very important to note that the regression equation only describes the relationship within the range of the observed x data. We should not use this equation to describe how birthweight and gestational age are related for ages of less than 35 weeks.

5.8.4 Using the regression line

We have used the regression equation to

1. **Describe** the general level of the dependent/outcome variable associated with each level of the independent/explanatory variable.

We can also use it to

2. **Predict** values of the dependent variable for new observations of the independent variable, within the range of the x data.

3. **Adjust** measurements of the dependent variable for the effects of the independent variable, before comparing individuals.

4. **Control** the dependent variable by changing the value of the independent variable.

For example,

- **Predict**: If another baby, not in the original data set, is to be born at 40 weeks, we predict that the weight will be $-1.4850 + 0.1155 \times 40 = 3.135$ kg. This is what you in fact did in exercise 5.8.1, and is our 'best guess' at the weight of this individual baby.

- **Adjust**: If we know the relationship between weight and height for men, we can take into account a man's height in deciding whether he is overweight.

- **Control**: If we know how blood pressure is related to dose of an antihypertensive therapy, we can determine the dose required to reduce blood pressure by a given amount.

5.8.5   Is the explanatory variable really associated with the outcome?

We can calculate a regression equation for any two continuous variables, so it is possible to come up with an equation even if the outcome is not in fact related to the explanatory variable. So how do we know if the explanatory variable really is associated with the outcome?

As a first step, we should always look at the data on a scatterplot. This will show whether there is any obvious non-linear pattern, in which case linear regression is not appropriate. It will also give an idea of whether there may be no relationship between the variables. This is subjective though – it is easier to see a relationship than the absence of one.

An objective way of investigating whether the outcome is really associated with the explanatory variable is to carry out an *hypothesis test*. We have said that to carry out regression, the two variables must simply be continuous and have an approximately linear relationship. However, to test hypotheses, we need to be able to assume that:

- The outcome y has a population with an approximately normal distribution.

- For each value of the explanatory variable x, the variation of y about the regression line is approximately the same.

These are reasonable assumptions to make in many situations – we shall comment on them further after looking at how to carry out an appropriate hypothesis test.

If the outcome and explanatory variables are really **not** associated, then the slope (b) of the regression line should be zero. However, we may happen to estimate a non-zero slope from the particular sample of data we have. So we want to test the null hypothesis H_0: slope $= 0$ in the population from which the sample was drawn. We can use the t-distribution for this hypothesis test.

Testing the null hypothesis of no association between y and x (H_0: slope $= 0$)

We calculate the test statistic

$$t = \frac{b}{SE}$$

where b is the estimated coefficient of x and SE is the standard error of b. The statistic is compared with the t distribution with $n - 2$ degrees of freedom to find the p-value of the test (n is the number of subjects).

If the assumptions given above are not satisfied, the estimate of the regression equation will not be seriously affected. What may happen is that the standard error and consequently the p-value will not be correct. So if it appears that the assumptions may not be satisfied, we should proceed with caution – particularly if the p-value is close to a critical value such as 0.05 – and seek advice if necessary. There are methods for checking these assumptions and dealing with departures from them, but they are beyond the scope of this book. The standard error can be calculated from a formula, but is usually obtained with computer software. For the regression of birthweight on gestational age, software gives:

	Coefficient	Standard error	t-value	p-value
Gestational age	0.11553	0.02210	5.23	0.000

You can see how the t-value is derived by dividing the slope (coefficient) by the standard error, as in the formula above. The p-value is stated as 0.000 due to the limit (3) on the number of decimal places in this output, but it is not in fact zero. We can, however, say that $p < 0.0005$. The conclusion is that there is very strong evidence of a relationship between the birthweight and gestational age of babies. The probability of the observed relationship arising if H_0 is true is very small.

5.8.6 How good is the regression model?

Once we have found the line of best fit, it is important that we assess how well this line fits the actual data (the ***goodness-of-fit*** of the model). This is a relatively straightforward concept in simple linear regression, but, as we shall see in Section 5.9, it becomes slightly more complicated when we include more than one independent variable in the model.

Calculating sums of squares

We estimated the line of best fit for our model (regressing birthweight on gestational age) by calculating the line that results in the smallest sum of squared differences between observed values and the line. In fact, there are several sums of squares that can be calculated to help us gauge the contribution of our model (gestational age) to predicting the outcome (birthweight).

Firstly, we can calculate the sum of squared differences for the most simple model available, the mean value of y (birthweight). Clearly, this is not a good model of a relationship between two variables. Using the mean as a model, we can calculate the squared differences between the observed values, and the values predicted by the mean and sum them. This sum of squared differences is known as the ***total sum of squares*** (SS_T) because it is the total amount of differences present when the most basic model is applied to the data.

Now, if we fit the model representing the line of best fit to the data, we can again work out the differences between this new model and the observed data. Although this regression line is ascertained by the method of least squares (as described previously), there will still be some inaccuracy represented by the differences between each observed data point and the value predicted by the regression line. As before, these differences are squared and then summed. The result is known as the ***sum of squared residuals*** (SS_R). This value represents the degree of inaccuracy when the best model is fitted to the data.

We can now use these two values (SS_T and SS_R) to calculate how much better the regression line (the line of best fit) is than just using the mean as a model. The improvement in prediction resulting from using the regression model rather than the mean is calculated by calculating the difference between SS_T and SS_R. This improvement is known as the ***model sum of squares*** (SS_M).

The following figure shows each of these sum of squares graphically (source: Field, A. (2001). *Discovering Statistics Using SPSS for Windows*. Sage: Thousand Oaks, CA).

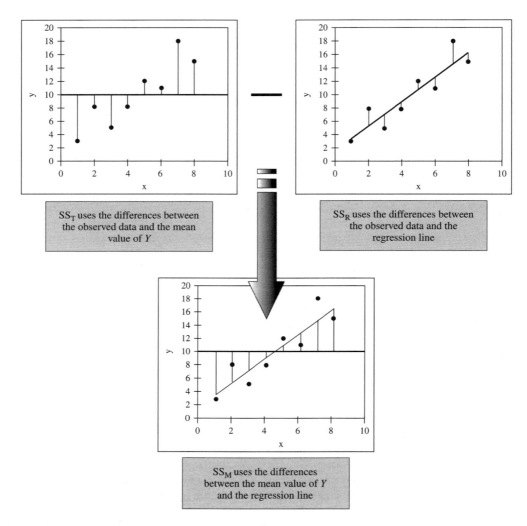

Source: Reproduced with permission from Field, A. (2001).

If the value of SS_M is large, then the regression model is very different from using the mean to predict the outcome variable. This implies that the regression model has made a substantial improvement to how well the outcome variable can be predicted. However, if the SS_M is small, then using the regression model is little better than using the mean.

Calculating R^2

A useful measure arising from these sums of squares is the proportion of improvement due to the model. This is calculated by dividing the sum of squares for the model (SS_M) by the total sum of squares (SS_T). The resulting value is called R^2 (multiplied by 100 to give a percentage). So, R^2 represents the amount of variation in the outcome explained by the model (SS_M) relative to how much variation there was to explain in the first place (SS_T).

$$R^2 = SS_M/SS_T$$

This concept of r^2 was introduced in Section 2.4 as the coefficient of determination when using Pearson correlation. This is equivalent to the R^2 described here for simple linear regression (one explanatory and one outcome variable).

Calculating the F-ratio

A second use of the sums of squares in assessing the regression model is through the F-test. Briefly, the test is based upon the ratio of the improvement due to the model (SS_M) and the difference between the model and the observed data (SS_R). In fact, rather than using the sums of squares themselves, we take the *mean sums of squares* (referred to as mean squares or MS). To work out the mean sum of squares, it is necessary to divide by the degrees of freedom.

For SS_M the degrees of freedom are the number of variables in the model, and for SS_R they are the number of observations minus the number of parameters being estimated: this will be the number of beta coefficients in the model (in the case of simple linear regression, this is just one) and the intercept (often referred to as the *constant*). The result is the mean squares for the model (MS_M) and the residual mean squares (MS_R). The F-ratio is a measure of how much the model has improved the prediction of the outcome compared to the level of inaccuracy of the model.

$$F = MS_M/MS_R$$

If a model is good, we expect the improvement in prediction due to the model to be large (so, MS_M will be large), and the difference between the model and the observed data to be small (so, MS_R will be small). In short, a good model should have a large F-ratio (greater than 1 at least). We can also obtain p-values to estimate the significance of the F-ratio with a computer, or by using tabulated critical values for the F-distribution for the relevant degrees of freedom. The F-distribution will be discussed further in Chapter 11).

5.8.7 Interpreting SPSS output for simple linear regression analysis

To demonstrate how we interpret the output from simple linear regression with SPSS, we will use the low back pain data set described in the Preface. For the current example, we will use two continuous variables from the data set: height and weight. The simple linear regression exercise will consider the effects of height on weight for the 765 employees comprising the data set. When carrying out linear regression analysis, SPSS generates four tables.

Table 1: variables entered/removed

The first table indicates what dependent variable has been selected (weight) and lists the independent variables (height) entered into the model to predict values of the dependent variable.

Variables Entered/Removed[b]

Model	Variables Entered	Variables Removed	Method
1	height in cms[a]		Enter

[a] All requested variables entered.
[b] Dependent Variable: weight in kgs

Table 2: model summary

The second table provided by SPSS is a summary of the model. This summary table provides the value of R and R^2 for the model that has been calculated. Because there is only one predictor (height), R represents the simple correlation between weight and height, that is the Pearson correlation coefficient introduced in Chapter 2 (Section 2.4).

Model Summary

Model	R	R Square	Adjusted R Square	Std. Error of the Estimate
1	.546[a]	.298	.297	10.3798

[a] Predictors: (Constant), height in cms

The Pearson correlation coefficient between height and weight is therefore 0.546, a relatively strong positive correlation. The value of R square (coefficient of determination) is 0.298, which tells us that height accounts for 29.8 per cent of the variation in weight. In other words, there might be many factors that can explain the variation in weight, but our model, which includes only height, can explain 30 per cent of this variation. Put another way, 70 per cent of the variation in weight cannot be explained by height alone.

Table 3: the ANOVA table

The next part of the SPSS output reports analysis of variance (ANOVA). The summary table shows the various sums of squares and the degrees of freedom (df) associated with each. From these values, the mean squares are calculated by dividing the sum of squares by the respective df. The most important part of the table is the F-ratio (the calculation of which is described in Section 5.8.6) and the associated significance value of that F-ratio.

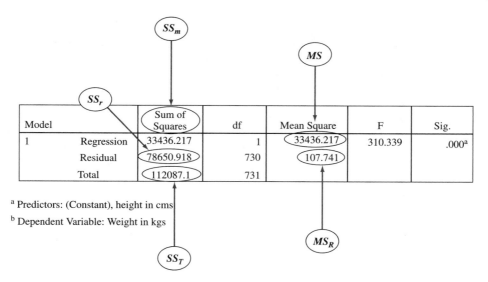

Model		Sum of Squares	df	Mean Square	F	Sig.
1	Regression	33436.217	1	33436.217	310.339	.000[a]
	Residual	78650.918	730	107.741		
	Total	112087.1	731			

[a] Predictors: (Constant), height in cms

[b] Dependent Variable: Weight in kgs

For these data, F is 310.339, which is significant at $p < 0.0005$. This result tells us that there is less than a 0.05 per cent chance that an F-ratio this large would happen by chance alone. Therefore, we can conclude that our regression model results in significantly better prediction of weight than if we used the mean value for weight.

Table 4: the coefficients table

The ANOVA table does not tell us about the individual contribution of variables in the model (although in simple regression, there is only one variable in the model and so we can infer that the variable is a significant predictor of weight). The coefficients table provides details of the model parameters (the beta coefficients, or the slopes of the regressions) and the statistical significance of these values.

Coefficients[a]

Model		Unstandardized Coefficients		Standardized Coefficients		
		B	Std. Error	Beta	t	Sig.
1	(Constant)	-34.659	5.818		-5.957	.000
	height in cms	.614	.035	.546	17.616	.000

[a] Dependent Variable: weight in kgs

We saw earlier that the intercept for the simple linear regression equation was denoted by the symbol α, also termed the constant. Note that (somewhat confusingly) in the SPSS output, this is labelled B for the constant, and has the value of -34.659. The slope of the regression is also labelled B, for the explanatory variable (height (cm)), and has the value 0.614. Thus, the regression equation is:

$$\text{Weight (in kg)} = -34.659 + 0.614 \text{ (height in cm)}$$

We can think of the beta coefficient (slope) as representing the unit change in the dependent variable (outcome) associated with a unit change of the independent variable. Therefore, if our predictor variable is increased by one unit (if height is increased by 1 cm), then our model predicts that weight will be increased by 0.614 kg.

A poor model will have a regression coefficient (slope) close to zero for the independent (explanatory) variable. A regression coefficient of zero means: (a) a unit change in the predictor variable results in no change in the predicted value of the outcome and (b) the gradient of the regression line is zero, implying that the regression line is flat. The coefficients table also provides the result of the hypothesis test (t-test) of whether the slope of the regression differs from zero, with the value of t and probability in the last two columns, respectively. This shows that the probability that this coefficient could have arisen by chance is <0.0005. This is very unlikely, and we can reject the null hypothesis of no association and conclude that height makes a significant contribution to predicting weight.

Finally, the coefficients table also shows 'standardised coefficients'. These are the beta coefficients (slopes) standardised so that the effect sizes of two or more explanatory variables (which are likely to have different units) can be directly compared.

Summary: simple linear regression

- An approximately linear relationship between two continuous variables can be summarised by the equation of a straight line.

- The most commonly used way of choosing a line which is 'close' to the observed data is least squares regression.

- We use the regression equation to:

  a) describe the relationship

  b) predict values of the dependent variable

  c) adjust values of the dependent variable for the effects of the independent variable

  d) control the dependent variable.

- The regression equation is only valid within the range of the observed x data.

- To test the null hypothesis that the dependent and independent variables are not related, we compare b/SE with the t distribution on $n-2$ degrees of freedom (n is the number of subjects).

- We can measure the goodness of fit of a linear regression model by calculating the R^2 value (the proportion of variation in the dependent variable explained by the independent variable(s)).

- We can also measure the goodness of fit of a linear regression model by calculating the F-ratio (a summary of how our much our model has improved the prediction of the dependent variable over the most basic model – the mean of the dependent variable).

5.9 Introduction to multiple linear regression

5.9.1 Principles of multiple regression

We have seen that we can use simple linear regression to summarise the relationship between an outcome (dependent variable) and a single explanatory (independent) variable. However, as we know from our discussion of confounding and the BRHS cohort studies, things are rarely so simple. The value of an outcome variable is usually affected by many factors, as we commented in the example of birthweight and gestational age – gestational age is only one of the factors associated with birthweight. To summarise the simultaneous relationship between a continuous outcome variable and a number of explanatory variables, we need to use multiple linear regression. The equation that allows us to study the effect on the outcome variable of a number of explanatory variables is as follows:

$$y = a + b_1 x_1 + b_2 x_2 + \cdots + b_k x_k$$

where x_1 is the first explanatory variable, x_2 is the second, and so on. When we have more than one explanatory variable, we can no longer think of the regression equation as a straight line: it is a mathematical description (a model) of the average relationship. However, this is still a linear relationship. The regression coefficients $b_1, b_2, \ldots, b_k$ are calculated from the data by a computer (it can be done on a calculator, but it is hard work!). For example, we may wish to explore how birthweight is related to gestational age *and* amount smoked during pregnancy. The regression equation is

$$\text{birthweight} = a + b_1 \text{ gestational age} + b_2 \text{ amount smoked}$$

where amount smoked is measured in suitable units, such as the number of cigarettes smoked per day.

5.9.2 Using multiple linear regression to study independent associations

Multiple regression allows us to look at relationships between variables, allowing for the effects of other variables. For example, the effect of smoking on birthweight, allowing for gestational age. In this way, we can investigate whether a risk factor is ***independently*** associated with an outcome, after allowing for the effects of a confounding factor. In order to illustrate how multiple linear regression works in practice, we will look at another example of linear regression analysis using SPSS. The example involves both simple (only one explanatory variable) and ***multivariate*** (involving several explanatory variables) linear regression. This example will be used now to describe the process, and to help familiarise you with the interpretation of the output from multiple linear regression analysis.

To illustrate the modelling of data by linear regression we will again use data from the low back pain data set, which includes 765 male and female employees aged 18–75 years working in a variety of manual occupational settings in northwest England.

5.9.3 An investigation of the effect of work stress on bodyweight

For this example, we are interested in identifying the relationship between a range of physiological variables and workplace exposures (independent variables) with recorded weight in kilograms (dependent variable or outcome). In particular we would like to measure the independent effect of stress in the workplace on bodyweight. Let us hypothesise that stress may increase body weight, though of course there may be a variety of mechanisms by which this might happen – for example stressed employees may eat more food or drink more alcohol. The variables in the low back pain data set that are of interest for this investigation include:

Dependent (outcome) variable
- *Weight* (kg) – continuous.

Independent (explanatory) variables (including potential confounders)
- *Stressful work* (4-point scale) – this is a categorical variable but will be treated here as a continuous variable in the linear regression (the increasing scale is proportional). In Chapter 6 we will look at an alternative method for including variables with more than two categories in regression, using so-called 'dummy variables' based on the response categories.
- *Height* (cm) – continuous.
- *Age* (years) – continuous.
- *Sex* – a dichotomous (categorical) variable.

Is there a univariate association?

Before constructing a multivariate model by multiple linear regression, we need to examine the association between the independent variable of interest (stressful work) and the dependent variable (weight in kilograms) by carrying out univariate (one independent variable) analysis by simple linear regression. The main SPSS output for this association is shown in the ANOVA and coefficient tables below:

ANOVA[b]

Model		Sum of Squares	df	Mean Square	F	Sig.
1	Regression	4358.946	1	4358.946	29.525	.000[a]
	Residual	108215.4	733	147.634		
	Total	112574.3	734			

[a] Predictors: (Constant), is work stressful
[b] Dependent Variable: weight in kgs

Coefficients[a]

Model		Unstandardized Coefficients		Standardized Coefficients		
		B	Std. Error	Beta	t	Sig.
1	(Constant)	62.075	1.113		55.750	.000
	is work stressful	2.496	.459	.197	5.434	.000

[a] Dependent Variable: weight in kgs

ANOVA table

As we discussed earlier, the ANOVA table gives an estimate of the *goodness-of-fit* of the model. The most important part of this table is the *F-ratio*, a measure of how much the model has improved the prediction of the outcome compared to the level of inaccuracy of the model (random error – think of this as being analogous to standard error). We saw that the F-ratio is calculated by dividing the mean squares for the model (MS_M – in this case 4358.946) by the residual mean squares (MS_R – in this case 147.634). In our simple model investigating the effect of stress on weight, the F-ratio is 29.525, which is significant at $p < 0.0005$. This result tells us that there is less than a 0.05 per cent probability that an F-ratio this large would happen by chance alone.

Coefficients table

The coefficients table provides details of the model parameters, that is, the beta values (slopes of the regressions) and their statistical significance. For stress, the beta coefficient is 2.496, with a highly significant p-value of <0.0005. Thus, as the explanatory variable (stress) is increased by one unit, our model predicts that the outcome (weight) will be increased by 2.496 kg. We can therefore conclude that, in a *univariate analysis*, stress is significantly associated with weight; the longer employees report working in a stressful environment during a shift, the heavier they weigh.

What about confounding?

To sum up, we have shown with the univariate linear regression that (i) stress at work is significantly associated with weight, and (ii) for each increase of one unit in the stress score, weight increases by 2.5 kg. This is an interesting finding, but it would be a mistake to conclude immediately that the relationship is causal. It seems likely that this association could – at least in part – be explained by confounding. For example, perhaps it is older people who are more prone to work stress, and weight does tend to increase with age. Or maybe men are more stressed in today's job market, and they are, on average, heavier than women.

In order to look at the *independent* effect of work stress on weight, adjusting for potential confounding, we can create a multivariate model by including the other independent variables in the linear regression. Before doing this, we would of course need to look at the univariate associations of all these other variables with weight: we will assume that height, age and sex are indeed associated with weight.

Briefly, then, our model will measure the independent effects of each independent variable (work stress, height, age and sex) on the dependent variable (weight in kilograms). The main SPSS output for this multiple linear regression model is shown in the ANOVA and coefficients tables below.

ANOVA table

We can see from the ANOVA table that the F-ratio for the model including the four independent variables is 124.773, which is again significant at $p < 0.0005$. This result tells us that there is less than a 0.05 per cent chance that an F-ratio this large would happen by chance alone. Therefore, we can conclude that our regression model results in significantly better prediction of weight (kg) than if we used the mean value of weight alone.

ANOVA[b]

Model		Sum of Squares	df	Mean Square	F	Sig.
1	Regression	45591.884	4	11397.971	124.773	.000[a]
	Residual	66228.340	725	91.349		
	Total	111820.2	729			

[a] Predictors: (Constant), is work stressful, SEX, AGE, height in cms
[b] Dependent Variable: weight in kgs

Coefficients[a]

Model		Unstandardized Coefficients		Standardized Coefficients		
		B	Std. Error	Beta	t	Sig.
1	(Constant)	−11.811	8.770		−1.347	.178
	height in cms	.470	.045	.418	10.507	.000
	AGE	.266	.029	.273	9.177	.000
	SEX	−6.059	1.020	−.232	−5.941	.000
	is work stressful	.552	.379	.044	1.455	.146

[a] Dependent Variable: weight in kgs

Coefficients table

The coefficients table provides details of the model parameters (the beta values) for the four explanatory variables together with their significance (p) values. Interestingly, following this *adjustment* for the effects of the other independent variables, the B (beta) value for stressful work is now considerably smaller: the gradient of the regression line being 0.552. This *adjusted regression coefficient* means that, if stress is increased by one unit, our model predicts that weight will be increased by 0.552 kg. We can also see from the table the p-value for stressful work has increased to 0.146 (the result is no longer statistically significant), whereas previously it was $p < 0.0005$.

This result illustrates the effects of *confounding* on the relationship between stress and weight. As we suspected, one or more of the other three variables (height, age and sex) explain much of the observed univariate association between stress and weight by their mutual association with both factors.

Confidence intervals (CIs) for the regression coefficients

Note that regression beta coefficients, including adjusted regression coefficients, should be quoted with 95 per cent CIs in the same way that we have emphasised previously for means, proportions, relative risks, etc. These can be calculated by the appropriate option in SPSS, but can also easily be derived from the standard errors in the coefficients table. Thus, for stress, the 95 per cent CI is:

$$\text{Beta } (0.552) \pm 1.96 \times \text{standard error } (0.379) = -0.191; \ 1.295$$

We are therefore 95 per cent confident that, after allowing for the effects of height, age and sex, in the population, this sample represents, for every increase in one unit of the stress at work score, the weight ranges from a decrease by 0.191 kg to an increase of 1.295 kg. The 95 per cent CI includes zero, so the result is not significant, consistent with the p-value being greater than 0.05.

5.9.4 Multiple regression in the cancer study

We will now return to the BRHS study of physical activity and cancer risk (paper A), to see how multiple regression was used to investigate the ***independent effect*** of physical activity on the risk of cancer after adjusting for a number of other factors. The method used is known as Cox regression, a type of multiple regression commonly employed in cohort studies where information is available on the time until an event (the cancer) occurs. We will study Cox regression in more detail in Chapter 8 on survival analysis, but for now we can interpret the results of analysis as described above in Sections 5.9.1–5.9.3 for multiple linear regression. Table 2 from paper A is reproduced again below (initially presented in Table 5.5.1).

Table 2 Physical activity and age-adjusted cancer rates/1000 person-years and adjusted relative risks for all cancers (excluding skin cancer) in 7,588 middle-aged British men

Physical activity	No.	Cases	Rates/1000 p-y	Relative risks (95% CI)	
				A	**B**
None/Occ	3017	424	8.4	1.00	1.00
Light	1749	234	7.8	0.93 (0.79, 1.09)	0.95 (0.80, 1.11)
Moderate	1196	163	8.1	0.95 (0.80, 1.14)	1.04 (0.86, 1.24)
Moderate-vigorous	1113	101	5.8	0.68 (0.54, 0.84)	0.78 (0.62, 0.97)
Vigorous	513	47	5.7	0.65 (0.44, 0.88)	0.76 (0.56, 1.04)
Test for linear trend				P < 0.0001	P = 0.02

A = age-adjusted
B = adjusted for age, cigarette smoking, BMI, alcohol intake and social class.

Self-Assessment Exercise 5.9.1

In Exercise 5.5.1, we compared the incidence rates of cancer among men taking vigorous exercise with those taking none/occasional exercise, and found this to be 0.68. We showed that this was the relative risk, and noted this was not adjusted for any confounding factors. We will now look at the results (relative risks) following adjustment with multiple regression (Cox regression in this study), shown in columns 5 (A) and 6 (B).

1. Why are the relative risks for none/occasional exercise equal to 1.00?

2. What is the relative risk (and 95 per cent CI) for vigorous exercise after adjustment only for age, shown in column 5 (A)? Interpret this result.

3. How does adjustment for all five potential confounding factors, shown in column 6 (B), affect the results? Does this alter your conclusion?

4. Is there any additional information in this table that might lead you to conclude that the association between exercise and reduced cancer risk is causal?

Answers in Section 5.10

Summary: multiple regression

- Multiple regression is used to summarise the relationship between a dependent (outcome) variable and a number of independent (explanatory) variables.

- Multiple linear regression allows us to determine the relationship between a continuous dependent (outcome) variable and a number of independent (explanatory) variables. These independent variables can be continuous or categorical.

- Regression coefficients should be quoted with the 95 per cent confidence interval.

- An important use of multiple regression is to adjust the estimated effect of a risk factor on an outcome for the effect of other potentially confounding factors, and hence derive an estimate of the independent effect of the exposure of interest.

- Other types of regression are commonly used (in simple or multiple forms), including logistic regression, where the dependent (outcome) is categorical (e.g. presence or absence of disease), and Cox regression, where the outcome is categorical and information is available on time until the event occurs. These methods will be studied in subsequent chapters.

5.10 Answers to self-assessment exercises

Section 5.1

Exercise 5.1.1

Research issues identified	Appropriate research method
• Increasing evidence that physical activity is associated with altered risk of total cancers and certain types of specific cancer.	Descriptive epidemiology and survey methods would be inadequate, as risk factors are thought to have an effect over an extended period of time and a survey would need to rely on recall of exercise patterns extending back many years.
• Data on physical activity and a number of types of cancer is limited. • Not clear about the amount and type of physical activity required to alter the risk of cancer.	Requires good, quantified evidence on risk factor effects: cohort study well suited.
Specified aims for BRHS • To examine the relationship between physical activity and incidence of total cancers and some site-specific cancers, and to assess the type and amount of activity required to achieve benefit.	Population-based cohort study is method of choice, at least for common cancers (we will see in Chapter 6 that for rarer conditions, case-control studies are usually more appropriate).

Section 5.2

Exercise 5.2.1

1. Middle-aged British men.

2. There are probably several reasons for this. The original aim of the study was to investigate cardiovascular risk factors and at the time the study was done, attention was being focused on heart disease in men rather than women since, at any given age, the incidence rates were higher for men. A very practical reason, which follows on from the last point, is that since the disease is rarer in women, a substantially larger sample would have been required to yield enough cases for useful analysis; that is, to achieve the necessary 'statistical power'. However, it is also true that the majority of epidemiological studies carried out at this time tended to exclude women, and it has been suggested that researchers assumed (incorrectly) that results would be equally applicable to both sexes.

3. The sampling frame was the updated age-sex registers of the selected general practices in the 24 towns.

4. Some of the points to consider are:

   • The practices were located in medium-sized towns, chosen purposefully according to set criteria to cover all regions of the country, but excluding rural and major urban populations.

   • The practices were selected from among all those in the town on the basis of certain criteria, and these may have favoured better organised practices.

- There were exclusions, but these were relatively few in number (6–10 per practice: 1.4 per cent to 2.4 per cent of the men selected from each practice population).

- From the randomly selected sample, 78 per cent responded. This would be considered a high response rate.

Thus, although the sampling frame was not random, it was designed to be representative, apart from excluding rural and major urban areas. The sample of men was selected randomly, exclusions werefew, and the response rate fairly high. Overall, this sample can be expected to be fairly representative of the population of middle-aged British men.

Section 5.3

Exercise 5.3.1

The following table summarises (question 1) the main components of blood pressure measurement, and (question 2) the possible sources of error:

Component of procedure	Source of error
Person taking the measurements (known as the *observer*)	(a) Training and knowledge of correct procedure, especially interpreting the sounds (Korotkow sounds) heard through the stethoscope.
	(b) Expectations of blood pressure level, e.g. that this would be higher in an overweight person.
	c) Awareness of the patient's disease state may influence the observations taken by the observer.
Machine used to take measurement	(a) Condition of machine, e.g. whether tubing leaks, etc.
	(b) How well *calibrated* the machine is; how accurately the machine records the true pressure can lead to error.
Circumstances in which measurement made	Subject's blood pressure is affected by anxiety, posture, recent exercise, etc.

Question 3. We noted in Chapter 4 that measurement error can be systematic (bias) or random. This distinction is very important in terms of the effect the error can have on the data, and in respect of what can be done to avoid or reduce the error. The table over the page identifies the ways in which the BRHS team minimised the possible sources of error and bias that could occur in measurement of blood pressure in the CHD arm of the study.

Exercise 5.3.2

Death certification should have been traceable on all men who died. There is a possibility, however, that cases could have been missed if cancer had been diagnosed but the death was due to another underlying cause. It is also possible that where the cause of death was due to a different underlying cause, such as a heart attack, for instance, the person had early stages of cancer but it was undiagnosed.

Type of error	Methods of minimising error in BRHS	Comment
Observer	(a) Diastolic taken at disappearance of sounds (phase V)	(a) This helps standardise readings, as diastolic (the pressure when the heart is between beats) is read by some people at phase IV (when sounds become muffled), and by others at phase V. There is usually about 5 mmHg difference, but it can be a lot more.
	(b) Training with audio tapes	(b) This type of training is a standard procedure.
	(c) Random allocation of observers to study subjects	(c) This allocation means that any observer bias will not, overall, be associated with important variables such as weight, alcohol consumption, etc.
	(d) Use of London School of Hygiene sphygmomanometer	(d) This sphygmomanometer was designed to prevent observers seeing the level of the mercury column (blood pressure level) until the procedure was completed. It also avoids the tendency to round levels to convenient numbers, e.g. 93 to 95, or 90 (this is called *digit preference*).
	(e) Adjustment for observer error in the analysis	(e) This involves statistical adjustment at the stage of analysis, and is referred to in paper B.
Machine error	Calibration	The settings of the machine are checked and adjusted at regular intervals.
Circumstances of measurement	(a) Subject seated with arm on cushion	(a) This helps to standardise posture, make the subject comfortable, and keep the arm at roughly the same position relative to the heart – all of which affect the recorded blood pressure.
	(b) Blood pressure measured twice	(b) Successive readings tend to fall, as the subject relaxes. The mean of two was used for analysis.

Cancer registration should include all diagnosed cases of cancer. This component of the system should therefore have picked up all known cancer morbidity among the sample. The postal questionnaires were used as a back-up to find any cases that had been missed or any very recently diagnosed cases that were not yet included on the registry database. It is not clear whether the responses given were validated with GP or hospital records, however.

On balance, the system for ascertaining cases appears to have been fairly thorough.

Section 5.4

Exercise 5.4.1

1. Paper A does not report that any additional information was collected on either exposure to risk factors (such as BMI and smoking) or the potentially protective effect of exercise. Under the heading of ascertainment of cases, we are informed that three further questionnaires were sent out in 1992, 1996 and 1998 asking about cancer diagnosis, but there is no discussion of changes in risk factors during the follow-up period, so the reader can assume that this information was only collected at the initial screening. A 5-year follow-up questionnaire was, however, used to reassess some risk factors (changes in smoking, drinking and economic status) for the heart disease component of the BRHS (see paper C, p. 368).

2. If those who took more exercise had been more likely to give up smoking during the follow-up period, smoking prevalence would have been relatively overestimated in the vigorous exercise group. The observed lower risk of cancer in the vigorous exercise group might then be at least partly due to a much larger true difference in smoking over the follow-up period than was apparent from the baseline data. We might note, however, that we would only expect to see this effect for cancers related to smoking, and there would need to be sufficient follow-up time for the growing difference in smoking rates to impact on new cases of cancer.

Section 5.5

Exercise 5.5.1

1. Incidence of cancer in the 'none/occasional exercise' group $= 8.4$ per 1000 person-years.

2. Incidence in the 'vigorous exercise' group $= 5.7$ per 1000 person-years.

3. Incidence in the 'vigorous exercise' group is 0.68 times that in the 'none/occasional exercise' group, that is, 32 % lower.

Exercise 5.5.2

1. The relative risk (RR) for ex-smokers $=$ incidence in exposed/incidence in unexposed $= 6.66/2.36 = 2.82$. RR for smokers $= 8.07/2.36 = 3.42$.

2. Interpretation: Smoking is clearly associated with an increased risk of IHD. What is surprising, is that ex-smokers had a RR that was not much less than current smokers (2.82 versus 3.42). This gradation of risk from never smokers, through ex-smokers to current smokers is an example of a *dose-response* relationship in which the greater the exposure to the risk factor (dose), the greater is the effect on outcome (response). This finding is one of a number of indications that an association may be causal, and we will return to this in Section 5.7.

3. The words we have used so far have been chosen carefully: thus, on the basis of the BRHS data studied so far, we have said that smoking appears to be *associated* with an increased risk of IHD, but we have not said it definitely causes it. We can see that the RR is quite large (around 3.5 for smokers), and also that there is some evidence of a *dose-response* relationship, both of which are suggestive of causation. Apart from chance effects, however, there is one other important explanation of an observed association such as this which we should start to consider. What if people who smoke more also tend to have higher cholesterol, take less exercise, and have higher blood pressure? Is it possible that it is these factors, and not the smoking, that are contributing to the IHD? This process is called *confounding*, which we will look at in more detail in Section 5.7.

Exercise 5.5.3

1. The group with the lowest level of exercise (none/occasional exercise) was taken as the reference group.

2. We do not have to use this group as the reference (any group could be used), but this choice seems entirely appropriate as we can see how increasing exposure to exercise is associated with a reduced risk of cancer. In addition, it is the largest group, so provides a well-estimated (more precise) reference for the comparisons.

Exercise 5.5.4

1. In Table 5.5.3 the variable *exercise* can take only take the values 'none/occasional' or 'vigorous' exercise. The variable *cancer* can take the value 'case' and 'non-case'. They are both **categorical** variables. (The physical index variable shown in Table 5.5.1 is an **ordered categorical** variable, with values that range from none/occasional exercise to vigorous exercise.)

2. and 3.

Exercise category	Cancer				
	Cases		Other men		Total
	No.	%	No.	%	
None/occ	424	**14**	2593	**86**	3017
Vigorous	47	**9**	466	**91**	513
Total	471	**13**	3059	**87**	3530

4. We see that the percentages of 'vigorous exercisers' who developed cancer (9 per cent) was less than the percentage of 'none/occasional' exercisers who developed cancer (14 per cent). We are interested in knowing whether this difference is because exercise and cancer are (inversely) associated, or whether it is just the result of chance – due to sampling error.

Exercise 5.5.5

1. Cancer is the outcome variable and exercise in the exposure variable.

2. The population of interest is all middle-aged British men.

Exercise 5.5.6

Table 5.5.4 Physical activity and cancer: expected frequencies

Physical activity	Cancer		Total
	Cases	Other men	
None/occ	402.55	2614.45	3017
Vigorous	68.45	444.55	513
Total	471	3059	3530

Exercise 5.5.7

Table 5.5.5 Physical activity and cancer: residuals

Physical activity	Cancer		Total
	Cases	Other men	
None/occ	21.45	−21.45	0.00
Vigorous	−21.45	21.45	0.00
Total	0.00	0.00	

Exercise 5.5.8

Table 5.5.6 Physical activity and cancer chi-squared table

Physical activity	Cancer		Total
	Cases	Other men	
None/occ	1.14	0.18	1.32
Vigorous	6.72	1.04	7.76
Total	7.86	1.22	9.08

Adding all four values in the cells $(1.14 + 0.18 + 6.72 + 1.04)$, we obtain 9.08, this being the value of the chi squared statistic.

Section 5.7

Exercise 5.7.1

Model 1: From the information given in this model, heavy alcohol consumption would confound the association between smoking and high blood pressure. In fact alcohol is a recognised cause of raised blood pressure, while smoking is not. Any observed association is due to confounding.

Model 2: From the information given in this model, cigarette smoking cannot confound the radon – lung cancer association. Although there is no question that smoking causes lung cancer, it is not associated with radon exposure; that is to say, people living in radon-exposed homes do not, on average, smoke any more than people living in homes that are not exposed to radon.

Model 3: This is a rather more complex situation, but such is life! Damp housing does cause respiratory illness, but that is not the whole story. People living in damp houses are in general poorer, and through this exposed to many other influences that can cause respiratory illness. These would include higher rates of smoking, work exposure, environmental pollution from traffic and industry, and so on. This is a situation where the observed association between damp housing and respiratory illness can be explained in two ways:

- In part a direct causal effect through mould, cold, damp air, etc.

- In part due to the association with poverty and the lifestyle, environmental and employment factors that come with that.

This situation is all too common in health research, and provides some insight into why establishing causation requires careful study design and interpretation.

Section 5.8

Exercise 5.8.1

1. The predicted values of birthweight are 2.79 kg for 37 weeks; 3.31 kg for 41.5 weeks.

2. These values should (and do) lie on the regression line.

3. It is not appropriate to use this regression relationship to calculate the birthweight of a baby of 28 weeks' gestation because we should never use regression to go beyond the range of the observed x variable data (in this case the x variable is gestational age).

Section 5.9

Exercise 5.9.1

1. The none/occasional exercise group is taken as the reference category, so the relative risk is quoted as 1.00. Note that this does not mean this level of exercise is associated with no risk of cancer: it simply means we can now compare other groups with this group, using the values of relative risk obtained for these from the regression analysis. Selecting this group as the reference is a sensible choice, as it makes the protective effect of higher levels of exercise easy to comprehend. A second, important reason for choosing the none/occasional group as the reference is that it is the largest, so that estimates of risk in this group are the most precisely estimated of all the groups.

2. The RR is 0.65, with a 95 per cent CI of 0.44–0.88. Thus, the estimated effect is a 35 per cent reduction in risk, and we can be 95 per cent confident that the population risk is reduced by 12–56 per cent. This interval does not include 1.00, so the finding is statistically significant at the 0.05 level. The effect of adjustment for age is small, reducing the relative risk estimate from 0.68 to 0.65.

3. Adjustment for all five potential confounding factors has more effect, attenuating the relative risk estimate to 0.76, equivalent now to a 24 per cent reduction in risk. The 95 per cent CI includes 1.00, and ranges from a 44 per cent reduction in risk to a 4 per cent increase in risk; hence, it is not significant at the 0.05 level. Thus, adjustment for all these other factors does suggest that part of the effect we originally observed was due to confounding. Although the result for vigorous exercise does not quite reach significance, we can see that the adjusted estimate for moderately vigorous exercise (which has larger numbers of subjects and hence

more 'power') is similar at 0.78, and the 95 per cent CI does not include 1.00. Overall, these results suggest that the finding of a protective effect of vigorous exercise is independent of confounding, and this is evidence in favour of causality.

4. The statistically significant test for trend provides evidence of a dose-response relationship, further evidence that the association is likely to be causal. The hypothesis test used (chi-squared for linear trend) will be discussed further in Chapter 11.

6

Case-control studies

Introduction and learning objectives

In Chapter 5, we noted that there are two commonly used, analytic, observational study designs, and we have studied the first of these – cohort studies. In this chapter we will look at the second design – the case-control study. Although more commonly used than the cohort design, case-control studies are in some respects more complex in terms of methods and interpretation. Your familiarity with cohort studies will help in understanding the strengths and limitations of case-control studies.

By the end of the chapter, you should be able to do the following:

- Describe the purpose and structure of a case-control study design, within an overall framework of epidemiological study designs.

- Give examples of the uses of case-control studies.

- Describe the strengths and weaknesses of case-control studies.

- Describe the most important types of bias that can arise with case-control studies, and how these can be minimised.

- Describe the purpose of using multiple controls in a case-control study.

- Describe the information required to calculate sample size, and interpret the output of sample size calculation with Epi Info (StatCalc).

- Describe how confounding can be avoided through matching.

- Describe the odds ratio (OR) as used in the analysis of a case-control study, and its relationship with relative risk.

- Calculate an OR in simple unmatched and matched case-control study analyses.

(*Continued*)

Quantitative Methods for Health Research   Nigel Bruce, Daniel Pope and Debbi Stanistreet
© 2008 John Wiley & Sons, Ltd

- Describe the approach used to calculate the OR in unmatched and matched case-control studies with multiple controls.

- Describe the various approaches to dealing with confounding in the analysis of a case-control study, including stratification and multiple logistic regression.

- Describe the use of, and principles underlying, multiple logistic regression, including the appropriate circumstances for use of unconditional and conditional methods.

- Calculate the adjusted OR from the logistic regression coefficient, and interpret the OR and 95 per cent confidence interval (CI).

Resource paper

We will explore case-control studies using material from the following paper. This describes a case-control study of pregnant women designed to investigate whether caffeine increases the risk of spontaneous abortion.

Paper A

Cnattingius, S., Signorello, L. B., Annerén, G. *et al.* (2000). Caffeine intake and the risk of the first-trimester spontaneous abortion. *N Engl J Med* **343**, 1839–1845.

Please now read the abstract for paper A given below.

Abstract

Background

Some epidemiologic studies have suggested that the ingestion of caffeine increases the risk of spontaneous abortion, but the results have been inconsistent.

Methods

We performed a population-based, case–control study of early spontaneous abortion in Uppsala County, Sweden. The subjects were 562 women who had spontaneous abortion at 6 to 12 completed weeks of gestation (the case patients) and 953 women who did not have spontaneous abortion and were matched to the case patients according to the week of gestation and area of residence (controls). Information on the ingestion of caffeine was obtained from in-person interviews. Plasma cotinine was measured as an indicator of cigarette smoking, and fetal karyotypes* were determined from tissue samples. Multivariate analysis was used to estimate the relative risks associated with caffeine ingestion after adjustment for smoking and symptoms of pregnancy such as nausea, vomiting, and tiredness.

Results

Among non-smokers, more spontaneous abortions occurred in women who ingested at least 100 mg of caffeine per day than in women who ingested less than 100 mg per day, with the increase in risk related to the amount ingested (100 to 299 mg per day: odds ratio, 1.3; 95 percent confidence interval, 0.9 to 1.8; 300 to 499 mg per day: odds ratio, 1.4; 95 percent confidence interval, 0.9 to 2.0; and 500 mg or more per day: odds ratio, 2.2; 95 percent confidence interval, 1.3 to 3.8). Among smokers, caffeine ingestion was not associated with an excess risk of spontaneous abortion. When the analyses were stratified according to the results of karyotyping, the ingestion of moderate or high levels of caffeine was found to be associated with an excess risk of spontaneous abortion when the fetus had a normal or unknown karyotype but not when the fetal karyotype was abnormal.

Conclusions

The ingestion of caffeine may increase the risk of an early spontaneous abortion among non-smoking women carrying fetuses with normal karyotypes.

∗ Further explanation of the term 'Karyotype' is given in section 6.2.1

6.1 Why do a case-control study?

6.1.1 Study objectives

We will begin our examination of case-control studies by establishing why the authors of this Swedish study chose this design to address their research question. This is described in the introduction section of paper A, reproduced below.

Introduction

Caffeine is a naturally occurring compound that is metabolized more slowly in pregnant women than in nonpregnant women.[1] Caffeine passes readily through the placenta to the fetus,[1] but the biologic mechanisms by which caffeine could induce a spontaneous abortion are not known.[2,3] The results of epidemiologic studies relating the ingestion of caffeine to the risk of spontaneous abortion have been inconclusive,[4–13] partly because the relation between the consumption of coffee (usually the primary source of caffeine), symptoms of pregnancy (such as nausea or aversion to the odour or taste of coffee), and fetal viability is complex. In response to such symptoms, many women decrease their ingestion of caffeine during pregnancy. Because the symptoms are more common among women with viable pregnancies than among those with nonviable pregnancies, the ingestion of caffeine in early pregnancy may reflect, rather than affect, fetal viability.[6,14]

Most previous studies have not included in their analyses data on symptoms of pregnancy,[4,5,8,11–13] and the few that have included these data have used fairly insensitive markers, such as the presence or absence of nausea or vomiting at any time during pregnancy.[6,7,9,10] Moreover, only one study with a sufficient sample size focused on the first trimester of pregnancy,[12] when changes in caffeine intake, pregnancy-related symptoms, and the majority of spontaneous abortions occur.

In epidemiologic studies, the range of caffeine ingestion has been narrow.[5–8,10,11,13] Moreover, the assessment of exposure has been suboptimal, with the reporting of caffeine intake occurring long after the period in question or with little regard to changes in ingestion during pregnancy.[4–6,8–10,12,13]

(Continued)

Finally, studies of caffeine ingestion and spontaneous abortion have, with one exception,[10] not distinguished between chromosomally normal and abnormal fetuses. In Sweden, the consumption of coffee is high, and health care coverage is nationwide; it was therefore possible to investigate whether caffeine is associated with an elevated risk of early spontaneous abortion in the general population. The current study was designed to analyze caffeine intake, smoking status, symptoms of pregnancy, and the risk of spontaneous abortion. In addition, fetal tissue, when available, was collected for chromosomal analysis.

 ### Self-Assessment Exercise 6.1.1

1. Make a list of all the research issues, including the limitations of previous studies, and the aim and objectives of the study noted in the Introduction to paper A.

2. Why do you think the authors chose to carry out a case-control study instead of a cohort study?

Answers in Section 6.6

6.1.2 Study structure

It is important to gain an overall understanding of the structure of a case-control study before we get into too much of the methodological detail. For the Swedish study, this is described in the methods section, part of which is reproduced below.

Study subjects

The study was conducted in Uppsala County, Sweden, from 1996 through 1998. Cases of spontaneous abortion were identified at the Department of Obstetrics and Gynecology of Uppsala University Hospital... During this period, we identified as potential case patients 652 women with spontaneous abortions who presented at the department at 6 to 12 completed weeks of gestation... 562 (86 percent) agreed to participate... The control subjects were selected primarily from the antenatal care clinics in Uppsala County. They were frequency-matched to the women who had had spontaneous abortions with regard to duration of gestation (in completed weeks) and area of residence (one of the five municipalities in the county). Of the 1037 women who were seeking antenatal care and were asked to participate, 953 (92 percent) agreed to do so.

Collection of Data

Three midwives conducted in-person interviews with the women with spontaneous abortion and the control subjects recruited among patients receiving antenatal care, using a structured questionnaire... All the women were asked to report specific sources of caffeine ingested daily on a week-by-week basis, starting four weeks before the last menstrual period and ending in the most recently completed week of gestation... We also collected data on other potential risk factors...

There are essentially four key steps in carrying out a case-control study:

- Identification of *cases*, that is, the people with the disease or outcome. In this study, cases were Swedish women with spontaneous abortions after 6–12 weeks' gestation, presenting to the hospital in Uppsala county.

- Identification of *controls*, that is, people who do not have the disease or outcome. In this study, they were women attending antenatal care. We will look at the technique of matching later (including frequency matching).

- Measurement of potential risk factors for spontaneous abortion among the cases and controls. In this study, the risk factor of interest was caffeine, and a range of other potential risk factors (including possible confounding factors) were also measured.

- Analysis of whether or not the *cases* were more likely to have been *exposed* to a risk factor than were the *controls*. In this study, we will want to see whether cases (those experiencing spontaneous abortion) had higher caffeine intake than controls.

The basic structure of a case-control study, using the exposure and outcome from the Swedish study, is illustrated in Figure 6.1.1. To summarise, study participants were selected in Uppsala

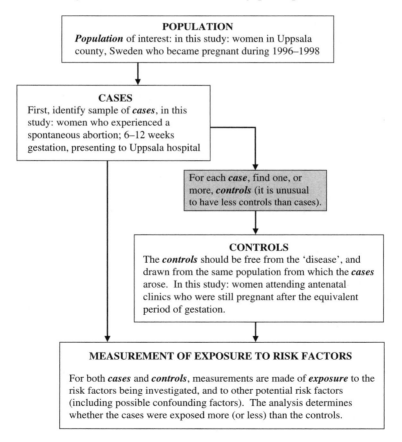

Figure 6.1.1   Overview of the structure of a case-control study, with exposure and outcomes drawn from the Swedish study (paper A)

County, Sweden from 1996 to 1998. *Cases* were women who had had a spontaneous abortion after 6–12 completed weeks' gestation and presented to the Obstetrics and Gynecology Department at Uppsala University Hospital, and who consented to take part ($n = 562$). *Controls* were pregnant women selected from antenatal clinics in Uppsala County who consented to take part ($n = 953$). Some matching of controls to cases was carried out, by which we mean that controls were selected to be similar to cases. In this study matching was done on two factors, namely duration of gestation (in completed weeks) and area of residence (county). This is done in order to reduce the effect of confounding, and we will look at the why and how of matching in some detail in Section 6.2.2. Finally, we can see that more than one control has been selected for each case; in fact, around twice as many. This is done to increase the statistical power of the study, and is considered further in Section 6.4 on sample size.

6.1.3 Approach to analysis

We have said that the approach to the analysis is to determine whether or not cases are more exposed to the risk factor(s) of interest than are the controls. This is illustrated diagrammatically in Figure 6.1.2. We will return to this concept in Section 6.3 when we look in detail at the analysis of case-control studies, and how the odds ratio *(OR)* is used to express this difference between cases and controls in the chances of being exposed. For the simplified example illustrated in Figure 6.1.2, we keep to the objective of paper A (risk factors for spontaneous abortion), but for ease of illustration restrict the study to just 30 cases and 30 controls.

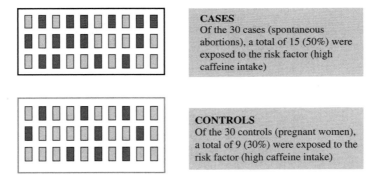

Figure 6.1.2 A hypothetical case-control comparison, investigating the association between exposure to a risk factor (high caffeine intake, compared with no/low intake) and spontaneous abortion

In this example, each square represents a woman, those in the upper box being cases (women experiencing a spontaneous abortion), and those in the lower box, controls (pregnancy continues). A darker shaded square means that the woman was exposed to the risk factor (high caffeine intake). A higher percentage of cases (50 per cent) were exposed to the risk factor than were controls (30 per cent). The analysis of a case-control study concentrates on quantifying this difference in exposure between cases and controls.

6.1.4 Retrospective data collection

The term *retrospective* is often associated with case-control studies, just as the term *prospective* is associated with cohort studies:

- *Retrospective* means looking backwards in time. If cases are identified now, the exposure must have occurred in the past. We must look backwards in time to find out about that exposure, either by asking the people concerned, or (if we are fortunate) finding sufficiently complete and valid records of that exposure.

- *Prospective*, a term we have already mentioned in respect of cohort studies, means looking forward in time. If a survey measuring exposure is done now, we await the occurrence of cases in the future.

These concepts are summarised in Figure 6.1.3;

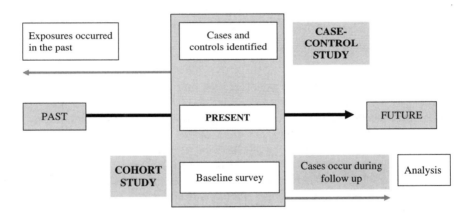

Figure 6.1.3 Time perspectives most commonly seen in case-control and cohort studies. These perspectives do not always apply, however, as explained below in the text

You may find examples of case-control analyses being carried out on data that have been collected prospectively, and cohort studies carried out retrospectively; for example:

- A case-control study analysis can be carried out within a prospective cohort study, perhaps for an outcome other than the main one for which the cohort study has been set up. Thus, as cases of this other outcome occur during follow-up these are selected (and become the cases for the 'nested' case-control study), and controls are selected from other study subjects in the cohort who remain free from that outcome. Information on exposure, other risk factors and confounders is available from the baseline survey.

- A cohort study can be carried out retrospectively if complete and accurate records exist of exposure, other risk factors and confounders for a cohort of people, such as employees of a large company, some of whom have now developed the disease or outcome of interest. In effect, information on a 'baseline' can be extracted from records, and since that information was recorded long before cases of disease appeared, there is no risk of bias from knowledge of who did or did not become cases (so long as data extraction is done 'blind' to this knowledge). Incidence rates for exposed and non-exposed can then be calculated as for a prospective cohort study.

However, most case-control studies are retrospective, and since many of the most important design issues we need to be concerned about arise from retrospective data collection, we will concentrate on this time perspective.

6.1.5 Applications of the case-control design

The case-control design can be used in a wide variety of circumstances, including:

- Understanding the cause of a disease or outcome of interest; for example, risk factors for cancer, death from violent injury, or (as in our example) spontaneous abortion.

- Measuring the effect of procedures or interventions; for example the effectiveness of breast-screening programmes.

- Investigation of disease outbreaks; for example, food poisoning.

Case-control studies are the design of choice for health outcomes with a long latency period – that is, the time period between exposure and onset of the disease (most cancers) – or that are relatively rare (many specific types of cancer, again). For very rare conditions, case-control studies may be the only option, as cohort studies would be impractical, if not impossible, within any reasonable timescale or budget. The obvious benefits of the case-control studies over alternative designs are the savings made in terms of cost and time. However, as we shall see later in this chapter, given the typically retrospective nature of the case-control study design, there are a number of important methodological issues that require careful attention in design and interpretation.

Summary

- The case-control design can provide strong, quantified evidence about the importance of risk factors or the effect of interventions, and is more practical than a cohort study where the outcome is (a) rare and/or (b) has a long latency period.

- A case-control study essentially involves:

  a) The identification of cases;

  b) The selection of controls, which may be matched to a greater or lesser extent (discussed further in Section 6.3);

c) The measurement of exposure to risk factors of interest, including possible confounders;

d) Analysis of any difference in exposure between cases and controls.

- Collection of data on the characteristics of cases and controls, including the exposure to risk factors, is usually done after the disease event has occurred. This is known as retrospective data collection, and is one of the reasons why case-control studies are more vulnerable to bias than cohort studies, where the events occur after the assessment of exposure and other variables (prospective data collection).

- There are sometimes circumstances in which assessment of exposure in a case-control study can be done prospectively.

6.2 Key elements of study design

6.2.1 Selecting the cases

Case definition and selection

We have noted that the first step in carrying out a case-control study is to identify the cases. As with cohort studies, it is very important to have a clear case definition, and to describe carefully how cases were selected. The following section from paper A describes how this case ascertainment was done in the Swedish study. Some additional background information on the terminology used for the assessment of chromosome abnormalities is provided after Exercise 6.2.1 below.

Study subjects

Cases of spontaneous abortion were identified at the Department of Obstetrics and Gynecology of Uppsala University Hospital, which is the only place in the county for the care of women with spontaneous abortions. During this period, we identified as potential case patients 652 women with spontaneous abortions who presented at the department at 6 to 12 completed weeks of gestation and whose pregnancies had been confirmed by a positive test.[15] Of these women, 562 (86 percent) agreed to participate. Among the 293 women in whom chorionic villi were identified in tissue obtained at curettage, karyotyping was successful in 258 (88 percent). Chromosomes were studied with the use of G-banding, and 11 cells in metaphase were routinely analyzed[16]; karyotyping was considered unsuccessful if fewer than 3 cells in metaphase were obtained. Karyotype analysis revealed that 101 fetuses (58 male and 43 female) were chromosomally normal and 157 (72 male, 63 female, 16 with triploidy, and 6 with tetraploidy) were abnormal. . . All potential control subjects underwent vaginal ultrasonography before the interview. If a nonviable intrauterine pregnancy was detected, the woman was recruited as a member of the group with spontaneous abortion (this occurred in 53 of the 562 case patients).

Self-Assessment Exercise 6.2.1

1. Describe how cases were defined.

2. Describe how and where cases were identified.

3. Comment on the overall quality of the case ascertainment.

Answers in Section 6.6

Notes on investigation of genetic karyotype

The karyotype describes the features of the chromosomes (genetic, DNA material) that were examined, where possible, at the time of the abortion. Triploidy means that there was an extra chromosome, and tetraploidy that there were two extra chromosomes. A fetus with this type of abnormality is at increased risk of spontaneous abortion. The authors included examination of chromosomal abnormalities, as only one previous study had done so, and it was felt important to distinguish possible effects of caffeine on genetically normal fetuses from those which were abnormal.

6.2.2 The controls

Selecting the control group

Having identified a total of 562 women who had experienced spontaneous abortions in the first trimester and who consented to participate in the study, the next step was to select the controls. Selecting the most appropriate groups of controls can be one of the most demanding aspects of a case-control study. We will look first at how this was done in the Swedish study and then consider some general points about control selection. The cases in the Swedish study were women who had experienced a spontaneous abortion in the first trimester, and who attended the Department of Obstetrics and Gynaecology at Uppsala University Hospital.

The single most important principle in control selection is that the controls should be representative of the population from which the cases have arisen, but without the disease in question. Let's see how this helps to understand the choice made in the Swedish study.

The first step is to ask ourselves from what population the cases arose from. The answer to this lies at the beginning of the excerpt on 'Study subjects' from paper A (above). The research team were dealing with all (or virtually all) spontaneous abortions for which medical care was sought in Uppsala County. The population from which these cases arose was therefore the Uppsala County population, but with the qualification that they were women who attended the hospital when they experienced a spontaneous abortion. Although it can be expected that most women in Sweden having a spontaneous abortion would attend the hospital, not all would. Furthermore, it is likely that those who do not attend would differ in some respects from those who do, so that the group attending the hospital will not be fully representative of the Uppsala County population.

Thus, we would be looking for a method that selected a group of control subjects representative of pregnant women from Uppsala County population, in the first trimester, and who consulted medical services in a way comparable with cases. Let's now look at the full description of how controls were selected for the Swedish study.

The control subjects were selected primarily from the antenatal care clinics in Uppsala County. They were frequency-matched to the women who had had spontaneous abortions with regard to duration of gestation (in completed weeks) and area of residence (one of the five municipalities in the county). Of the 1037 women who were seeking antenatal care and were asked to participate, 953 (92 percent) agreed to do so. All potential control subjects underwent vaginal ultrasonography before the interview. If a nonviable intrauterine pregnancy was detected, the woman was recruited as a member of the group with spontaneous abortion (this occurred in 53 of the 562 case patients).

In Uppsala County, there are approximately 3 legally induced abortions for every 10 completed pregnancies, and some of these terminated pregnancies would have resulted in spontaneous abortion if the pregnancy had continued. To limit bias in the selection of control subjects, women with induced abortions were added to the control group. In total, 310 women who had undergone induced abortions were asked to participate, and 273 (88 percent) agreed to do so. In these supplementary analyses, women with induced abortions were added to the control group according to the distribution of the length of gestation of induced abortions in Uppsala County during the study period.

 Self-Assessment Exercise 6.2.2

1. How well does the selection of controls meet the principle we specified, that is, they should be representative of the population from which the cases have arisen, but without the disease in question?

2. Comment on the addition of induced abortions to the control group. What effect might this have on the results?

Answers in Section 6.6

Bias arising from control selection

The discussion in the answer to question 1 from Exercise 6.2.2 (above) illustrates some of the complex issues that may need to be considered in selecting controls. In order for these problems with control selection to bias the results of the study (the relationship between caffeine and spontaneous abortion), one or more of the factors that determine who gets into the case and control groups needs to be associated with the exposure. We have already suggested that attendance at antenatal clinics in the first trimester is related to socio-economic factors and these in turn could well be related to caffeine intake.

Let's also consider another situation. A case-control study in a developed country is investigating lung cancer in men aged 40–65, and cases have been recruited from a hospital. Since this is a very serious disease in relatively young people, we can assume that virtually all cases in the population will end up in hospital, so although the cases are recruited from hospital, they are effectively representative of all cases in the population. Therefore, following our principle for control selection, we should select controls to represent the population of males less than 65 years of age. One approach would be to select controls through general practice lists, probably matching a few variables such as age and area of residence. It might appear counter-intuitive to use general practice-based controls for cases selected as inpatients, but it does follow logically from the need to ensure that controls arise from the same population as cases.

If, on the other hand, hospital controls were sought, we would have to ensure that (a) there were no health-care access issues that might prevent the controls being representative of the population, and (b) that the disease condition for which they were admitted was not related to lung cancer risk factors (e.g. smoking). Sometimes, if it is difficult to decide on which approach will deliver the most appropriate controls, more than one control group can be used. If the results using (for example) hospital and general practice-based control groups differ markedly, further investigation would need to be made into which approach is providing the less biased finding.

We have mentioned matching on a number of occasions, and will now look at this aspect of case-control design in more detail.

Matching

You will recall the importance of **confounding** when it comes to interpreting associations between **risk factors** and **outcomes**. The figure below shows the model of confounding (introduced in Chapter 5). It has been adapted here to consider the possible causal effect of caffeine ingestion on spontaneous abortion in the first trimester, and the role of confounding due to pregnancy symptoms such as nausea (which are associated with the viability of the fetus) (Figure 6.2.1).

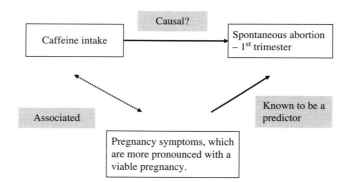

Figure 6.2.1 Diagram summarising how pregnancy symptoms (nausea, etc.) could confound the relationship observed between caffeine intake and spontaneous abortion

In this model, pregnancy symptoms such as nausea (a) can discourage a woman from drinking coffee, and (b) are associated with a healthy fetus. If this is the predominant mechanism at work, it could be the symptoms that are mainly responsible for any observed association between higher caffeine intake and adverse pregnancy outcome (spontaneous abortion), and not the caffeine itself. Thus, any observed association between high caffeine intake and spontaneous abortion could be explained by a lack of aversive symptoms resulting from an already non-viable fetus.

Matching overcomes confounding by preventing it from occurring in the first place. This is done by making cases and controls similar with respect to potential confounding factors. In the Swedish study, matching was not carried out specifically on symptoms, as this would have been very impractical, and we will see how the authors dealt with this in the analysis. Matching was, however, done on gestational age, which can confound the relationship between caffeine and spontaneous abortion because gestational age and caffeine intake are related, and gestational age is an important determinant of the risk of spontaneous abortion.

By matching the cases and controls for gestational age, we know that any effect of this factor on (a) caffeine intake and (b) risk of spontaneous abortion is the same in both cases and controls. Thus, let's say woman A (a case) has a spontaneous abortion at 11 weeks, and was taking an average of 250 mg of caffeine per day. If she is matched to a control with the same gestational age, we have removed the possibility that any association subsequently observed between caffeine intake and being a case is due to any relationship between caffeine intake and gestational age.

One effect of matching is to remove the possibility of studying the association between the variable matched (e.g. gestational age) and the outcome (e.g. spontaneous first trimester abortion). This does not matter because the association is well established and was not one of the research questions for the Swedish study. There are a number of related issues that are worth considering at this point, and these are explored through the following self-assessment exercise.

 Self-Assessment Exercise 6.2.3

1. The other factor matched for in the Swedish study was area of residence. What confounding factor, or factors, were the authors trying to avoid by doing this?

2. If matching helps prevent confounding, why do you think the team did not match for a lot more possible confounding factors?

Answers in Section 6.6.

In this study, the research team did not *individually match* controls to cases but instead used *frequency matching*. Controls 'were frequency-matched to the women who had had spontaneous abortions with regard to duration of gestation (in completed weeks) and area of residence (one of the five municipalities in the county)'. With frequency matching (group matching) controls are selected according to the proportion of all cases that are in categories of the matching variable (e.g. county of residence). Thus, if 6 per cent of women are of gestational age 10 weeks and live in County X, then the research team will ensure that 6 per cent of controls have the same gestational age and county. This differs from *individual matching*, in which controls are selected individually for each case by the matching variables. In that case, if a case is from County Y and 9 weeks' gestation, a control will be sought with the same characteristics. The choice of individual or frequency matching will involve consideration of study precision and the practicalities of matching, further exploration of which are beyond the scope of this book.

Implications of matching for analysis

We have already said that matching should be done judiciously, and not overdone. Some studies do not match at all, and deal with the problem of confounding entirely at the stage of analysis.

A study that has not been matched will be subjected to **unmatched analysis**. A matched study will normally be analysed by **matched analysis**, as this is more efficient, but unmatched analysis can also be used. We will study both of these analysis methods in Section 6.3.

Multiple controls

We saw in paper A that approximately two controls were selected for each case. The reason for selecting multiple controls is to increase the **statistical power** of the study $(1 - \beta)$, a concept introduced in Chapter 5. We could of course do this just by increasing the total number of cases and keep to a 1:1 ratio of cases and controls. However, in many situations, cases are harder to identify than controls, so it is simpler and cheaper to increase power by increasing the ratio of controls to cases. We will look in more detail at the multiple control selection in paper A, when considering **sample size** in Section 6.4.

6.2.3 Exposure assessment

Assessing the level of exposure to the risk factor(s) under study can also be a challenging component of case-control studies, not least because this is often done **retrospectively**. The following section of paper A describes how exposure data were collected for the Swedish study.

Collection of data

Three midwives conducted in-person interviews with the women with spontaneous abortion and the control subjects recruited among patients receiving antenatal care, using a structured questionnaire, and two doctors conducted interviews with the control subjects in whom abortions had been induced. Ninety percent of the case patients were interviewed within two weeks after the diagnosis of spontaneous abortion, and all were interviewed within seven weeks. All control subjects were interviewed in early pregnancy, within six days after their completed week of gestation used in matching. To avoid delay and to limit non-participation, 50 women who had had spontaneous abortion and 5 control subjects were interviewed by telephone.

All the women were asked to report specific sources of caffeine ingested daily on a week-by-week basis, starting four weeks before the last menstrual period and ending in the most recently completed week of gestation. Sources of caffeine included coffee (brewed, boiled, instant, and decaffeinated), tea (loose tea, tea bags, and herbal tea), cocoa, chocolate, soft drinks, and caffeine-containing medications. Respondents were offered four cup sizes from which to choose (1.0 dl, 1.5 dl, 2.0 dl, and 3.0 dl). Weekly consumption of soft drinks was estimated by the women in centiliters. We estimated the intake of caffeine using the following conversion factors: for 150 ml of coffee, 115 mg of caffeine if it was brewed, 90 mg if boiled, and 60 mg if instant; for 150 ml of tea, 39 mg if it was loose tea or a tea bag and 0 mg if herbal tea; for 150 ml of soft drinks (cola), 15 mg; for 150 ml of cocoa, 4 mg; and for 1 g of chocolate (bar), 0.3 mg. A few medications included 50 to 100 mg of caffeine per tablet.[17] Of all caffeine ingested, coffee accounted for 76 percent, tea for 23 percent, and other sources for 1 percent. None of the women ingested decaffeinated coffee predominantly. The mean daily amount of caffeine ingested was calculated from the time of estimated conception (two weeks after the last menstrual period) through the most recently completed week of gestation.

Plasma cotinine was measured by gas chromatography with use of N-ethylnorcotinine as an internal standard.[18] Blood samples for the measurement of cotinine were obtained from the case patients at the time of spontaneous abortion and from the control subjects at the time they were interviewed. We defined smokers as women who had a plasma cotinine concentration of more than 15 ng per milliliter[19]; for 23 women whose plasma cotinine values were missing, we used self-reported daily smoking during all weeks of pregnancy.

We determined scores for symptoms related to pregnancy for each week of gestation by assigning a score for nausea (0, never; 1, sometimes but not daily; 2, daily but not all day; 3, daily all day), vomiting (0, never; 1, sometimes but not daily; 2, daily), and fatigue (0, no; 1, yes but with unchanged sleeping habits; 2, yes with slightly changed sleeping habits; 3, yes with pronounced change in sleeping habits). We then calculated the average weekly score for each symptom. We also collected data on other potential risk factors.

 Self-Assessment Exercise 6.2.4

1. Make brief notes on how caffeine intake, pregnancy symptoms and smoking status were determined.

2. What aspects of these methods do you think could have led to bias?

Answers in Section 6.6.

6.2.4   Bias in exposure assessment

Having worked through Exercise 6.2.4, we can appreciate the problems of bias that can occur due to *retrospective* data collection. The critical issue, however, is whether the nature and extent of error in obtaining this information differs between cases and controls, as it is this difference that will lead to bias. Highlighted here are three important possible sources of bias in exposure assessment.

Recall bias

When asking people in these studies to recall their exposure to a given risk factor, there is always the possibility that the experience of having the disease (being a case) will alter people's actual knowledge of exposure, or the importance that they attach to it. This can happen because during the course of treatment the person (case) may have been asked questions about relevant exposure, or may be aware of media coverage of emerging theories or 'scares' about what causes the disease. Hence, when asked about the exposure, their description of their own level of exposure may well differ considerably from that of a control, even if in reality there is no difference between them in level of exposure.

Interviewer bias

In many case-control studies, including the Swedish study, much of the information is collected by interview. In a retrospective study where cases have already occurred, an interviewer setting out to collect information from the subjects will quite often know who is a case and who is a control. This would likely have been true for the interviewers in the Swedish study. We have seen in Chapter 5 on cohort studies how, even with training and checking, *observer bias* can still occur. Interviewers, knowing whether they are talking to a case or control, could allow their own knowledge of the disease to interfere with objectivity in eliciting information about exposure. Even if the interviewer cannot be 'blinded' to whether the interviewee is a case or a control, it may well be possible to downplay knowledge of the hypothesis under test, or to embed this among a number of topics (possible risk factors) being investigated so that it is not obvious which exposure the research team is most interested in.

Bias from records

Given the problems associated with individual recall of exposure, it would be ideal if valid and unbiased information could be retrieved from records, such as medical case notes or employment records. The key question to ask in this situation is whether the fact of being a case could have influenced the information in the records, in a way that differs from records of people used as controls. This becomes less likely the longer the period is between the time the record was made and the appearance of the illness, or some 'early sign' of that illness. In addition, such records may not have recorded the information exactly as required by the study, and some may be incomplete, but these problems are less likely to lead to serious bias.

The following exercise presents some case-control study scenarios. See whether you can spot potential sources of bias affecting the assessment of exposure to risk factors.

 Self-Assessment Exercise 6.2.5

Study	Hypothesis under study	Methods of assessing exposure
1	Investigation in the USA of whether the oral contraceptive pill (OCP) causes breast cancer.	Telephone interview of women (cases and controls), to determine history of type and duration of OCP use.
2	Investigation of efficacy of BCG vaccine in preventing tuberculosis in a developing country.	District-based clinic records of BCG vaccination.
3	Investigation of whether low birthweight is associated with poor educational performance at age 10 years in the UK.	Health-care records.

Answers in Section 6.6.

Summary

- Eligible cases must be clearly defined, and ascertained as completely as possible.

- Controls should be representative of the same population from which the cases arise, and free from the disease in question.

- Matching helps to overcome the problem of confounding, but not all case-control studies are matched. If matching is not carried out, confounding must be dealt with in the analysis.

- It is possible to over-match in a case-control study. It is therefore wise, and more practical, to match for a few key confounders, the effects of which are known already, and which are not strongly associated with the potential risk factors under study.

- Obtaining information about exposure to risk factors must usually be done retrospectively in a case-control study. This makes the study vulnerable to recall bias, interviewer bias, and bias from inconsistent records.

- If possible, the interviewer should not know whether the subject is a case or a control, but in practice this is often difficult or impossible to achieve.

- If possible, the interviewer should not be aware of the hypotheses under investigation, e.g. which risk factors are being studied as possible causes, or at least be unaware of which of a number of risk factors is the subject of the main study hypothesis.

6.3 Basic unmatched and matched analysis

6.3.1 The odds ratio (OR)

In the analysis of cohort studies, we introduced the concept of *relative risk* (RR), describing it as a means of expressing the way in which the risk of disease varies according to the level of exposure to a risk factor. We defined RR as (incidence of disease in *exposed* group) ÷ (incidence of disease in *unexposed* group). So, to calculate the RR, we need to know incidence rates in exposed and unexposed groups. We saw that a cohort study provides these incidence rates, but in most cases the case-control design does not. This is because the group of exposed people (to deal with that group first) are made up of some cases and some controls, and they are not usually a representative sample of all exposed people in the population. The same can be said of the unexposed group. The exception to this is a population-based case-control study where all or a known fraction of cases in the population are obtained together with a representative sample of controls (we discussed in Section 6.2 the extent to which the Swedish study is a true population case-control study).

In most case-control studies we do not have incidence rates, and therefore need another means of expressing and quantifying the concept of relative risk. This is provided by the *odds ratio* (OR). The OR compares the odds (chances) of a case being exposed to the risk factor with the odds of a control being exposed.

Calculation of the *OR* – simple unmatched analysis

As we noted previously, the Swedish study incorporated frequency matching for (a) duration of gestation and (b) area of residence. When matching has been used, it is more efficient – although not required – to use analysis that takes account of that. This is known as ***matched analysis***, and we will look at the techniques for this in Section 6.3.2. For now, we will look at how to calculate the OR in ***unmatched analysis*** using the results from the Swedish study. Let's start with a simple example. Illustrated below is the hypothetical case-control comparison introduced in Section 6.1 (Figure 6.1.2). This was based on the Swedish study, but with just 30 cases and 30 controls.

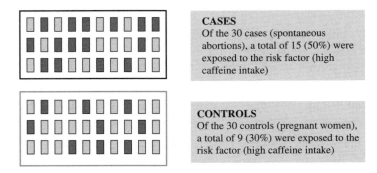

CASES
Of the 30 cases (spontaneous abortions), a total of 15 (50%) were exposed to the risk factor (high caffeine intake)

CONTROLS
Of the 30 controls (pregnant women), a total of 9 (30%) were exposed to the risk factor (high caffeine intake)

Figure 6.1.2 Hypothetical case-control comparison investigating the association between exposure to a risk factor (high caffeine intake versus no/low intake) and spontaneous abortion

This diagram can be summarised in a 2×2 contingency table as in Table 6.3.1.

Table 6.3.1 Outcome of hypothetical case-control study

	Cases	Controls
Exposed	15 (*a*)	9 (*b*)
Not exposed	15 (*c*)	21 (*d*)
Total	30	30

The OR is calculated as the odds of being exposed if a case (a:c) divided by the odds of being exposed if a control (b:d) and, by transformation, can be expressed as follows:

$$OR = \frac{a/c}{b/d} = \frac{(a) \times (d)}{(b) \times (c)}$$

Inserting the figures from Table 6.3.1, we get $(15 \times 21) \div (15 \times 9) = 2.33$. So the OR is 2.33. What does this mean? It means that the odds of exposure to the risk factor (caffeine intake) among the cases (spontaneous abortion) is 2.33 times greater than among the controls (pregnant women). It is a good approximation to the RR, and for all practical purposes we can take it to be that.

Interpreting the OR:

- An OR greater than 1 indicates the odds (or risk) of disease is greater among those who are exposed – that is, a positive association between risk factor and disease.

- An OR less than 1 indicates a reduced odds (or risk) of disease among the exposed – a negative association, or protective effect.

- An OR equal to 1 indicates no association between exposure to the risk factor and disease.

The 95 per cent CI for the OR

A **CI** to estimate the true OR in the population should be presented, giving more information than simply quoting the sample OR. This is usually obtained by computer (e.g. with SPSS), although an approximation can be calculated quite easily, as illustrated in the reference section below.

 RS - Reference section on statistical methods

We can estimate the standard error and hence CI using the *log* of the OR (we will return to the use of $\log_e$ OR later when we look at logistic regression methods for case-control studies in Section 6.5). The standard error of the log OR is:

$$\text{SE}\,[\log_e(\text{OR})] = \sqrt{\frac{1}{a} + \frac{1}{b} + \frac{1}{c} + \frac{1}{d}}$$

Using the data from Figure 6.1.2

	Cases	Controls
Exposed	15 (a)	9 (b)
Not exposed	15 (c)	21 (d)
Total	30	30

we obtained an OR of 2.3333 (truncated to 2.33 for ease of interpretation). The log OR is therefore $\log_e(2.33) = 0.8459$ with the standard error being

$$\text{SE}\,[\log_e(\text{OR})] = \sqrt{\frac{1}{15} + \frac{1}{9} + \frac{1}{15} + \frac{1}{21}} = \sqrt{0.2921} = 0.5404$$

Provided the sample is reasonably large, we can assume that the log OR comes from a normal distribution and thus the approximate 95 per cent CI is:

$$\log_e(\text{OR}) \pm 1.96 \times \text{SE}(\log_e(\text{OR})) =$$

$$0.8459 - 1.96 \times 0.5404 \text{ to } 0.8459 + 1.96 \times 0.5404 =$$

$$-0.2133 \text{ to } 1.9051$$

To get a CI for the OR itself we must take the antilog:

$$e^{-0.2133} \text{ to } e^{1.9051} = 0.81 \text{ to } 6.72$$

Hence, from the data in Figure 6.1.2, we get an OR of 2.33 with a CI of 0.81 to 6.72. We should note that this CI is not symmetrical around the OR, reflecting the multiplicative nature of the latter (OR for the same risk $= 1.0$, for half the risk $= 0.5$, while OR for twice the risk $= 2$, etc.). As with RR, a CI around an OR estimate that includes 1 is not statistically significant. Hence, we cannot be sure (at the 95 per cent confidence level) that our sample OR of 2.33 represents a true increase in risk in the population.

 RS - ends

OR and RR – how similar?

What we have arrived at is the same concept of RR that we used to express and quantify the findings of the cohort study. It is true that this is an approximation of true RR, and is calculated differently, but it is the same concept nonetheless. It can be shown theoretically that the OR is a good, unbiased estimate of the RR when the prevalence of the disease in the population is low. In practice, however, it has been found that the OR is a good approximation to the RR even if the disease is not particularly rare, and is very commonly taken to be equivalent.

We will now apply the ideas and techniques discussed in the preceding section to the results of the Swedish study, by looking at the associations between smoking, caffeine intake and spontaneous abortion. Table 6.3.2, reproduced from Table 1 of paper A, illustrates these results:

Table 6.3.2 Characteristics of the women with spontaneous abortion (case patients) and the control subjects*

Characteristic	Case Patients (n = 562)		Control Subjects (n = 953)	
	No.	**%**	**No.**	**%**
Smoking status				
Nonsmoker	401	71	811	85
Smoker[1]	115	20	121	13
data missing on 46 cases				
and 21 controls				
Mean daily intake of				
caffeine during pregnancy[2]				
0–99mg	116	21	307	32
100–299mg	210	37	378	40
300–499mg	140	25	184	19
$\geq$ 500mg	96	17	84	9

* Because of rounding, not all percentages total 100.
[1] The criterion for classification as a smoker was a plasma cotinine value above 15ng per millilitre or daily smoking during pregnancy.
[2] Intake was estimated on a week-by-week basis from the estimated date of conception to the end of the last completed week of gestation before the interview.

Self-Assessment Exercise 6.3.1

1. Using the data in Table 6.3.2 relating to smoking status among cases and controls, construct a contingency table similar to Table 6.3.1.

2. Using this table, calculate the OR for smoking status (smoker = exposed), as we did in Section 6.3.2 (we are ignoring matching for now).

3. Interpret this OR.

4. Using the formula for the ***standard error*** of the log of the OR (described in the previous reference section on statistical methods), a 95 per cent CI for the OR was calculated of 1.45–2.55 (use the formula to calculate this yourself if you wish). How does this help your interpretation of the OR?

5. Now repeat steps 1–4, comparing the highest level of caffeine intake (≥500 mg/day), as the exposed group, with the lowest level of caffeine intake (0–99 mg/day), as the unexposed reference group. The 95 per cent CI for the OR is 2.11–4.35.

Answers in Section 6.6

6.3.2 Calculation of the *OR* – simple matched analysis

OR with one control per case

We noted previously that when matching has been incorporated into the design of a case-control study it should be taken into consideration when the analysis of the study data is carried out. The authors of the Swedish study did not present a simple ***matched*** analysis in paper A, but went straight on to report the multivariate analyses which take account of confounding. We will discuss these methods in Section 6.5, but for now we will look at simple matched analysis.

A simple matched analysis of a case-control study uses data from cases and controls as ***matched pairs***. In the example below, Table 6.3.3, in the analysis, there are two categories of matched pair we have 180 matched pairs, that is, 180 cases, each one of which has been matched to one control.

Table 6.3.3   Matched Pairs in a case-control study.

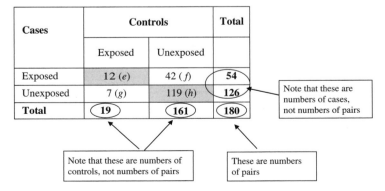

In the analysis, there are two categories of matched pair.

- One category consists of pairs of cases and controls that both have the same exposure status: either both exposed [group (e), $n = 12$ in this example] or both unexposed [group (h), $n = 119$]. These are the shaded cells of Table 6.3.3, and are known as *concordant pairs*.

- In the other category of case-control pairs, the exposure status differs: either the case is exposed and the control unexposed [group (f), $n = 42$], or vice versa [group (g), $n = 7$]. These are the non-shaded cells of Table 6.3.3, and are known as *discordant pairs*.

In a case-control study, we are interested in the association between exposure and the disease, so the concordant pairs (same exposure status) will not tell us anything. We therefore do not include them in the calculation of the OR, because they would only dilute the effect, and make the analysis less efficient. In this simple matched analysis, the OR is calculated by dividing the number of matched discordant pairs (different exposure status):

$$\text{OR} = \frac{\text{Number of pairs with case exposed and control unexposed}}{\text{Number of pairs with case unexposed and control exposed}} = f/g$$

So in this example, the OR $= 42 \div 7 = \mathbf{6.00}$. If we had ignored the matching in the analysis, we would have the following data (Table 6.3.4), and the OR $= (54 \times 161) \div (126 \times 19) = \mathbf{3.63}$. The estimate of the OR from the matched analysis differs considerably from the estimate based on the unmatched analysis of the same data. Ignoring matching will *bias* the estimate of the OR towards unity (1.00); that is, it dilutes the observed effect.

Table 6.3.4   Unmatched analysis of matched design (see Table 6.3.3 for data)

	Cases	Controls
Exposed	54	19
Not exposed	126	161
Total	180	180

More than one control per case

If we have two controls matched to each case, we cannot summarise the data in a 2×2 table. We need to take account of eight possible outcomes for each set of three subjects (one case and two matched controls), as shown below.

Case	Control 1	Control 2	Frequency
Exposed	Exposed	Exposed	n_0
Exposed	Exposed	Not exposed	n_1
Exposed	Not exposed	Exposed	n_2
Exposed	Not exposed	Not exposed	n_3

Not exposed	Exposed	Exposed	n_4
Not exposed	Exposed	Not exposed	n_5
Not exposed	Not exposed	Exposed	n_6
Not exposed	Not exposed	Not exposed	n_7

The estimate of the OR is still based on the ratio of discordant sets, and in this case is:

$$OR = (n_1 + n_2 + 2n_3)/(2n_4 + n_5 + n_6)$$

The sets of subjects who are all exposed, n_0, or all not exposed, n_7, do not tell us about the effect of exposure – these are the concordant sets. This can be extended to more than two matched controls per case, but becomes a lot more complicated. If there are three controls per case, there are $2^4 = 16$ possible outcomes; four controls per case results in $2^5 = 32$ possible outcomes; and so on.

6.3.3 Hypothesis tests for case-control studies

Simple unmatched analysis (chi-squared test)

If a 95 per cent CI for the OR does not include 1.0, it shows there is a statistically significant association at the 5 per cent significance level. A test of the ***null hypothesis*** that the population OR is equal to 1.0 (i.e. there is no association), and a p-value, is another way of measuring the strength of evidence against the hypothesis. Returning to our hypothetical example of an unmatched study from Section 6.3.1, we had (Table 6.3.1):

	Cases	Controls	Total
Exposed	15	9	24
Not exposed	15	21	36
Total	30	30	60

We are investigating the association between two categorical variables, women who have had a spontaneous abortion compared to currently pregnant women (case or control) and the risk factor (high caffeine intake). As we saw in Chapter 5 on cohort studies, the appropriate hypothesis test for this type of comparison is the chi-squared test. Recall that the null hypothesis can be stated in a number of equivalent forms, including:

H_0: there is no association between spontaneous abortion and caffeine intake.

H_0: the probability of exposure to caffeine intake is the same for cases and controls.

A further equivalent form which is meaningful in the context of a case-control study is:

H_0: the OR for caffeine intake and spontaneous abortion in the population is 1.0.

The OR from Table 6.3.1 is 2.33 suggesting an increased risk of spontaneous abortion among those exposed. We also calculated the 95 per cent CI (0.81–6.72), and found that this was quite wide and included the value of 1.0 (no increased risk). To complete the picture, we now need the chi-squared statistic.

Using the procedure to calculate the chi-squared statistic that we introduced in cohort studies (Chapter 5; Section 5.5.3), we get a chi-squared value of 2.50 on one degree of freedom, with a corresponding p-value is $p = 0.11$. Therefore, the value of the test statistic is not significant at the 5 per cent level, and we do not have statistical evidence that spontaneous abortion is associated with current caffeine intake in pregnancy. This is consistent with our conclusion from the 95 per cent CI.

So, although an OR of 2.33 appears to indicate an increased risk, it is in fact, in this small sample, consistent with no association. In other words, this could be a chance finding, or the study is too small (there is insufficient power) to detect what is in fact a real effect (a type II error). A somewhat larger sample with the same OR would have shown a significant result and a 95 per cent CI that did not include 1.0. Clearly, we cannot estimate the OR very precisely from this small sample.

Simple matched case-control study (McNemar's test)

To consider the hypothesis test for a matched study, we will return to the example from Section 6.3.2. We had 180 matched pairs, resulting in the following table (Table 6.3.3 in Section 6.3.2):

Cases	Controls		Total
	Exposed	**Unexposed**	
Exposed	12 (e)	42 (f)	**54**
Unexposed	7 (g)	119 (h)	**126**
Total	**19**	**161**	**180**

The OR was calculated as $f/g = 42/7 = 6.00$. To test the null hypothesis that the population OR is 1, we need a test appropriate for matched pairs. This is called the **McNemar's test**. The test statistic is

$$\chi^2 = \frac{(f-g)^2}{f+g}$$

which is compared to the chi-squared distribution with one *degree of freedom* to find the p-value. In this example, the value of the test statistic is

$$\frac{(42-7)^2}{42+7} = 25.00$$

and the p-value is $p < 0.0005$. The result is highly significant: there is strong evidence of an association between the disease and the risk factor, and the OR of 6.00 shows that exposure substantially increases the risk of disease.

Summary

- Most case-control studies do not allow calculation of incidence rates in the exposed and unexposed populations that are required for the calculation of the RR: as a result, the OR is used, and in most situations is a good, unbiased estimate of the RR.

- The analysis of a case-control study should be appropriate to the study design: matched analysis should be used for a matched design.

- A matched study can be analysed unmatched, but this is generally less efficient and will bias the OR towards 1.0 (no effect).

- For a simple unmatched case-control study, the chi-squared test is used to test the hypothesis of no association between the disease and a single risk factor.

- For a simple matched case-control study, the McNemar's test is used to test the hypothesis of no association between the disease and a single risk factor.

6.4 Sample size for a case-control study

6.4.1 Introduction

We have already looked at sample size calculation for a cohort study and have seen why this is such an important step in the design. It is equally important for case-control studies. An estimation of sample size was not given in paper A, so we will calculate this based on reasonable assumptions of what would be needed for this particular study.

With cohort studies, the RR was the key measure of outcome that we used for estimating sample size. For a case-control study it is the OR, and we need to decide on a value for the OR that we want to be fairly confident of being able to detect (that is, demonstrate as statistically significant). Based on results in 6.5.3 of paper A, we shall calculate sample size so that we have sufficient *power* to detect as *statistically significant* an OR of at least 2.0 for spontaneous abortion, when comparing the highest level of caffeine intake ($\geq 500 \, \text{mg/day}$) to the lowest. Let's now look at the information we need to proceed with the sample size calculation.

6.4.2 What information is required?

In order to determine the required sample size for a case-control study, we need:

- (As noted already) a decision about the OR that we wish to be able to detect. We have decided on an OR of 2.0.

- Knowledge of the *prevalence* of the risk factor in the population, and in our example the risk factor is caffeine intake of $\geq 500 \, \text{mg/day}$. First, we need to identify a source of information about this. As a general rule, one would try to find previous studies that provide estimates of the population prevalence of exposure. We can use paper A as a source and, provided the disease is not common, the prevalence of exposure in the control group will provide a reasonable estimate of population prevalence (also assuming the controls are fairly representative of the population). From Table 6.3.2, Table 1 from paper A, we see that the prevalence of high caffeine intake ($\geq 500\,\text{mg/day}$) in controls is approximately 9 per cent.

- A decision on the ratio of controls to cases. As we have seen in the Swedish study, approximately two controls were selected for each case. We will start by using that assumption, and then find out what happens if we adjust this ratio.

- A *significance level* for the appropriate hypothesis test, here taken at 0.05 (and used in most studies).

- A level of statistical *power*, here taken at 80 per cent.

The last two points are exactly the same assumptions as we used for cohort studies.

6.4.3   An example of sample size calculation using Epi Info

As with cohort studies, we will demonstrate the sample size calculation for a case-control study using StatCalc from Epi Info statistical software. The program for calculating sample size in case-control studies requires all of the information listed in Section 6.4.2, but in the format set out in Table 6.4.1. The values based on our assumptions for the Swedish study have been entered in the right-hand column. These were a significance (α) value of 0.05 (Epi Info refers to $1 - \alpha$., hence $1 - 0.05 = 0.95$, or 95 per cent), a power ($1 - \beta$) of 80 per cent, a control to case ratio of 2:1, an expected frequency of exposure (caffeine intake of $\geq 500\,\text{mg/day}$) in controls of 9 per cent, and an OR of 2.0.

Table 6.4.1   Information for sample size in case-control study (Epi Info (Stat Calc))

Information needed for sample size calculation	Values for this example
Probability that if two samples differ, it reflects a true difference in the two populations (confidence level or $1 - \alpha$)	95.00% (equivalent to the α value of 0.05)
Probability that if two populations differ, the two samples will show a 'significant' difference (power or $1 - \beta$)	80.00%
# not ill (controls)/# ill (cases) (1 means equal sample sizes)	2:1
Expected frequency of exposure in not ill group (controls)	9%
Please fill in the closest value to be detected for one of the following:	
• OR – closest to 1.00	2.00
• % exposure among the ill (cases) closest to % for not ill (controls)	(automatic when OR completed)

There are two different approaches to calculating sample size for case-control studies, and these depend on whether we are using a matched or an unmatched design. A matched design will require fewer participants because the variation between cases and controls is likely to be less due to the matching for potential confounders. Although the Swedish study did carry out some matching (controls were frequency matched to cases with regard to gestation period and area of residence), we will use the unmatched approach for this example. Calculation for the unmatched design is often used even if some matching has been carried out, as this provides a more conservative estimate of the required sample size. The output from the Epi Info (Stat Calc) program looks like what is shown in Table 6.4.2.

Table 6.4.2 Example of output from sample size calculation for an unmatched case-control study (Epi Info)

```
C:\WINNT\System32\cmd.exe                                              _ □ ×
 EpiInfo Version 6            Statcalc              November 1993

     Unmatched Case-Control Study (Comparison of ILL and NOT ILL)
            Sample Sizes for 9.00 % Exposure in NOT ILL Group

                    NOT ILL    Exposure   Odds        Sample Size
  Conf.    Power    :ILL       in ILL    Ratio    NOT ILL     ILL    Total
 95.00 %  80.00 %    2:1       16.51 %    2.00      484       242     726

 90.00 %    "         "      1            @          392       196     588
 95.00 %    "         "                              484       242     726
 99.00 %    "         "       Change values for     696       348    1,044
 99.90 %    "         "       inputs as desired,     994       497    1,491
 95.00 %  80.00 %    "        then press F4 to       484       242     726
   "      90.00 %    "     E  recalculate.           646       323     969
   "      95.00 %    "                               796       398    1,194
   "      99.00 %    "                             1,124       562    1,686
   "      80.00 %   1:1                              334       334     668
   "        "       2:1                              484       242     726
   "        "       3:1                              633       211     844
   "        "       4:1                              784       196     980
   "        "       5:1                              930       186    1,116
   "        "       6:1                            1,080       180    1,260

 F1-Help                       F5-Print    F6-Open File    F10-Done
```

Conf means confidence; that is, $1 - \alpha$

So what does Table 6.4.2 show? The first row of figures, gives the sample size for the data we entered (Table 6.4.1). The rest of the table give sample sizes for various permutations of the values, although the OR has not been changed. Thus, we need at least 242 cases and 484 controls for a study with 80 per cent power to detect an OR of 2.0, where exposure in the controls is 9 per cent, with a significance level of 0.05, and a 2:1 ratio of controls:cases. In fact the Swedish study (paper A) had more than enough cases (562) and controls (953) to meet these sample size requirements. We note, however, that the Swedish study carried out analyses within strata (e.g. of smoking), effectively reducing the available sample size for any one stratum. Among smokers, for example, there were only 115 cases and 121 controls (Table 6.3.2, reproduced from paper A).

Moving down Table 6.4.2, we can see how the sample size increases as the significance level is decreased from 0.1 (90.00 per cent) to 0.01 (99.00 per cent). We can also see how the sample size increases as the power is increased from 80 to 99 per cent. The lowest portion of the table shows the sample size for varying control:case ratios. For the same level of significance and power as in the first row (our original calculation), using a 5:1 ratio results in only about 186 cases being required compared to 334 for the 1:1 ratio. That would be a great help if cases were very hard to recruit, but note that 930 controls are required. We can also see how the law of 'diminishing returns' operates as the ratio of controls:cases increases. Essentially, it would rarely be worthwhile in a case-control study to select more than four controls per case.

Clearly, the decision about what is the appropriate ratio for any given study will depend on a balance of factors, including ease of finding cases and controls, complexity and cost of obtaining data on exposure and confounding factors in cases and controls, level of matching required, and so on. The StatCalc program can also illustrate what happens with a larger number of cases than controls, but that will not be considered further here.

Summary

- Sample size calculation is as important in case-control studies as it is with other study designs.

- Information on the prevalence of exposure in the population is required, and ideally should be available from prior studies, or may have to be estimated.

- Judgement is required to decide what size effect (OR) should be detected.

- Increasing the number of controls relative to cases is a practical way of increasing power if cases are difficult to identify.

- Increasing the number of cases relative to controls can also be done to increase power, if appropriate, although this is less commonly seen.

- Sample size calculation is only approximate, and allowance must always be made for lack of response, and problems of data collection that might mean not all cases and controls can be used.

6.5 Confounding and logistic regression

6.5.1 Introduction

In a case-control study, confounding can be dealt with at the design stage, the analysis stage, or both. We saw earlier in Section 6.2.2 how *matching* can be used in the study design to avoid the effects of *known* confounding variables, and noted that the Swedish study used frequency matching to match for gestation age and area of residence. Another approach employed in the design stage to deal with confounding is *stratification*. This was used in the Swedish study, and is discussed in the next section. Lastly (and in many ways the most important), we can *adjust* for confounding at the analysis stage by using either post-stratification or multiple logistic regression. Adjustment in analysis is often combined with matching. Logistic regression is discussed in Section 6.5.3.

6.5.2 Stratification

Stratification during study design

Stratification is a way of eliminating confounding through the study design, by using a stratified sampling procedure. The population is divided into strata (groups) according to one or more confounding factors, and predetermined numbers of cases and controls are selected from each stratum. For example, in an investigation of whether there is a relationship between regular alcohol consumption and myocardial infarction (MI), smoking is suspected of being a confounding factor. Smoking is known to be a cause of MI, and smoking is commonly associated with regular alcohol consumption:

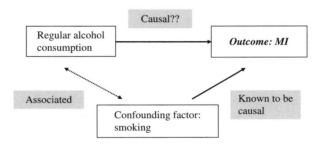

We can eliminate the confounding effect of smoking by selecting cases and controls from each of the two groups: smokers and non-smokers. That is, we *stratify* on smoking. The analysis must be appropriate to the design of the study, so we need to use a *stratified analysis*. We will explore this through the following example and exercise. Suppose that we select cases and controls from among 100 smokers (stratum 1), and from among 100 non-smokers (stratum 2), making 200 study subjects in total. We obtain the following results with unequal numbers of cases and controls, as it was easier to find cases of MI among smokers:

		Non-smokers		Smokers	
		Cases of MI	Controls	Cases of MI	Controls
Regular	Yes	11	15	54	36
alcohol	No	29	45	6	4
		40	60	60	40

 ### Self-Assessment Exercise 6.5.1

1. Calculate the ORs for (a) non-smokers and (b) smokers, and comment on the results.

2. If we had ignored the stratification, we would have the following combined table.

		Cases of MI	Controls
Alcohol	Yes	65	51
	No	35	49
		100	100

Calculate the OR for this combined table, and compare this with the ORs you obtained in question 1. Interpret what you find.

Answers in Section 6.6

Although stratification was carried out in the Swedish study for both smoking (for an example see Table 6.3.2 in paper A) and karyotype the recruitment of cases and controls was not carried out in advance for this purpose in the way that it is was for our example here. The authors ensured that they had the information required to carry out stratification (by asking about smoking and testing for plasma (blood) cotinine, and by carrying out chromosome analysis), but they only carried out stratification in the analysis. We will now consider this approach.

Post-stratification

As with matching, stratification requires that potential risk factors be identified and used during the selection of cases and controls. It is possible, however, to carry out a stratified analysis when the sample was not stratified. This is called ***post-stratification***, and can be used to take account of possible confounders – provided information on these factors has been collected. A disadvantage of post-stratification is that there is no guarantee that all the strata will contain enough cases and controls for calculation of the OR.

Stratification results in a series of ORs, one from each stratum. For example, if we were to study smoking in categories of never-smokers, ex-smokers and current smokers, we would have three ORs. These ORs are of individual interest but we generally want an overall summary measure of association with the risk factor as well. This is a ***pooled*** or ***adjusted*** OR, adjusted for the effects of the stratifying factor(s).

A pooled, adjusted OR is obtained by the Mantel–Haenszel method, which combines the ORs from each stratum. Although not difficult to calculate, it becomes tedious for more than a few strata. This technique will not be further described in this book.

Returning to the Swedish study, and the stratified results (for an example, see Table 2 of paper A), we notice that stratum ORs are not pooled, but reported separately throughout. The reason for this is that, according to the authors, there is evidence of an effect in non-smokers, but not smokers. This is due not to confounding by smoking, as the stratification has removed that, but to an apparent ***interaction*** (also termed ***effect modification***). It is not clear whether smoking genuinely modifies (reduces or eliminates) the risk of caffeine for spontaneous abortion, or whether, in this study, the powerful effects of smoking on this outcome simply mask any effect of caffeine (see Discussion of paper A).

6.5.3 Logistic regression

Introduction

Confounding may be dealt with at the analysis stage by the method of ***logistic regression***. The application of this technique of regression is similar, in principle, to that we described for simple and multiple linear regression in Chapter 5 on cohort studies. The main difference lies in the way we deal with the fact that in case-control studies the outcome is categorical ('case' or 'not case'), and not a continuous variable such as bodyweight, as we used for the example in Chapter 5. The implications of this, and how logistic regression deals with it, are discussed in Section 6.5.3 below.

In other respects, the application of the method is similar. We will enter explanatory variables (exposures of interest and confounding variables) and model these to obtain adjusted ORs which show the independent effect of each risk factor, adjusted for the other variables in the regression. In the same way that we can carry out simple linear regression to produce an unadjusted (univariate) relative risk, we can do the same with simple logistic regression, although this will just produce the OR that we calculated in Section 6.3.

We have seen, and emphasised, that it is not usually practical to match on more than a few factors, so the effects of confounders frequently need to be taken into account in the analysis, irrespective of whether matching has been used in the design. Additionally, factors used to match cases and controls cannot be investigated as risk factors, so if we want to investigate whether a factor is associated with the disease, we should not match for it. Thus, for various reasons, the majority of case-control studies require some adjustment for confounding in the analysis. In many studies, most (if not all) adjustment for confounding is carried out during analysis.

Two forms of logistic regression are commonly used. These are **unconditional** for unmatched, and **conditional** for matched study designs. We will look at these two forms, and the other issues discussed above in more detail in the remaining parts of this section, but will start with a brief overview of why we need a different type of regression for the categorical outcomes used in case-control studies.

The logistic regression model

Having a categorical outcome presents a problem for regression, which has as one key assumption a **linear association** between the explanatory variable(s) and the outcome. In practice, therefore, to carry out regression with the OR, we need to derive some form of **continuous outcome**. This is done by using – as the outcome – the (natural) logarithm of the **odds** of being a case rather than a control. The log adds provides an appropriate mathematical transformation that gives a continous linear function and therefore meets the characteristics required for logistic regression analysis. The rationale for logistic regression goes like this:

1. In a given study population, if we call the probability of being a case p, then the probability of being a control (not a case) is $1 - p$. Therefore, the **odds** of being a case is $p/(1-p)$.

2. If we take the logarithm of this, we have the log odds, which (as argued in (1) above) is $\log(p/(1-p))$.

3. This can have any value, positive, negative or zero. So we have turned a categorical outcome into a continuous variable, and we can now apply multiple-regression methods.

The equation for simple logistic regression, that is, with one explanatory variable, is:

$$\log(p/(1-p)) = \alpha + \beta x$$

And, the equation for multiple logistic regression, where we want to look at the independent effects of a number of explanatory variables on the outcome, is:

$$\log(p/(1-p)) = \alpha + \beta_1 x_1 + \beta_2 x_2 + \cdots$$

We are almost ready now to look at an example of multiple logistic regression, but there is one more complication to address – how to represent categorical explanatory variables in the regression equation where these have more than two categories. We do this with 'dummy' variables.

Dummy variables

The independent (explanatory) variables may be either continuous (e.g. blood pressure), or categorical (e.g. smoking status). Continuous variables present no problem, as we saw in the example used for multiple linear regression in Chapter 5. For categorical variables, we need to distinguish between those which have two categories (e.g. sex) and those that have more than two (e.g. never smoker; ex-smoker; light current smoker; heavy current smoker).

Variables with two categories

We need only one variable in the regression equation to represent a categorical variable with two categories. Thus, to include the variable for sex with categories 'male' and 'female', we can use one variable coded, for example, as 0 = male and 1 = female.

Variables with more than two categories

We can include these categorical variables in the regression model in one of two ways:

- By the use of **dummy variables**, that is, newly created variables, each of which can have the value 0 or 1 (explained below).

- As a continuous variable if the category values are ordered, and it is reasonable to assume that these values differ in a proportionate way.

Dummy variables are used when a categorical variable with more than two levels cannot be treated as continuous. As we will see from the example in Section 6.5.4, programmes like SPSS create dummy variables automatically when such variables are specified as categorical. It is useful to see how dummy variables work, and the following example based on the Swedish study illustrates this.

Let us consider the risk factor, 'daily intake of caffeine' (Table 6.3.2 reproduced from paper A). There are four possible values for this variable: '0–99 mg', '100–299 mg', '300–499 mg' and '≥ 500 mg'. The intervals between these categories are not consistent (and the upper limit for ≥ 500 mg is undefined), so in order to include this risk factor in a multivariate analysis, we will need to define dummy variables. In general, we require one less dummy variable than the number of categories, so we will need three: let these be called status 1, status 2 and status 3, and note that each can only take the values 0 and 1.

Status 1 will have the value 1 if daily caffeine intake is 100–299 mg and 0 if caffeine intake does not fall into this category. Status 2 will have the value 1 if caffeine intake is 300–499 mg and 0 if caffeine intake does not fall into this category. Status 3 will have the value of 1 if caffeine intake is ≥ 500 mg and 0 if caffeine intake does not fall into this category. This means that daily caffeine intake of 0–99 mg will have a value of 0 for status 1 (caffeine intake is not 100–299 mg), 0 for status 2 (caffeine intake is not 300–499 mg) and 0 for status 3 (caffeine intake is not ≥ 500 mg). The three dummy variables therefore distinguish the four categories:

Daily caffeine intake	Status 1	Status 2	Status 3
0–99 mg	0	0	0
100–299 mg	1	0	0
300–499 mg	0	1	0
≥ 500 mg	0	0	1

The value '0–99 mg', having the value 0 for all three dummy variables, is the ***reference category*** to which each of the others will be compared.

We will now look at an example of multiple logistic regression to see how all this works in practice.

6.5.4 Example: multiple logistic regression

In order to illustrate how multiple logistic regression works in practice, we will now look at an example using our data set investigating occupational risk factors for back pain, analysed using SPSS. This example will be used now to describe the process, step by step, and to familiarise you with the interpretation of the output from logistic regression analysis.

Investigating the effect of psychosocial work environment on low back pain

For this example, we will treat the back pain data set as if it were an unmatched case-control study. In total there were 765 employees. Of these, 198 (25.9 per cent) had back pain (cases), and 567 (74.1 per cent) did not have back pain (controls). Therefore, there are approximately three controls for each case, but they are not matched.

We are interested in identifying the relationship between psychosocial work environment, defined as self-reported psychological demands associated with manual work, and low back pain. In particular we would like to investigate the independent effects of (a) work speed (whether workers find their work hectic or too fast), (b) work monotony (whether workers find their work unstimulating), and (c) work stress (whether the work carried out by employees causes them anxiety or stress).

The study hypothesis is that a poor psychosocial work environment, in terms of these three psychological demands, may increase muscular tension through psychological stress, which in turn increases the risk of low back pain. The ***variables*** in the database that are of interest for this investigation include:

- The outcome (dependent) variable: this is low back pain, a categorical variable with two values (dichotomous) of 'no low back pain' and 'low back pain'.

- A number of explanatory (independent) variables, listed in Table 6.5.1.

Is there a univariate association with psychosocial work environment?

Before constructing a multivariate model we should examine the association between the independent variables of interest (representing psychosocial work environment) and the dependent variable (low back pain) by carrying out univariate logistic regression.

When we carry out logistic regression with SPSS, the first table to take note of is the *categorical variables codings* table that displays how categorical variables are coded into dummy variables.

Table 6.5.1 Features of explanatory variables to be included in the logistic regression

Domain	Variables	Type of variable
Psychosocial work environment	• Hectic work • Monotonous work • Stressful work	The main variables for exposure of interest. These are categorical variables with four-point response scales (1 = never, 2 = occasionally, 3 = half the time, 4 = always). Each will require three dummy variables in logistic regression.
Psychological distress	• General Health Questionnaire	A continuous variable relating to a score on a questionnaire measuring psychological distress. The score ranges from 12 (no distress) to 48 (severely distressed). This variable will be included in the logistic regression as a possible confounder of the relationship between psychosocial working environment and low back pain.
Demographic characteristics	• Age (years) • Sex	Age is a continuous variable, and sex is a dichotomous (categorical) variable. These variables will be included in the logistic regression as possible confounders. Neither requires any special treatment for the regression.

We noted earlier that with four categories, we would need three dummy variables. These dummy variables are created automatically in SPSS when we specify 'hectic work' as a categorical variable and define the reference group (in this case 'never'). When the regression is run, the SPSS output includes the following table.

Categorical Variables Codings

			Parameter coding		
		Frequency	**(1)**	**(2)**	**(3)**
is work hectic?	never	31	.000	.000	.000
	occasionally	319	1.000	.000	.000
	half the time	223	.000	1.000	.000
	always	191	.000	.000	1.000

We can see that three dummy variables have been created based on the response categories of 2 (occasionally), 3 (half the time) and 4 (always). Thus, the reference category (never) has values of zero (.000 in the table), zero, zero for each dummy variable. The 'occasionally' category has values of one (1.000 in the table), zero, zero, and so on. Similar tables would be constructed for 'monotonous' and 'stressful' work.

Goodness of fit – how good is the model?

The next important output from SPSS to take note of is the Omnibus Tests of Model Coefficients (OTMC) table. In a similar way to the ANOVA table in linear regression (see Section 5.8 of Chapter 5 on cohort studies), the OTMC table gives an estimate of the 'goodness of fit' of the model. The *chi-square* value for the model is interpreted in a similar way to the *F-ratio*; a measure of how much the model has improved the prediction of the outcome compared to the level of random error of the model (think of this as being analogous to standard error). If the model is a good one, then we expect the improvement in prediction due to the model to be large and the difference between the model and the observed data to be small. In short, a good model should have a large chi-square, relative to the degrees of freedom (the number of degrees of freedom is derived from the number of observations and the number of explanatory variables). Thus, the chi-squared statistic should be significant, and 0.05 is taken as the conventional level of probability for this purpose.

The OTMC table for 'hectic work' in univariate analysis looks like this, and shows the chi-square, degrees of freedom, and the significance (p-value).

Omnibus Tests of Model Coefficients

		Chi-square	df	Sig.
Step 1	Step	8.366	3	.039
	Block	8.366	3	.039
	Model	8.366	3	.039

We can see that the chi-squared value for this **univariate model** is statistically significant ($p < 0.05$), so there is less than a 5 per cent chance that a chi-squared value this large would have arisen by chance alone. We can conclude that the univariate logistic regression model with 'hectic work' predicts low back pain significantly well. Similar univariate analyses for the two other variables shows that these models are also significant.

Univariate effect estimates

The final output in this univariate analysis is the variables in the equation table, interpreted in much the same way as the coefficients table when carrying out linear regression in SPSS, but with one important difference. Whereas with linear regression the **beta coefficient** gave us a direct estimate of the effect of any given variable, in logistic regression the beta coefficients are **log odds** and, as such, are difficult to interpret as they stand. To obtain the **OR** for the outcome (low back pain) with exposure to any given variable it is therefore necessary to take the exponential of the beta coefficient. This is given automatically by SPSS in the variables in the equation table,

Variables in the Equation

		B	S.E.	Wald [+]	df	Sig.	Exp(B)
Step 1[a]	HECTIC[*]			7.789	3	.051	
	HECTIC(1)	.676	.552	1.498	1	.221	1.965
	HECTIC(2)	.954	.556	2.945	1	.086	2.597
	HECTIC(3)	1.128	.558	4.087	1	.043	3.088
	Constant	−1.908	.536	12.699	1	.000	.148

[a] Variable(s) entered on step 1: HECTIC.
[*] This row corresponds to the full (4 category) variable for hectic work and therefore has 3 (n–1) degrees of freedom.
[+] The Wald Statistic is the chi-squared value under the null hypothesis of no significant effect under 1 degree of freedom. It is calculated as β (beta) divided by S.E. (standard error of beta).

in the right-hand column with the heading Exp(B). The SPSS table providing the output for the univariate logistic regression analysis of the 'hectic work' variable is shown below:
It is possible to specify calculation of CIs for the ORs (Exp(B)) in SPSS (not shown in this univariate analysis). However, we can see from the model investigating the association between 'hectic work' and low back pain that the OR increases with the amount of time employees spend carrying out work they believe to be too hectic.

For employees who report their work to be occasionally too hectic or fast the *OR* (Exp(B)) is 1.97, with a p-value (Sig) of 0.221. This OR of 1.97 means that employees are twice as likely to experience low back pain if they 'occasionally' carry out work that is too hectic or fast relative to those who 'never' carry out such work – the *reference category*, although as this result is non-significant we cannot exclude chance as an explanation. We then see that the OR for low back pain increases to 2.6 for employees carrying out hectic work 'half the time' and to 3.09 for employees who 'always' report their work as being too hectic or fast, relative to those who 'never' report such work. However, only the association between low back pain and the fourth level (work is hectic/too fast 'always') compared to 'never' has achieved statistical significance ($p < 0.05$). Analysis of 'monotony' and 'stress' shows similar progressive increases in the OR across categories, with generally smaller p-values (results are more significant).

Assessment of potential confounders

We now need to take into account the effect of confounding factors. The first step is to explore the relationship between possible confounding factors that we know to be associated with the exposure variable (e.g. hectic work environment), and the outcome (low back pain). The potential confounders we are interested in are shown in Table 6.5.2.

Table 6.5.2 Confounding factors for consideration in multiple regression analysis for psychosocial work environment and low back pain

Variable	Reason for consideration as a potential confounding variable
Psychological distress	In this data set, there is a strong, positive relationship between hectic work environment and psychological distress as measured by the General Health Questionnaire score. Such distress has been observed to be related to the experience of pain.
Sex	In this data set there is a weak relationship between female sex and reporting a hectic work environment, with slightly more women than men reporting the most frequent category. Females have been found to report a greater amount of low back pain than males.
Age	Although in this data set there is a rather weak, but positive, association with hectic work environment, there is generally such a strong relationship between age and almost all symptoms and health problems that it would be very unwise not to include age in our model.

With the variable for psychological distress (GHQ score) care needs to be taken when considering whether it is a confounder of the relationship between psychosocial working environment and low back pain. This is because it could be argued that psychological distress is on the 'causal pathway' from psychosocial working environment to the experience of low back pain (as described in Chapter 5, Section 5.7.2). If this is the case, when we adjust for GHQ we might eliminate the association between psychosocial working environment and low back pain. For the purpose of this example, however, we will assume that GHQ score is not a major factor in the causal pathway between psychosocial working environment and low back pain.

The summary table (variables in the equation table in SPSS) describing the association between the first of the potential confounding factors ('psychological distress', that is, GHQ score) and low back pain is shown below:

Variables in the Equation

		B	S.E	Wald	df	Sig.	Exp(B)
Step 1[a]	PSYCHO	.094	.018	26.248	1	.000	1.098
	Constant	−3.225	.438	54.244	1	.000	.040

[a] Variable(s) entered on step 1: PSYCHO

We can see from the table that the association between psychological distress and low back pain is highly significant ($p < 0.0005$). The OR [Exp(B)] for this association is 1.098. For each unit increase in psychological distress score the increased risk of having low back pain is 9.8 per cent.

Note here though, that ORs operate in a multiplicative way, so that the increase in risk associated with a 2-point increase in the GHQ score is $1.098 \times 1.098 = 1.206$ (a 20.6 per cent increase), and a 3 point increase is associated with a $1.098^3 = 1.324$ (32.4 per cent) increase. We can therefore conclude that psychological distress is associated with low back pain, at least in univariate analysis. Similar univariate analyses show that 'sex' was marginally significantly associated with the outcome (OR = 1.6 for females compared to males; $p = 0.06$), and that 'age' is more strongly associated (OR = 1.02 per year; $p = 0.013$). For simplicity, in this example, we will include only 'psychological distress' and 'age' as confounders in the multivariate analysis, excluding 'sex' from the model (although often a more conservative cut-off of $P < 0.1$ is used for inclusion of a variable as a confounder in a model).

The multivariate model

Our multivariate model will determine the independent effects of each explanatory variable on the outcome (low back pain). The SPSS output for this multiple logistic regression model is now described, starting with the Omnibus test for the overall model.

Omnibus Tests of Model Coefficients

		Chi-square	df	Sig.
Step 1	Step	59.436	11	.000
	Block	59.436	11	.000
	Model	59.436	11	.000

The OTMC table tells us how good the model is. We can see from the table that the logistic regression model incorporating the five explanatory variables (the three exposure variables and the two confounders identified in the univariate analysis above) significantly predicts the variation in low back pain in our study sample. The chi-squared value for the model is 59.436 on 11 degrees of freedom and we are more than 99.9 per cent ($p < 0.0005$) certain that obtaining a value this large has not been due to chance. Therefore, we can conclude that our regression model predicts low back pain significantly well.

The variables in the equation table provide details of the model parameters (the beta values and the exponential of these values (ORs)) for the five explanatory variables together with their significance (p) values. For this table we have also specified the inclusion of 95 per cent CIs.

Variables in the Equation

		B	S.E.	Wald	df	Sig.	Exp(B)	95.0% C.I.for EXP(B)	
								Lower	Upper
Step 1[a]	HECTIC*			.869	3	.833			
	HECTIC(1)	.415	.575	.520	1	.471	1.514	.490	4.674
	HECTIC(2)	.476	.581	.672	1	.412	1.610	.516	5.027
	HECTIC(3)	.516	.585	.780	1	.377	1.676	.533	5.271
	MONOT*			10.716	3	.013			
	MONOT(1)	.277	.306	.819	1	.365	1.319	.724	2.401
	MONOT(2)	.761	.311	5.976	1	.015	2.140	1.163	3.937
	MONOT(3)	.777	.306	6.458	1	.011	2.176	1.195	3.963
	STRESS*			10.096	3	.018			
	STRESS(1)	.590	.254	5.393	1	.020	1.805	1.096	2.971
	STRESS(2)	.911	.298	9.371	1	.002	2.487	1.388	4.457
	STRESS(3)	.749	.312	5.764	1	.016	2.115	1.147	3.898
	PSYCHO	.078	.019	16.539	1	.000	1.081	1.041	1.122
	AGE	.016	.007	4.924	1	.026	1.016	1.002	1.030
	Constant	−4.972	.789	39.688	1	.000	.007		

[a] Variable(s) entered on step 1: HECTIC, MONOT, STRESS, PSYCHO, AGE.

* These rows correspond to the full (4 category) variable for psychosocial working environment and therefore have 3 (n–1) degrees of freedom.

The effect of adjustment

Interestingly, following this *adjustment* for the effects of other variables, the ORs (Exp(B)) for the three levels of 'hectic work' (compared to the 'hectic' reference category) are all attenuated and none achieve statistical significance. This latter observation is confirmed by the 95 per cent confidence limits that span unity; for example, taking the highest level for 'hectic work' (comparing 'always' with 'never' finding work hectic) the OR estimate is 1.68 but might be as small as 0.53 or as large as 5.27.

This important result illustrates the effects of *confounding* on the relationship between 'hectic work' and low back pain. One or more of the other four variables (stressful work, monotonous work, psychological distress and age) must explain part of the univariate association that we observed between 'hectic work' and low back pain by their mutual association with both factors.

In contrast, the univariate associations observed for monotonous and stressful work persist in the multivariate analysis, after adjustment for the other explanatory variables. As such, these psychosocial work factors are *independently* associated with low back pain (this would lend weight to our assumption that GHQ score was not a major factor in the 'causal pathway' between psychosocial working environment and low back pain). The two levels for monotonous work representing 'half the time' and 'always' are associated with more than a twofold increase in the risk of low back pain relative to 'never' finding work monotonous. The 95 per cent CIs for these ORs do not span unity and the estimates are therefore significant.

Similarly, all three levels for stressful work are significantly associated with low back pain, with ORs ranging from 1.81 for 'occasionally' finding work stressful to 2.49 for finding work stressful 'half the time'. Again, the 95 per cent CIs for the ORs do not span unity and these estimates are therefore significant.

Finally, we can also see from the table that the significant associations observed for the two potential confounders (psychological distress and age) in the univariate analysis have persisted in the multivariate analysis. The ORs are similar to the univariate analysis and the 95 per cent CIs do not span unity. As such, psychological distress and age can also be interpreted as being *independent predictors* of low back pain.

In this example, we have seen how multiple logistic regression is carried out and interpreted. In fact, this was a general form known as unconditional logistic regression, which (as mentioned previously) is the appropriate method for unmatched case-control studies. We will now look at the method for matched studies, and finally review the results of regression analysis in the Swedish study.

6.5.5 Matched studies – conditional logistic regression

The form of (multiple) logistic regression used to analyse matched case-control studies is called *conditional logistic regression*. The outcome is now defined to be the difference in disease status for each case-control pair. Each x variable for each matched pair is the difference between the value of the variable for the case and the value of the variable for the control. This is the analytic procedure used in the Swedish study (paper A). While a different statistical procedure is used to carry out conditional logistic regression (which we will not consider further in this book), interpretation of the output from the analysis is essentially the same.

6.5.6 Interpretation of adjusted results in Swedish study

We will now consider analysis of the Swedish study that uses conditional multiple logistic regression to study the effect of caffeine on spontaneous abortion, independent of confounding. This brief section from the methods section of paper A describes the statistical approach used:

Statistical Analysis

Data were analyzed with the use of conditional logistic-regression analysis, matched for the week of gestation and area of residence . . . Variables were included in the multivariate analyses if they were judged, a priori, to be potential confounders or if they changed the estimates of the effect of caffeine by more than 5 percent . . .

The following table (Table 6.5.3 including data and information extracted from Table 6.5.3, paper A) provides information about which variables were included in the regression models, and the adjusted ORs (and 95 per cent CIs) for levels of caffeine intake. We have already discussed (in Section 6.5.2) the reasons why the table is stratified by smoking status.

Table 6.5.3 Adjusted odds ratios for spontaneous abortion associated with ingestion of caffeine during pregnancy among smokers and non-smokers*

| Variable | Smokers | | Non-smokers | | | |
| | All | | All | | 'no aversion to coffee' | |
	OR	95%CI	OR	95%CI	OR	95%CI
Daily intake of caffeine						
0–99mg	1.0		1.0		1.0	
100–299mg	0.9	0.3–2.5	1.3	0.9–1.8	1.8	1.2–2.7
300–499mg	1.7	0.6–4.6	1.4	0.9–2.0	2.7	1.7–4.5
≥ 500mg	0.7	0.3–1.9	2.2	1.3–3.8	4.1	2.1–8.1

* Data on smoking status were missing for 46 case patients and 21 controls. The odds ratios have been adjusted for age; number of previous pregnancies; history of spontaneous abortion; consumption of alcohol during pregnancy (yes vs. no); and the presence or absence of nausea, vomiting, and fatigue as symptoms of pregnancy.

 Self-Assessment Exercise 6.5.2

1. Describe how the authors of the Swedish paper decided on which factors were potential confounders for the association between caffeine ingestion and spontaneous abortions.

2. For the following variables, note whether each was entered into the regression as (a) continuous, (b) dichotomous categorical, or (c) categorical with more than two categories requiring use of dummy variables:

   - age
   - alcohol consumption in pregnancy
   - caffeine intake
   - pregnancy induced symptoms.

3. Describe the relationship between caffeine intake and spontaneous abortions for *smokers*.

4. Describe the relationship between caffeine intake and spontaneous abortions for *all non-smokers*.

5. Describe the relationship between caffeine intake and spontaneous abortions in the women with 'no aversion to coffee'. Why do you think the authors carried out a separate analysis on this group.

Answers in Section 6.6

With this exercise we have seen how multiple logistic regression has been used to identify the independent effect of caffeine on spontaneous abortion. The analysis in (paper A) above also includes post-stratification on smoking status, but the results in the two strata (smokers and non-smokers) were not combined due to the possibility of an effect–modification (interaction), such that the risk of spontaneous abortion associated with caffeine is not seen among smokers.

Summary: confounding and logistic regression

- Confounding can be dealt with in the design of the study, the analysis of the study, or (commonly) both.

- Design methods that help to reduce confounding include matched and stratified designs. Stratification can also be carried out during analysis.

- The analysis should be appropriate for the study design: matched analysis for a matched design, stratified analysis for a stratified design.

- Confounding can be dealt with in analysis by using multiple unconditional logistic regression (for unmatched studies), or conditional multiple logistic regression (for matched studies)

- Multivariate logistic regression analysis allows the OR for a putative risk factor to be estimated, independently of the effect of other explanatory variables, including confounders.

6.6 Answers to self-assessment exercises

Section 6.1

Exercise 6.1.1

1. Research issues, including limitations of other studies, and aims

- Caffeine is metabolised more slowly in pregnant women than in non-pregnant women, and passes readily through the placenta to the fetus.

- Results from epidemiological studies relating caffeine ingestion to the risk of spontaneous abortion have been inconclusive. The authors speculate that this might be due to the complex relationship between coffee consumption, symptoms of pregnancy and fetal viability. For example, women with viable pregnancies are more likely to have pregnancy symptoms (e.g. nausea/aversion to strong tastes and smells) and therefore will avoid the primary source of caffeine intake – ingestion of coffee. Most studies have not included analysis of pregnancy symptoms.

- Also, most studies have not looked at the first trimester of pregnancy, when changes in caffeine intake, pregnancy symptoms and the majority of spontaneous abortions occur.

- Exposure measurement of caffeine intake in previous studies has been suboptimal:

  o reporting of caffeine intake after the outcome (spontaneous abortion)

  o changes in caffeine ingestion during pregnancy not considered

  o differences between chromosomally normal and abnormal fetuses not considered.

  Aim and objectives are not specified as such. The overall aim is to determine whether caffeine increases the risk of spontaneous abortion. The specific objectives can be identified as:

- To study the relationship between caffeine intake, smoking status, symptoms of pregnancy and the risk of spontaneous abortion.

- To determine the effect of genetic abnormality on the effect of intake on spontaneous abortion, by carrying out a chromosomal analysis (where fetal tissue is available).

3. Choice of study design

A cohort study design is likely to have been impractical. In order to obtain the main benefit of a cohort design, namely the prospective time frame and assessment of exposure prior to occurrence of the spontaneous abortion, a population sample of women 'at risk' of becoming pregnant would need to be recruited, their caffeine intake assessed and the sample followed up until sufficient numbers had become pregnant and completed the first trimester. It would be unsatisfactory to recruit pregnant women, as the spontaneous abortion may occur very early in the pregnancy, and many women would not bring their pregnancy to the attention of the health system until well into (and not infrequently after) the first trimester. A very large sample (cohort) would therefore be required, and the cost and difficulty of assessing caffeine intake (including changes that might be occurring during the first trimester) would be immense.

Section 6.2

Exercise 6.2.1

1. Case definition

   - Patients attending a clinic for the care of women with spontaneous abortions.

   - Patients were women presenting to the clinic at 6–12 completed weeks of gestation.

   - Pregnancies had been confirmed by a positive test.

   - Patients were then invited to participate in the study.

   - In addition, the control subjects underwent vaginal ultrasonography (ultrasound scan). If a nonviable intrauterine pregnancy was detected, the woman was recruited as a case (group with spontaneous abortion).

2. How cases were found

   Cases of spontaneous abortion were identified at the Department of Obstetrics and Gynaecology of Uppsala University Hospital, and all women were invited to participate.

3. Quality of case ascertainment

   - The cases were clearly defined, and a high proportion (86 per cent) of eligible women agreed to participate. Even though this is quite a high rate of consent to the study, it would have been useful to find out whether those declining to participate differed from those agreeing to participate in terms of exposure status, or other factors that might be related to spontaneous abortion.

   - The Department of Obstetrics and Gynecology of Uppsala University Hospital is the only place in the county for the care of women with spontaneous abortions.

   - The inclusion as cases of women with non-viable pregnancies on ultrasound can also been seen as strengthening the methods, as this ensured that these women were not misclassified as controls. Some of the non-viable pregnancies would probably subsequently be experienced as spontaneous abortions, though not all.

   - Overall, case ascertainment appeared to be thorough and well described, although some further consideration of the complexity of finding all cases of first trimester spontaneous abortion and pregnancy loss is discussed further in Section 6.2.2 on control selection.

Exercise 6.2.2

1. The controls should meet the principle fairly well, but it is worth reflecting a little more on the two groups. The cases represent the proportion of all women experiencing a spontaneous abortion who then attended hospital, which is likely to be the majority in a country such as Sweden; hence it should be representative of the population of all cases of spontaneous abortion. The controls were (mainly) women attending for antenatal care in the first trimester: however, not all women attend during the first trimester, and those that do not, on average, tend to differ on a range of socio-economic and lifestyle factors from those who do (and they may also differ by caffeine intake). So, while it is possible that there are some differences in the populations represented by cases and controls, these are probably not major. Without further information,

however, we cannot assess the extent of any such differences – particularly in respect of patterns of caffeine intake or other risk factors – for the interpretation of study results.

2. The assumption, with the induced abortions, is that these would have remained viable pregnancies and have therefore been added to the controls. A small proportion may, if allowed to continue, have become non-viable and/or spontaneously aborted, but the effect of this would be to misclassify cases as controls, and dilute any effect of the risk factor in the analysis. Thus, if there is any error (bias), it is a conservative direction; that is, it would under-estimate rather than exaggerate the effect of the risk factor.

Exercise 6.2.3

1. This could cover many specific factors including those related to socio-economic conditions, and possibly environmental exposures such as air pollution from industry, etc.

2. There are two important reasons for not matching for too many factors:

    - It would not be practical. If there is a long list of factors that have to be matched, it would be very difficult and time-consuming to find a control that meets all of the criteria for each case.

    - It is quite possible to over-match in a case-control study. If one or more of the variables used for matching are strongly associated with the risk factor being studied, this could inadvertently lead to matching (at least in part) of the risk factor being studied. In Figure 6.1.2, we saw that the purpose of the case-control study design is to measure the difference in exposure to the risk factor between cases and controls. If by matching we end up making the cases and control more similar with respect to that risk factor, the very difference we are trying to measure will be reduced. It would be (in Figure 6.1.2) like reducing the percentage of shaded squares from 50 per cent to 45 per cent among cases, and increasing it from 30 per cent to 35 per cent among controls, weakening the association. It is therefore wise, and more practical, to match for a small number of key confounders (two or three at most), the effects of which are known already, and which are not associated with the risk factor of interest. Later in this chapter we will look at how other confounding factors can be dealt with in the analysis.

Exercise 6.2.4

Assessment of risk factors, and comments on possible bias, are provided in the table below:

Risk factor	How assessed	Comment on possible bias
Caffeine intake	Three midwives and two doctors collect information.	Well-trained interviewers using a standard questionnaire may result in minimal bias, but there are some issues here to consider. In particular, we note that doctors carried out some of the interviews, in fact all of the induced abortion controls, of which 273 participated – a substantial number. It is quite possible that interview techniques of midwives and doctors differ. Interviewers may also introduce bias by eliciting information differently from cases and controls if they are aware of the patient's case/control status (very likely) and of the hypothesis.

Patient recall.	It is difficult to assess how accurate recall of all caffeine intake will be, going back as far as 4 weeks prior to the last menstrual period (hence 3–4 months, or more, for some women). The authors tried to minimise this by completing the interviews as quickly as possible. Inaccurate recall could simply add 'noise' (random error) in equal measure to both cases and controls: the key issue is whether the two groups may recall differently. Although possible, we are not provided with any further information to assess recall bias.
Caffeine intake calculated from estimated cup sizes.	Standard measures were used to assess the amount of caffeine ingested from recall of quantities of various drinks consumed. The use of these same standard methods for cases and controls should help to minimise bias.
Pregnancy symptoms — Three midwives and two doctors collect information	As for caffeine intake (above).
Patient recall.	Women may well (and quite reasonably) associate presence or absence of symptoms with the occurrence of the abortion, seeking explanation, or for other reasons. We might expect, however, that women seeking explanation would associate (and hence report) more symptoms with the loss of the pregnancy, and this runs counter to the relationship described in the paper.
Smoking status — Measured from plasma cotinine, and questionnaire.	The principal measure was by plasma cotinine concentration, using gas chromatography and N-ethylnorcotinine as an internal standard. This objective measure of smoking, with quality control, should be free of measurement bias. On the other hand, it is a short-term measure of exposure to cigarettes, carried out after the 'disease event'. Cases are probably more likely to alter their smoking habit as a reaction to the abortion than controls. This is another limitation of retrospective exposure assessment in case-control studies.

Exercise 6.2.5

Study	Potential for bias in the assessment of exposure to risk factor
1	Although there is a risk that telephone interviews could exclude certain groups of the population, in the USA virtually everyone would have had a telephone (the issue of use of mobile phones rather than land lines may be a complicating factor). There are two other potential sources of bias to consider:

• Would the interviewers have known whether they were talking to a case (with breast cancer) or a control (disease free)? If so, could that knowledge have influenced the way in which they elicited the information about OCP use? If so, that would lead to interviewer bias.

• Is it possible that the cases, as a result of their experiences and awareness since diagnosis, would be able to give a more detailed history of OCP use, or perhaps exaggerate their OCP compared to controls? If so, this would be recall bias.

(Continued)

Study	Potential for bias in the assessment of exposure to risk factor
2	Since it is based on records, we might expect no reason for a difference between cases (children with TB) and controls (disease free) in the recording of this information. However, there are likely to be quite a lot of children with poor records, or no records at all. It is likely that children who are more susceptible to TB live in areas or circumstances where record keeping is poorer. This would lead to bias: for example, we might have a situation in which (assuming BCG was effective in this population) disease-free controls that had in fact been vaccinated did not have this event recorded. This would lead to the study underestimating the efficacy of the vaccine.
3	Birthweight is recorded fairly accurately in the records of virtually every child born in the UK, and this would have been true 10 years ago. Furthermore, there is no reason to think that cases (children subsequently performing poorly in school at age 10 years) would have any less adequately recorded data than the controls. It is difficult to see how this method of exposure assessment could result in bias in the case-control comparison.

Section 6.3

Exercise 6.3.1

1. It is very useful to go through the process of setting out the data in this way:

	Cases (spontaneous abortions)	Controls (pregnant women)
Exposed (smokers)	115	121
Not exposed (non-smokers)	401	811
Total	516	932

2. OR $= (115 \times 811) \div (121 \times 401) = 1.9222$, which can be rounded to 1.92.

3. The OR is interpreted as follows: the odds of being a smoker are 1.92 times greater in cases (women who have had a spontaneous abortion) than controls (currently pregnant women). As the OR is used to approximate the relative risk, we can interpret the OR as indicating that women who smoke are 1.92 times more likely to have a spontaneous abortion than women who do not smoke.

4. The CI gives us an estimate of the precision of our sample OR in relation to the true population OR. As the CI does not include 1.0 (no increased or decreased risk), we can be 95 per cent confident that our sample OR of 1.92 represents a true increase in risk in the population. Or put another way, we are 95 per cent confident that the risk in the population of spontaneous abortions among women who smoke in pregnancy, compared to those that do not, lies in the range 1.45–2.55.

5.

Caffeine intake	Cases (spontaneous abortions)	Controls (pregnant women)
Exposed (≥ 500 mg)	96	84
Not exposed (0–99 mg)	116	307
Total	212	391

The OR $= (96 \times 307) \div (84 \times 116) = 3.0246$, which rounds to 3.02. The odds of having the highest daily mean level of caffeine relative to the lowest level of caffeine are more than three times (OR $= 3.02$) greater in cases (women who have had a spontaneous abortion) than controls (currently pregnant women). Alternatively, expressed as the estimate of relative risk, we can say that women ingesting more than 500 mg of caffeine daily during pregnancy are more than three times more likely to have a spontaneous abortion than women whose daily amount of caffeine is less than 100 mg. The interpretation of the 95 per cent CI (2.11–4.35) is similar to that in no. 4 above, noting that the interval does not include 1.0. Although the interval is not that narrow, neither is it very wide, and the lower limit of the interval is above 2.0. Overall, the 95 per cent CI tells us that this is a reasonably precise estimate, and we can be 95 per cent confident that the risk of spontaneous abortion associated with this level of caffeine intake is at least twice that associated with the lowest intake group.

Section 6.5

Exercise 6.5.1

1. For non-smokers OR $= 1.14$, (and $\chi^2 = 0.0780$, $p = 0.78$); for smokers OR $= 1.00$, (and $\chi^2 = 0.0000$, $p = 1.0$). Both of these OR values are close to (one is equal to) 1.0, and, not surprisingly, neither reaches statistical significance. Thus, having eliminated the effect of smoking, we see that there is no association between alcohol and MI.

2. If we had ignored the stratification in the analysis (or had not stratified, but obtained these same data), the result would be as follows: OR $= 1.78$, $\chi^2 = 4.023$, $p = 0.0449$. This OR is (just) significant at the 5 per cent level, so we would conclude that there is a positive association between MI and alcohol. Ignoring the stratification, or failing to take smoking into account in some way, gives a misleading result due to confounding by smoking. While the figures in this example are made up, the results are consistent with research findings.

Exercise 6.5.2

1. The authors used two approaches to identify potential confounders to include in the multivariate analysis.

   - First, they used an 'a priori' approach. Thus, they chose to include variables that they had prior reason to believe would confound the relationship between caffeine intake and the occurrence of a spontaneous abortion. One example would be the presence of pregnancy-related symptoms. The authors described in the introduction how women with viable pregnancies would be more likely to have pregnancy symptoms (e.g. nausea/aversion to strong tastes and smells) and would therefore be more likely to avoid the primary source of caffeine intake – ingestion of coffee.

- Secondly, they included variables as confounders if 'they changed estimates of the effect of caffeine by more than 5 per cent'. This implies that they carried out separate regression models including each potential confounder together with caffeine ingestion to see whether the relationship between caffeine ingestion and spontaneous abortion was altered by this inclusion. If the OR for caffeine intake and spontaneous abortions was changed by 5 per cent, the variable was deemed to be a confounder.

Variable	How entered in regression
Age	A continuous variable, which would most likely have been entered into the regression as such (the alternative would be to use age categories, but this is likely to be less efficient when the continuous variable can be used).
Caffeine intake	Caffeine intake, as we have seen, was arranged into four categories, with the lowest (0–99 mg) as the reference category. This would have necessitated three dummy variables.
Alcohol consumption in pregnancy	Alcohol consumption was entered as 'yes' versus 'no'; hence, it is a dichotomous categorical variable without the need for a dummy variable.
Pregnancy-induced symptoms	Symptoms of pregnancy were also treated as dichotomous categorical variables; for example, 'presence' or 'absence' of nausea.

3. We can see from 6.5.3 that there appears to be no relationship between caffeine intake and spontaneous abortion in smokers. For each increasing level of caffeine intake relative to the reference level (0–99 mg), the 95 per cent CIs are wide and include 1.0.

4. When we look at all non-smokers, we can see that there is clear evidence of a relationship between increasing caffeine intake and spontaneous abortions. The OR increases with increasing levels of caffeine (relative to the reference category of 0–99 mg). However, only the association between the highest level of caffeine ingestion (≥ 500 mg) is significantly associated with spontaneous abortions; we can be 95 per cent confident that the true OR for the association between a high caffeine intake (≥ 500 mg) relative to no/low caffeine intake (0–99 mg) and spontaneous abortion lies in the range 1.3–3.8. For intermediate levels of caffeine ingestion (100–200 mg and 300–499 mg), the CIs include 1.0. Nevertheless, there is some evidence here of a *dose-response* relationship, which we identified as one of the Bradford Hill guidelines that help us judge whether an observed associated is causal (see Section 5.7, Chapter 5).

5. When we restrict the analysis to women who had 'no aversion to coffee', the relationship between caffeine ingestion and spontaneous abortion is more pronounced with a clearer dose-response relationship than was seen for all smokers (see above). Indeed, the intermediate levels of caffeine intake (100–299 and 300–400 mg) are both significantly associated with an increased risk (95 per cent CIs do not include 1.0), so we can be much more confident about this dose-response relationship. The highest level of caffeine intake (≥ 500 mg) is now associated with more than a fourfold increase in the risk of spontaneous abortion.

You may wonder why the authors did not just add the variable 'aversion to coffee' to the conditional logistic regression model instead of carrying out a separate analysis. The reason is that there was a very strong inverse association between aversion to coffee and caffeine ingestion (the stronger the aversion, the less the caffeine intake), and this is illustrated in paper A. Where two variables are very strongly associated, the inclusion of one in the regression equation may effectively take account of the other variable, and therefore make it very difficult to study the true independent effects of either. This separate analysis is another example of post-stratification, since, in the 'no aversion to coffee' group, there can be no opportunity for confounding by this symptom.

7

Intervention studies

Introduction and learning objectives

The study designs that we have examined so far have relied on going to existing data sources or on collecting new information on risk factors, health status and events, and then analysing the associations. In essence we have been 'observing' what is going on out there, albeit in quite sophisticated ways – especially with the case-control and cohort studies. The key point here is the observation: what we have not done is deliberately change things, or 'experiment'. The study designs examined so far are therefore described as ***observational***. We will now go on to look at ***experimental*** research. The most important new feature of experimental designs is that we deliberately intervene to alter the level of the factor(s) that we think could affect health. This has important consequences for the strength of the study design, but also for the ethical implications of the research.

We will begin our exploration of experimental studies with a relatively simple intervention – a drug. Once you are familiar with the basic design features of a randomised trial, with blinding and placebo control, we will look at studies where the interventions being tested are rather more complex and cannot easily be tested with this ideal design. This is important because many aspects of health care and health promotion present considerable challenges for the trial design. We will also look at sample size calculation for two-group trials (and other two-group comparisons), how to deal with any imbalance in confounding factors following randomisation and a special type of randomised trial known as the cross-over trial.

Learning objectives

By the end of this chapter you should be able to do the following:

- Describe the purpose and structure of intervention study design, within an overall framework of epidemiological study designs.
- Describe what is meant by eligibility (inclusion) and exclusion criteria in the context of an intervention study.
- Describe the purpose of randomisation and how this can be done in practice.

(Continued)

Quantitative Methods for Health Research   Nigel Bruce, Daniel Pope and Debbi Stanistreet
© 2008 John Wiley & Sons, Ltd

- Describe the purpose and technique of blinding and the methods for achieving some degree of blinding in situations where the nature of the intervention cannot be concealed.

- Describe what is meant by the term 'placebo control' and why this is used.

- Describe what is meant by the term 'analysis by intention to treat' and explain why this is important.

- Carry out an appropriate statistical analysis of a two-group trial with either a categorical or continuous outcome variable(s).

- Describe the main strengths and weaknesses of intervention studies.

- Describe the important ethical issues in designing and carrying out an intervention study including informed consent.

- Describe what information is required to calculate the sample size of a two-group trial and carry out this calculation (with formulae provided).

- Identify situations where paired data are generated and describe in general terms the methods for analysis of paired data.

- Describe how to deal with imbalances in randomisation by using multiple-regression methods in the analysis of a trial.

- Describe the strengths and weaknesses of a wider range of intervention study designs including cluster randomised trials, community-based interventions, cross-over trials and quasi-experimental designs.

Resource papers

We will explore intervention studies through the following four papers:

Principal references

Paper A

Bollinger, C. T. *et al.* (2000). Smoking reduction with oral nicotine inhalers: double blind, randomised clinical trial of efficacy and safety. *Br Med J* **321**, 329–333.

Paper B

Day, L. *et al.* (2002). Randomised factorial trial of falls prevention among older people living in their own homes. *Br Med J* **325**, 128–134.

Supplementary references

Paper C

Elley Raina, C. *et al.* (2003). Effectiveness of counselling patients on physical activity in general practice: cluster randomised controlled trial. *Br Med J* **326**, 793–799.

Paper D

Biglan, A. *et al.* (2000). A randomised controlled trial of a community intervention to prevent adolescent tobacco use. *Tob Control* **9**, 24–32.

7.1 Why do an intervention study?

7.1.1 Study objectives

> The best way to prevent the detrimental health consequences of cigarette smoking is to quit, and efforts to date have focused on this strategy. Many smokers, however, find it impossible to quit, even with help, because of their dependence on nicotine, which is a highly addictive psychoactive drug. (Bollinger *et al.* (paper A))

Smoking is one of the most important contributors to the global burden of disease (World Health Organisation 2002). Primary prevention (ways of preventing people from adopting tobacco smoking) is the priority, but we also need to help smokers to quit. As the above quotation from paper A emphasises, many smokers find this desperately difficult so finding effective ways to assist them is very important. The first exercise will help you understand why the authors chose an intervention study design.

Please now read the following which is the abstract from paper A:

Abstract

Objectives: To determine whether use of an oral nicotine inhaler can result in long term reduction in smoking and whether concomitant use of nicotine replacement and smoking is safe.

Design: Double blind, randomised, placebo controlled trial. Four month trial with a two year follow up.

Setting: Two university hospital pulmonary clinics in Switzerland.

Participants: 400 healthy volunteers, recruited through newspaper advertisements, willing to reduce their smoking but unable or unwilling to stop smoking immediately.

Intervention: Active or placebo inhaler as needed for up to 18 months with participants encouraged to limit their smoking as much as possible.

Main outcome measures: Number of cigarettes smoked per day from week six to end point. Decrease verified by a measurement of exhaled carbon monoxide at each time point compared with measurement at baseline.

Results: At four months sustained reduction of smoking was achieved in 52 (26%) participants in the active group and 18 (9%) in the placebo group ($P < 0.001$; Fisher's test). Corresponding figures after two years were 19 (9.5%) and 6 (3.0%) ($P = 0.012$).

Conclusion: Nicotine inhalers effectively and safely achieved sustained reduction in smoking over 24 months. Reduction with or without nicotine substitution may be a feasible first step towards smoking cessation in people not able or not willing to stop abruptly.

Self-Assessment Exercise 7.1.1

Why do you think the research team opted to carry out an intervention study to test this approach to smoking reduction, rather than a case-control or cohort study?

Answers in Section 7.7

7.1.2 Structure of a randomised and controlled intervention study

Figure 7.1.1 illustrates the generalised structure of a randomised controlled trial with two groups. One feature to note is that intervention trials have much in common with cohort studies and many

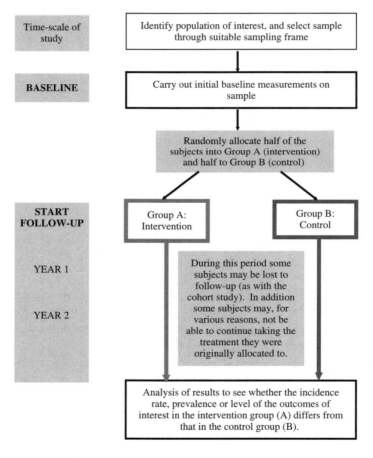

Figure 7.1.1 Generalised structure of a randomised, controlled trial with two groups (testing an intervention, in comparison with a control), and – in the case of this example – a 2-year follow-up period. Randomisation, blinding and the use of placebo will be examined in Section 7.2

of the methodological issues that we examined in Chapter 5 apply equally to intervention studies. Make sure that you have understood the design in Figure 7.1.1 before doing the next exercise.

The methods used for the study by Bollinger *et al.* (paper A) include the following features: (a) randomisation, (b) double blinding and (c) placebo control. You may already know something about what these terms mean, but we will study each in more detail shortly, together with the reasons for incorporating these aspects of study design. Later in this chapter, we will look at intervention studies for which it is not possible to include some or any of these design features and consider the implications for interpretation of the results.

At this stage, it is useful to look at the rationale and structure of intervention trial design in what might be termed its purest form, the ***randomised blind (placebo) controlled trial*** (RCT), of which paper A is an example. This is important because the randomised controlled trial is often regarded as the 'gold standard' when it comes to providing evidence about the ***efficacy*** of preventative measures or health care. Exercise 7.1.2 will introduce you to the design of this study. Please now read the following excerpt, which includes parts of the methods section of paper A relating to study design, participants and the treatment investigated:

Methods

Study design

Smokers were recruited into this two centre, double blind, placebo controlled, randomised clinical trial through newspaper advertisements that asked for healthy smokers who were unwilling or unable to quit but were interested in reducing their smoking. All participants were given information about possible ways to achieve this goal. Smoking cessation was recommended as the ultimate goal throughout the study.

Participants

Participants in the trial had to be at least 18 years of age, smoke 15 or more cigarettes a day, have a carbon monoxide concentration in exhaled air $> 10\,ppm$, have smoked regularly for three or more years, have failed at least one serious attempt to quit within the past 12 months, want to reduce smoking as much as possible with the help of the nicotine inhaler, be prepared to adhere to the protocol and be willing to provide informed consent. Exclusion criteria were current use of nicotine replacement therapy or any other behavioural or pharmacological smoking cessation or reduction programme, use of other nicotine containing products or any condition that might interfere with the study. The ethics committees of the universities of Basle and Lausanne approved the study.

Treatment

Independent pharmacists dispensed either active or placebo inhalers according to a computer generated randomisation list. All smokers received information about the general implications of smoking and its effects on health. Participants were asked to reduce the number of cigarettes smoked daily as much as possible and an initial reduction of 50% was suggested. The active treatment comprised nicotine replacement through an inhalation device (Nicorette Inhaler, Pharmacia and Upjohn).[12,13] The inhaler consists of a plastic mouthpiece into which a disposable cartridge containing $10\,mg$ nicotine and $1\,mg$ menthol is inserted. At room

(Continued)

temperature the total available nicotine content is 4-5 mg per cartridge. The inhaler delivers about 13 μg of nicotine per puff (average puff volume of 50 ml), which means that about 80 puffs are required to obtain 1 mg nicotine. The placebo inhalers were identical in appearance and contained only menthol. Both treatment groups were allowed to use the inhalers as needed, with the recommendation to use between six and 12 cartridges over 24 hours. Participants were encouraged to decrease use of the inhaler after four months but were permitted to continue treatment for 18 of the 24 months in the study.

 Self-Assessment Exercise 7.1.2

According to information in the abstract (Section 7.1.1) and the methods section (above) of paper A:

1. What were the objectives of this study?

2. From what population was the study sample selected?

3. How was the study sample selected? Comment on how suitable you think this sample is for addressing the objectives of the study

4. What were the intervention and control treatments?

Answers in Section 7.7

Summary

- Intervention studies provide a very powerful research design.

- The process of selecting a sample and following up the groups has much in common with cohort studies.

- As with any research design, practical considerations (time, money, design feasibility, etc.) influence the choice of population from which the sample is drawn and hence the generalisability of the findings.

7.2 Key elements of intervention study design

7.2.1 Defining who should be included and excluded

We have seen that the population for this study was residents in the areas of Basle and Lausanne, Switzerland, qualified by the requirement that they were smokers who were willing or unable to quit. Furthermore, since recruitment was via newspaper adverts, the population was also defined as people who read newspapers or would otherwise see (or be told about) this type of advert: this probably includes most of the adult population, but we cannot be sure of this.

The next step is to establish exactly what factors determined whether a subject was included (eligible) in the sample, and who was excluded, known as *eligibility* and *exclusion criteria*. The next exercise looks at these criteria.

Self-Assessment Exercise 7.2.1

Using the information from the abstract (Section 7.1.1) and methods (Section 7.1.2) of paper A:

1. List all the criteria used to determine whether or not a subject took part in the trial.

2. Was the selection of study subjects through a random sampling procedure, or by some other means of selection?

3. How representative do you think the study subjects are of smokers aged 18 and over in Switzerland?

Answers in Section 7.7

7.2.2 Intervention and control

Defining the intervention

In our exploration of intervention studies we will consider a range of interventions, from single medications such as the nicotine inhaler (paper A), through complex care packages for the prevention of falls among the elderly delivered through primary care, to a community-wide health promotion programme on smoking.

For now though we will keep to the nicotine inhaler study. The intervention is simple and clearly defined: use, as needed, of an inhaler that delivers about $13\,\mu g$ of nicotine per puff (methods section of paper A, Section 7.2.1). You will have noted that the nicotine inhaler (and the 'placebo' inhaler) also contained 1 mg of menthol – we will return to the reason for this in the next section.

A trial should be designed, as far as possible, with a view to wider implementation of the intervention. The intervention being tested and the circumstances in which the trial is done (e.g. the sample, exclusions, etc.) should be as close as possible to the setting in which it is hoped the intervention would ultimately be applied.

In the case of paper A, if the trial is successful and the scientific community recommend that the inhaler should be used for smokers 'unable or unwilling to quit' the intervention would be applied to the general population in pretty much the same way as it was in the trial. This means that the researchers are testing an intervention that is delivered, packaged and used almost exactly as it would be if recommended for the general population. This is not always the case with trials. The practical demands of carrying out a successful trial can require that the intervention has to be defined and/or delivered in a way that differs from what would be routine practice.

We noted, however, that the sample in this study was selected to ensure good compliance – indeed that was one of the eligibility criteria. As a result we might conclude that the findings would be most relevant to well-motivated subjects.

What should the intervention be compared with?

A crucial question arises as to what the new intervention should be compared with. In the case of this study (paper A), a *placebo* was used. This is a chemically inert substance designed to be indistinguishable from the intervention treatment. So, in this case, the nicotine inhaler is being compared with nothing, although it was a special kind of nothing. We will look at what is special about placebo after this next exercise.

 Self-Assessment Exercise 7.2.2

Again using information from the abstract of paper A (Section 7.1.1):

1. Make brief notes on exactly what the nicotine inhaler was being compared with.

2. In what circumstances do you think it is appropriate to compare a new intervention with no active treatment (whether this is nothing at all, or a placebo)?

Answers in Section 7.7

Why placebo?

It is worth restating the very important point that emerges from this exercise: ethical practice requires that the control (comparison) group be offered the best existing treatment that is in routine use. If there is no known effective treatment then the controls can be given no active treatment. If practical, this 'no active treatment' may be given as a placebo.

Why should the research team go to the trouble of providing an inactive intervention that appears identical to the real nicotine inhaler? They do so because of the *placebo effect*. The fact of being given something, especially something that looks like a medication, can influence the way people perceive their health and may in some circumstances actually directly affect health outcomes. So part of the effect of an active drug is this influence on perception and part is due to the pharmacological effect of the chemicals on the body (in the case of nicotine, reducing the craving for a cigarette). In order to identify the effect that is only due to the pharmacological effect of the drug, a placebo is introduced as the comparison:

INTERVENTION	PLACEBO CONTROL
Placebo effect	Placebo effect
Pharmacological effect of the active drug	

Both intervention and control groups experience an identical placebo effect. Any observed difference in outcome must therefore be due to the pharmacological effect of the active drug. While it is relatively easy to produce a placebo for a drug, it is much more difficult for other types of intervention. We will return to this issue later in the chapter.

7.2.3 Randomisation

Purpose

One of the most important design features of the trial is the randomisation of study subjects to receive either the intervention or the control 'treatment'. The great value of this randomisation is that, if successful, it avoids the effects of *confounding* factors.

Confounding can operate in a trial just as it does in other study designs we have looked at. Suppose that in the smoking cessation study, subjects were allocated to intervention and control groups in a non-random way and as a result those using the active inhaler were lighter smokers than those on placebo. All other things being equal we would expect the reduction in smoking to be greater in the nicotine inhaler group before taking account of any beneficial effect of the drug. This of course would be highly misleading.

Randomisation balances the two groups in terms of social, demographic, lifestyle, and other personal characteristics that could have a bearing on the outcome. This is the really big advantage of the randomised intervention design. Until now we have generally had to try to measure confounding factors, and adjust for their influence in the analysis. The one exception was the *matching* process in the case-control design, where we selected cases and controls in a way that avoided confounding factors, although this could be applied to a quite limited number of factors. The great strength of the randomised trial is that we can arrange the comparison between the intervention and control groups in a way that avoids the influence of confounding factors. This also includes confounders that we do not know about and would therefore not even measure, or match for, in other types of study. In Section 7.3 we will look at how we assess whether the randomisation has been successful.

Method of randomisation

You will encounter a variety of methods of actually carrying out the randomisation. The most important point is to ensure that the randomisation process is not influenced by the characteristics and circumstances of the subject being allocated. In the current study randomisation was done with a computer-generated list held by independent pharmacists (see excerpt on methods, Section 7.1.2).

In many clinical trials subjects are entered into the study as they present for treatment with the requisite sample size being built up over a period of months or years. A common procedure in this situation would be to have pre-randomised numbered envelopes available to the doctor or surgeon carrying out the treatments. When the next eligible person presented, the next envelope would be opened: this would inform the doctor about which treatment that person was to receive. The critical feature of this procedure is that the decision is taken in advance, so this cannot be influenced by the immediate circumstances of the person presenting for treatment.

7.2.4   Outcome assessment

The definition and assessment of outcomes is as important in intervention studies as in other study designs and we will look at how this was carried out in the nicotine trial. Please now read the following excerpt taken from the methods section of paper A describing assessment and measures of outcome:

Methods

Assessment

After the initial telephone screening and baseline assessment participants were reassessed at the clinic after one, two, three and six weeks and three, four, six, 12, 18 and 24 months. Counselling on smoking reduction was provided at each visit. Admission criteria and demography, including the Fagerström test for nicotine dependence, reasons for reducing smoking and medical and smoking history were assessed at baseline. At all key visits (baseline and months four, 12, and 24) we measured expired carbon monoxide concentrations, symptoms of withdrawal, smoking status, respiratory function, blood pressure, pulse, weight, plasma cotinine concentration, haematological variables and concentrations of blood lipids and fibrinogen. We also assessed smoking status, intention to quit, compliance, concomitant medications, adverse events and quality of life (with the SF 36 questionnaire).[15] Reported adverse events and plasma cotinine concentrations served as a basis for the safety analysis of concomitant smoking and nicotine replacement therapy.

Measures of outcome

The primary efficacy measure (success) was defined as self reported reduction of daily cigarette smoking by at least 50% compared with baseline from week six to month four, the duration for which the study was powered. This reduction was verified by decreased carbon monoxide concentrations at week six and months three and four. Results up to 24 months are presented in this paper. Smoking cessation was defined as not smoking from week six and a carbon monoxide concentration < 10 ppm at all subsequent visits. Smoking reduction and cessation are also presented with verification of carbon monoxide concentrations at each time point (point prevalence).

Self-Assessment Exercise 7.2.3

According to the above information from the methods section of paper A:

1. What is the main outcome (measure of success)?

2. How was this validated?

3. What other key outcome was assessed?

Answers in Section 7.7

7.2.5 Blinding

Blinding means preventing a person involved in the study from knowing which treatment a subject is receiving. In respect of this, there are essentially three groups of people involved in trials that can be blinded:

- the subjects, who therefore do not know whether they are taking the intervention or control treatment;

- the research team who are involved in data collection and analysis;

- the staff carrying out the treatments and patient care, which may include at least some of the research team.

You will encounter the terms, *single blinding, double blinding* (and *triple blinding*). These terms refer to blinding of one, two (or all three) of the groups described here.

 Self-Assessment Exercise 7.2.4

Using the information from the abstract (Section 7.1.1) and methods (Sections 7.1.2 and 7.2.4) of paper A:

1. Make brief notes on the blinding applied to these three groups: subjects, researchers and health-care staff.

2. List some of the reasons why you think blinding is important for each of these three groups.

3. Drawing (if you wish) on your own field of interest, describe one intervention that could not easily be blinded.

Answers in Section 7.7

7.2.6 Ethical issues for intervention studies

Earlier in this chapter we emphasised the importance of ethical practice in trials, particularly in respect of the randomisation and the choice of the control 'treatment'. We also noted that it is necessary to obtain *informed consent* from the subject before randomisation occurs. In paper A, informed consent was obtained, and ethical approval gained from the university ethics committees.

Trials, by their very nature, involve an experimental situation with something being done to the study subjects. This is very different from the study designs we have considered previously, which have involved *observing* the level of exposure in the past, now or in the future. While this observation (e.g. the sampling, measurement and follow-up work) must be done in an ethically appropriate way, in trials the experimental nature of the study demands extra attention to ethical practice.

Summary

- Clarity about criteria for inclusion in (eligibility), and exclusion from, the trial is very important for those involved in carrying out the study and also for applying the results.

- It is important to think about whether the form of the intervention is typical of what would be generally applied. If not, the trial may have little practical relevance.

- On ethical grounds, the comparison group should be offered the best existing (routine) treatment and, if there is no evidence of an effective existing treatment, this can be no treatment. Where practical, 'no treatment' can be offered as a placebo.

- Blinding reduces the possibility of bias in assessing outcomes, side effects, etc., and can be applied to (a) the study subjects, (b) the research team and (c) health-care staff involved in the care of subjects.

- Where the intervention is such that it cannot be blinded, it is important to maintain as much objectivity as possible in the outcome assessment. This can be done by involving staff who are kept unaware of the treatment allocation (for example, in analysis of laboratory specimens and of outcome data), and by using investigations (for example, breath carbon monoxide (CO)) which are less likely to be influenced by knowledge of the treatment.

- Good ethical practice is vital for all research on human populations, and this is particularly important in trials due to their experimental nature. All subjects must give informed consent before they are randomised to intervention or control groups.

7.3 The analysis of intervention studies

7.3.1 Checking the success of randomisation

The usual way to assess how well the randomisation process has balanced confounding factors is to tabulate *baseline* information about a range of these variables (age, sex, smoking habits, etc.) for the intervention and control groups. That is, we look at values for these variables before the intervention has been implemented according to the groups to which subjects were then randomised. This has been done in Table 1 from paper A, reproduced in Table 7.3.1 below.

Table 7.3.1 Baseline demographic characteristics including smoking status and history. Values are expressed as means (SD); range (Table 1 from paper A)

	Placebo ($n = 200$)	Active ($n = 200$)
No. of men	104	86
Age (years)	45.8 (10.5): 22–77	46.4 (10.5); 23–79
Weight (kg)		
Women	62.9 (10.6); 48–109	64.0 (11.2); 43–120
Men	81.5 (12.3); 57–121	80.1 (12.6); 58–130
Age when started smoking (years)	17.1 (2.7); 11–35	18.2 (4.4); 12–45
No. of cigarettes smoked/day	30.3 (12.1); 15–70	28.2 (11.4); 15–70
Exhaled CO concentration (ppm)	27.1 (11.1); 10–61	27.1 (11.5); 10–61
FTND score	5.6 (2.0); 1–10	5.5 (2.1); 1–10

CO = carbon monoxide; FTND = Fagerström test for nicotine dependence.

We can see from this that the groups are very similar for most variables, although there are some differences – particularly in the percentages of men receiving each treatment ($104/200 = 52$ per cent placebo; $86/200 = 43$ per cent active). The placebo group began smoking at a slightly younger age and smoked slightly more, but had identical breath CO and almost identical FTND (nicotine dependence) scores. These findings suggest that the placebo and intervention groups were similarly addicted and certainly the nicotine groups did not have any marked advantage. We will look at these findings in some more detail in the next exercise and consider what implications they might have for analysis of the trial.

 Self-Assessment Exercise 7.3.1

1. From the data in Table 7.3.1 (Table 1 from paper A), construct a 2×2 contingency table to illustrate the distribution of men and women in the two groups and add column percentages in each of the four cells.

2. What hypothesis test would you use to assess whether this difference is likely to have arisen by chance? Carry out the test if you wish (the result is given in the answers).

3. Do you think that the randomisation in this study has worked adequately? Can you think of any other issues that should be taken into account in making this assessment?

Answers in Section 7.7

So what should be done if it is decided that there is a significant imbalance in the two groups? First, some effort should be made to establish why this has happened – for example, is it just chance or can some systematic problem with the randomisation be identified?

Assuming there are no concerns about serious bias in the randomisation process, allowance can be made for the imbalance by adjusting the intervention effect on the outcome by multiple regression (linear for continuous outcomes, logistic for categorical). The application of these methods is essentially as has been described for cohort and case-control studies. For the current study, the (main) outcome is smoking reduction, a categorical variable which therefore requires logistic regression. The intervention will be entered in the model as a categorical explanatory variable: this has only two values of intervention and control, so dummy variables are not required. In addition, other explanatory variables which might be confounding the effect of the intervention (due to imbalance in randomisation) will be included, such as gender (categorical variable with two values: male/female), age when started smoking, and number of cigarettes smoked per day (both continuous variables).

Adjustment was not carried out in the nicotine inhaler study, however, presumably because the authors did not feel that, overall, there was any important imbalance in the randomisation.

7.3.2 Loss to follow-up

It is inevitable that some subjects will be lost to follow-up. Figure 7.3.1 is reproduced from paper A and provides detailed information on the numbers in each group that withdrew for various reasons. Inclusion of this type of flow chart in reports is increasingly considered to be good practice, especially for cohort studies and trials where dropouts can be expected.

Note that there were more withdrawals from the placebo group, particularly for the 'not willing to participate' category. If a substantial proportion of the sample is lost to follow-up, this could lead to bias, particularly if the extent and nature of these losses differ between intervention and control groups.

7.3.3 Compliance with the treatment allocation

Another issue which arises during the follow-up period of a trial is that some of the intervention group subjects (for whatever reason) might stop, or change, the 'treatment' to which they were allocated, while some of those in the control group might start, or change, the 'treatment' to which they were allocated (which may be nothing/placebo). This issue, and the consequences it has for analysis, is explored in Exercise 7.3.2 and in Section 7.3.4. Please now read the following excerpt that relates to treatment compliance and review Table 7.3.2 from the results section (Table 2 from Paper A).

Results

Treatment compliance
Inhaler use decreased over time, as expected. Of participants present at week six, 222/368 (60%) used the inhaler every day. Corresponding figures after four, 12 and 18 months were 146/318 (46%), 39/331 (12%) and 30/289 (10%), respectively. Participants in the active treatment group used an average of 4.5 cartridges a day after two weeks and 2.6 a day after 18 months; they reduced their cigarette intake significantly more than participants in the placebo group from week two onward. Table 2 shows inhaler use and reduction in the number of cigarettes smoked and exhaled carbon monoxide concentration in daily users for both the active and the placebo groups.

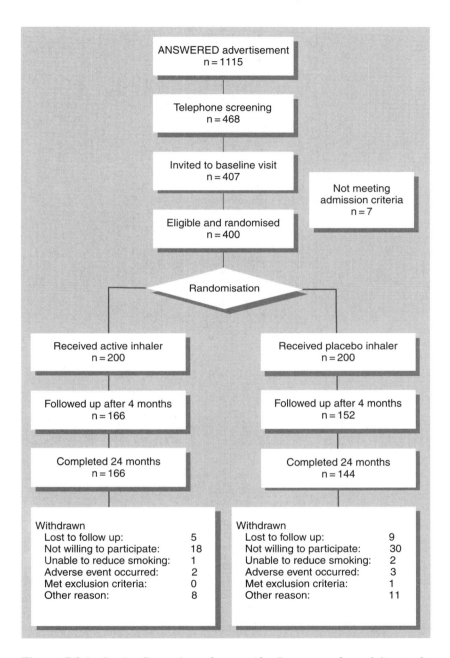

Figure 7.3.1 Study flow chart (paper A): Progress of participants in trial of oral nicotine therapy as aid for reduction in cigarette smoking. *Source*: Reproduced from Bollinger *et al.*, p. 331.

Table 7.3.2 Number of inhalers used, reduction in number of cigarettes smoked and exhaled CO concentration in participants using inhaler every day; active and placebo treatment groups. Values are expressed as means (SD) and range (Table 2 from paper A)

Time point	Intervention group				Placebo group			
	No of subjects	No of inhalers/day	Cigarettes /day as % of baseline	CO as % of baseline value	No of subjects	No of inhalers /day	Cigarettes /day as % of baseline	CO as % of baseline value
1 week	169	4.3(2.1);1–12	53(19.9);4.3–105	79.8(34.3);12.5–208	162	4.4(2.0);1–12	56.4(18.3);9.5–100	83.4(30.6);29–171
2 weeks	168	4.5(2.0);1–10	48.5(20.0);0.0–100*	73.6(31.4);11.1–182	164	4.9(2.0);1–12	54.7(18.9);0.0–104*	82(37.9);13.6–255
6 weeks	117	4.3(2.1);1–12	45.1(23.8);0.0–100†	68.4(31.4);11.1–155‡	104	4.7(2.0);1–14	55.8(18.2); 1.9–100†	84.1(50.0);16.1–450‡
4 months	84	3.9(2.0);1–10	42.7(24.3);0.0–100§	58.3(32.1);5.6–141§	62	4.0(1.9);1–10	52.0(21.7);0.0–100§	71.1(26.5);12.5–170§
12 months	27	3.5(1.9);1–7	32.6(27.3);0.0–83¶	63.7(42.4);14.3–180	12	2.8(2.1);0–6	56.3(33.4);0.0–133¶	83.9(61.4);9.8–250
18 months	22	2.6(1.7);0–6	36.2(29.6);0.0–100**	71(58.8);7.9–222	8	3.9(2.5);1–8	67.2(27.8);20–100**	81.7(41.4);50–177

P values (Wilcoxon's rank sum test) for difference between intervention and placebo: *p = 0.004; †p = 0.003; ‡p = 0.01; §p < 0.001; ¶p = 0.03;**p = 0.02
Source: Reproduced from Bollinger *et al.*, p. 331.

Self-Assessment Exercise 7.3.2

Based on the information from the previous text excerpt from paper A (Results; treatment compliance):

1. Overall, what happened to inhaler use over the course of the study?

2. From Table 7.3.2 (above), describe inhaler use in the intervention and control groups.

Answers in Section 7.7

7.3.4 Analysis by intention to treat

Table 7.3.2 presents data for only those subjects who used their inhalers every day. You may think it would be best to use these subjects for the main analysis. However, in the description of the statistical analysis (on p. 330 of paper A) we learn that;

> The primary analysis is an intention to treat analysis, including all participants who were randomised and received medication.

This means that the main analysis compares the outcomes for all subjects allocated to the intervention group with all those allocated to the control group, no matter what their compliance with treatment was. Why have the authors taken this approach? To understand the reasons for this, it is useful to consider what might at first be thought of as a more efficient approach to the analysis by doing one of the following:

- Exclude anyone from the analysis who did not comply with the treatment that they were originally allocated; or

- Analyse the outcomes for intervention group subjects who stopped using the active inhaler as if they were controls (e.g. add them to the control group) and vice versa for the control group subjects who started to use the active inhaler.

Unfortunately both of these approaches can lead to bias. The problem is that the intervention group subjects who stop taking the treatment are unlikely to be representative of the whole intervention group. If these people are excluded, or analysed as controls, the two groups (intervention and control) will no longer be balanced for confounding factors, and this was the whole point of the randomisation. The same argument applies to studies in which controls who start the intervention treatment (for example, in a study where controls become ill and need to have additional treatment), as they too are unlikely to be representative of all controls. Analysis should therefore be by *intention to treat*. As noted above, this means carrying out the analysis with subjects in the group to which they were originally allocated, even if they are no longer complying with the treatment for that group. This avoids potentially serious bias and is regarded as the most appropriate method of analysis.

One consequence of using an intention to treat approach is that any real treatment effect will be diluted by having to keep non-complying intervention and control subjects in their original groups. This is unfortunate, but at least the effect detected is (a) if anything an underestimate of the true effect and (b) not biased by the non-compliers. Another important point about analysing in this way is that it gives a more realistic idea of the effect that the treatment will have in practice, allowing for the fact that some people will not be willing or able to comply with treatment as intended.

7.3.5 What is the effect of the intervention?

To decide whether the intervention has any meaningful effect on the outcome, we need to measure the effect and then test whether the effect is statistically significant. The **hypothesis test** we use must be appropriate to the question of interest and the type of data: for example the **chi-squared test** for a categorical outcome or the **t-test** for a continuous outcome.

Table 7.3.3 Efficacy results measured as sustained and point prevalence reductions in smoking and point prevalence abstinence rates according to treatment with oral nicotine inhaler (active treatment) or placebo (Table 3 from paper A)

Definition	Time point (months)	No (%) with active treatment	No (%) with placebo	Odds ratio (95% CI)	P value (Fisher's test)
Sustained					
Reduction*	4	52 (26.0)	18 (9.0)	3.65 (2.04 to 6.19)	< 0.001
	12	26 (13.0)	8 (4.0)	3.59 (1.65 to 7.80)	0.002
	24	19 (9.5)	6 (3.0)	3.39 (1.39 to 8.29)	0.012
Point prevalence					
Reduction†	4	83 (41.5)	44 (22.0)	2.52 (1.63 to 3.87)	< 0.001
	12	59 (29.5)	43 (21.5)	1.53 (0.97 to 2.40)	0.085
	24	55 (27.5)	46 (23.0)	1.27 (0.81 to 2.00)	0.357
Abstinence‡	4	13 (6.5)	4 (2.0)	3.41 (1.16 to 10.01)	0.044
	12	16 (8.0)	12 (6.0)	1.36 (0.63 to 2.95)	0.557
	24	21 (10.5)	17 (8.5)	1.26 (0.65 to 2.47)	0.609

* Sustained reduction in number of cigarettes smoked daily by at least 50% from week 6, verified by decreased carbon monoxide concentrations compared with baseline.
† Point prevalence reduction of cigarettes smoked daily by at least 50% at months 4, 12 and 24, verified by decreased carbon monoxide concentrations compared with baseline.
‡ No cigarettes smoked, verified by carbon monoxide concentrations < 10 ppm at months 4, 12 and 24.
Source: Reproduced from Bollinger *et al.*, p. 332.

In the simplest case we want to determine whether there is a difference between the intervention and control groups in terms of the outcome measure(s) used. The hypothesis underlying our decision is the ***null hypothesis***, the opposite (or negation) of the research question; that is, that there is no difference between the two groups. In the nicotine study (paper A) the main effect (primary efficacy measure) is a ***categorical*** outcome because the effect is measured by counting the number of people in each group who have reduced smoking sufficiently to meet the success criterion. In this case, therefore, the appropriate hypothesis test is the ***chi-squared*** test, so long as the assumptions for this test are met. This approach to the analysis is explored in Exercise 7.3.3. Please now review Table 7.3.3, reproduced from the results section of paper A (Table 3 of paper A).

 Self-Assessment Exercise 7.3.3

1. We will look first at the primary efficacy measure, reported in Table 7.3.3.

   a) Create a 2×2 table for sustained reduction at 24 months (note, the total numbers that you will need are shown in the flow chart from paper A (Section 7.3.2)).

   b) The authors use the Fisher's exact test. Can you find any reason why the chi-squared test should not be used for this hypothesis test?

   c) Interpret the odds ratio (OR) and 95 per cent confidence interval (CI).

2. If you had wanted to compare the mean breath CO in the two groups (at any particular follow-up visit), what hypothesis test would you have used?

Answers in Section 7.7

7.3.6 Drawing conclusions

Based on our assessment of this trial (paper A), what can we conclude? Do our conclusions differ from those of the authors?

 Self-Assessment Exercise 7.3.4

1. Do you agree with the authors' main conclusion, as stated in the Abstract from paper A (Section 7.1.1), that the nicotine inhaler led to sustained reductions in smoking over 24 months?

2. Assuming you do agree with this conclusion, to what population(s) do you think the findings would apply?

Answers in Section 7.7

7.3.7   Safety management and trial administration

There are a number of other aspects of trial management that may have a bearing on the analysis. Some trials will arrange to have a *Data Safety Monitoring Board* (DSMB), which operates independently of the main research group. The DSMB is charged with keeping progress of the trial under review, looking particularly for adverse events. This function is in keeping with the ethical imperative that flows from the fact that the trial involves deliberately altering the management of the human subjects involved. If the DSMB is concerned about these events, it may require further investigation and possibly discontinuation of the trial.

This independent group may also carry out an *interim analysis*, breaking the randomisation code (in a blind study) to determine whether a large enough effect from the intervention can be reliably determined before the anticipated end of the study. If so, the DSMB may judge that it is unethical to continue withholding the intervention treatment (and associated benefits) from the control group and ask for the trial to be stopped.

Other recent developments in management and reporting of trials include prior registration as a condition of publication (see Chapter 9, Section 9.1.5), and guidelines for the standardisation of reporting of trials – the so called Consolidated Standards of Reporting Trials or CONSORT statement: see www.consort-statement.org.

Summary

- Randomisation is carried out to balance the distribution of confounding factors in the intervention and control groups. It is important to check how well this has been achieved.

- It is important to define the outcome measure clearly and how it will be assessed.

- Loss to follow-up should be kept to a minimum. The methods for achieving this and the consequences of substantial and/or unrepresentative loss from the groups are essentially the same as for cohort studies.

- It is inevitable that some of the intervention and control subjects will stop or change the treatment that they were originally allocated to. The extent of the compliance with treatment should be assessed.

- In order to avoid bias arising from the unrepresentative nature of non-compliance the appropriate method of analysis is by intention to treat.

- Results should be presented with a CI (and a p-value) from the hypothesis test.

- If, despite randomisation, there are imbalances in important confounding factors, these can be addressed in the analysis by multiple-regression techniques.

- Some trials engage an independent DSMB to check for adverse events and to carry out interim analysis to determine whether the trial should be stopped early to allow controls to benefit from the intervention.

7.4 Testing more complex interventions

7.4.1 Introduction

The intervention we have considered so far was rather simple: taking a nicotine inhaler as needed. No other procedure or supporting advice was tested as part of the intervention: although counselling was available, the effect of this was not being tested. RCTs of drugs are extremely important; however drug interventions are very simple by comparison with the majority of 'treatments' that are used in health care, health promotion and public health. We will see that, when testing these more complex treatments, it is often far more difficult to adhere to the **gold standard** of the blinded, randomised, placebo-controlled trial.

In this section we will start to look at a study describing a trial of a complex intervention, but which nevertheless has adhered as closely as possible to the ideal of the RCT. It also introduces a **factorial design** which involves testing more than one intervention at a time and allows us to determine whether an intervention is more effective in combination than when applied in isolation. This is known as an **interaction**, or alternatively as an **effect modification**. We will now look at the key design elements of this through Exercise 7.4.1, based on paper B.

Note that **factorial design** and **sample size** will be discussed in later sections of this chapter and survival analysis in Chapter 8.

 Self-Assessment Exercise 7.4.1

Using the information in the abstract and following excerpts (including Figure 7.4.1) from the methods section of paper B:

1. List (a) the eligibility criteria for inclusion, and (b) the exclusion criteria.

2. How representative of people over 70 years of age was the sample of people who were randomised?

3. Briefly describe the intervention and control 'treatments'. Don't go into the details of the factorial design allocation, as we will deal with that later, just focus on the types of intervention treatment and control group management.

4. How generally applicable do you think the intervention treatment would be?

5. Does the treatment of controls conform to the ethical requirement we identified in Section 7.2 of this chapter?

6. Which of the three groups involved in the trial (subjects, research team and health-care staff) were blinded to the intervention?

Answers in Section 7.7

Abstract

Objective: To test the effectiveness of, and explore interactions between, three interventions to prevent falls among older people.

Design: A randomised controlled trial with a full factorial design.

Setting: Urban community in Melbourne, Australia.

Participants: 1090 aged 70 years and over and living at home. Most were Australian born and rated their health as good to excellent; just over half lived alone.

Interventions: Three interventions (group based exercise, home hazard management and vision improvement) delivered to eight groups defined by the presence or absence of each intervention.

Main outcome measure: Time to first fall ascertained by an 18 month falls calendar and analysed with survival analysis techniques. Changes to targeted risk factors were assessed by using measures of quadriceps strength, balance, vision, and number of hazards in the home.

Results: The rate ratio for exercise was 0.82 (95% confidence interval 0.70 to 0.97, p = 0.02), and a significant effect (p < 0.05) was observed for the combinations of interventions that involved exercise. Balance measures improved significantly among the exercise group. Neither home hazard management nor treatment of poor vision showed a significant effect. The strongest effect was observed for all three interventions combined (rate ratio 0.67 (0.51 to 0.88, p = 0.004)), producing an estimated 14.0% reduction in the annual fall rate. The number of people needed to be treated to prevent one fall a year ranged from 32 for home hazard management to 7 for all three interventions combined.

Conclusions: Group based exercise was the most potent single intervention tested and the reduction in falls among this group seems to have been associated with improved balance. Falls were further reduced by the addition of home hazard management or reduced vision management, or both of these. Cost effectiveness is yet to be examined. These findings are most applicable to Australian born adults aged 70–84 years living at home who rate their health as good.

Methods

Inclusion and exclusion criteria

Participants had to be living in their own home or apartment or leasing similar accommodation and allowed to make modifications. Potential participants were excluded if they did not expect to remain in the area for two years (except for short absences); had participated in regular to moderate physical activity with a balance improvement component in the previous two months; could not walk 10–20 metres without rest, help, or having angina; had severe respiratory or cardiac disease; had a psychiatric illness prohibiting participation; had dysphasia; had had recent major home modifications; had an education and language adjusted score > 4 on the short portable mental status questionnaire[5]; or did not have the approval of their general practitioner.

(Continued)

Recruitment

... When compared with data from the national census and health survey for Australians aged over 70 living at home, the study group differed as follows: a higher proportion (46.0% v 42.8%) were aged 70-74 years and a lower proportion (7.3% v 9.8%) aged over 85 years old; a higher proportion (77.3% v 66.7%) were Australian born; a higher proportion (53.8% v 32.7%) were living alone; and a lower proportion (46.8% v 52.3%) were married. Study participants rated their health status considerably higher (very good to excellent, 62.6% v 30.7%), and a higher proportion (13.8% v 9.0%) reported taking antidepressant and hypnotic medication.

Interventions

We sent all participants a letter outlining their assigned interventions advising of necessary actions. Strength and balance—Participants attended a weekly exercise class of one hour for 15 weeks, supplemented by daily home exercises. The exercises were designed by a physiotherapist to improve flexibility, leg strength, and balance and 30-35% of the total content was devoted to balance improvement. Exercises could be replaced by a less demanding routine, depending on the participant's capability. Transport was provided where necessary. Home hazards—Home hazards were removed or modified either by the participants themselves or via the City of Whitehorse's home maintenance programme. Home maintenance staff visited the home providing a quotation for the work, including free labour and materials up to the value of $A100 (£37; $54; €60).

Vision—If a participant's vision tested below predetermined criteria and if he or she was not already receiving treatment for the problem identified, the participant was referred to his or her usual eye care provider, general practitioner, or local optometrist, to whom the vision assessment results were given. Participants not receiving the vision intervention were provided with the Australian Optometrist Association's brochure on eye care for those aged over 40.

Assessment

Participants received a home visit by a trained assessor, who was initially blinded to group assignment. After informed consent was obtained, a baseline questionnaire was completed covering demographic characteristics; ability to perform basic activities and instrumental (more complex) activities of daily living[9]; use of support services; social outings and interests; the modified falls efficacy scale[10]; self rated health; and falls and medical history. Current prescription and over the counter drugs were recorded from containers at the participants' homes. The targeted risk factors were assessed by using the methods outlined in table 1. Participants were then assigned (by computer generated randomisation) to an intervention group by an independent third party via telephone.

After 18 months the risk factor assessments were repeated in a proportion of participants (n = 442) randomly selected by an assessor blinded to the intervention group (we used only a proportion of the participants because resources to reassess the whole study group were not available and this assessment was of secondary importance to the study's main goal).

Strength and balance were also measured at the final exercise class of the first 177 participants to complete the 15 week programme, 79 of whom were among the 442 subsequently selected for final reassessment.

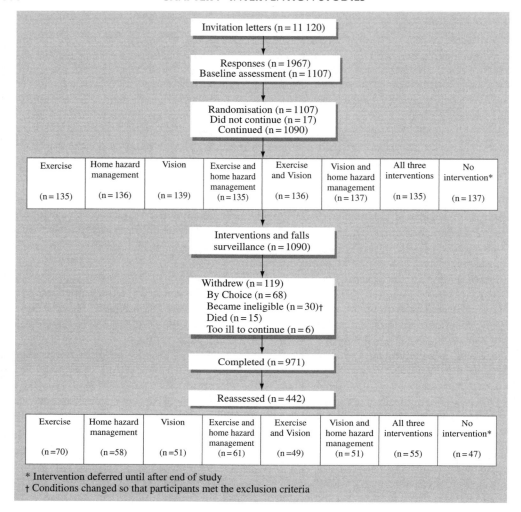

Figure 7.4.1 Flow chart showing stages in study protocol and numbers of participants
(Figure 1 from paper B)
Source: Reproduced from Day *et al.*, p. 129.

Summary

- Testing more complex interventions makes it more difficult to adhere to the 'pure' RCT design.

- Placebo control is especially difficult to achieve in these circumstances.

- Blinding may be difficult to achieve, but some degree of blinding of the assessment is usually possible and should be attempted.

7.5 How big should the trial be?

7.5.1 Introduction

The approach usually taken to determine the sample size for an intervention study involves the comparison of two groups. Indeed, the methods described here apply to any situation in which you wish to calculate sample size for comparing two groups; for example, information on smoking (the variable of interest) in men and women (the two groups) obtained through a survey.

We have previously discussed the two main types of data for statistical analysis, *categorical* and *continuous*, and the fact that we use different formulae for calculating *standard error* for these two types of data. Since standard error forms the basis of the sample size calculation we need to deal with categorical and continuous data outcomes separately.

7.5.2 Sample size for a trial with categorical data outcomes

The following description from the falls prevention trial (paper B) indicates the information that is required for sample size calculation with a categorical outcome.

> To detect a 25% relative reduction (or more) in the annual fall rate, with 5% significance level and power of 80%, 914 individuals were needed . . . The calculation assumed a non-intervention annual rate of 35 per 100 people, and a main effects two-group comparison for each intervention. Allowing for a 20% dropout rate, 1143 subjects were needed. (paper B, p. 129)

The outcome is *categorical* because the subjects are classified as either (i) experiencing a fall or (ii) not experiencing a fall. Thus, the information required is as follows:

- P_1: The percentage (or proportion) of people with the characteristic in the control group. In this study the characteristic is falling (over 1 year). The rate of falls in the non-intervention population is taken as 35 per 100 per year; hence, P_1 is 35 per cent.

- P_2: The percentage (or proportion) of people we expect to have the characteristic in the intervention group. Here the authors are designing the study to detect (at least) a 25 per cent reduction in the fall rate so P_2 is 26.25 per cent (note: this is a 25 per cent (one quarter) reduction on a rate of 35 per cent). In choosing these values the authors are making a decision about the difference $(P_1 - P_2)$ that they regard as important to be able to detect.

- The significance level chosen for the hypothesis test. In this study the chosen significance level is 5 per cent.

- The power of the study. Here 80 per cent (or 0.8) power is chosen.

With this information we can calculate the number of people needed in each group (intervention and control) using the following formula:

Number n required per group is

$$n = \frac{(P_1(100 - P_1) + P_2(100 - P_2))}{(P_1 - P_2)^2} \times f(\alpha, \beta)$$

where P_1 is the percentage with the characteristic in the control group and P_2 is the percentage we wish to detect in the intervention group with a power of $1 - \beta$ at the α significance level.

The value of $f(\alpha, \beta)$ used in the formula depends on the significance level α of the statistical test and the power β required. Table 7.5.1 below provides a range of values of $f(\alpha, \beta)$, with those that are commonly used in bold.

Table 7.5.1   Values of $f(\alpha, \beta)$ for different significance levels and powers (Reproduced from Pocock, 1984)

		Power $(1 - \beta) \times 100\%$			
		95%	**90%**	**80%**	50%
Hypothesis test	10%	10.8	8.6	6.2	2.7
significance level	**5%**	13.0	**10.5**	**7.9**	3.8
$\alpha(\times 100\%)$	2%	15.8	13.0	10.0	5.4
	1%	17.8	14.9	11.7	6.6

Inserting the figures we now have into the formula yields the following:

$$
\begin{aligned}
n(\text{per group}) &= \frac{(35 \times (100 - 35) + 26.25 \times (100 - 26.25))}{(35 - 26.25)^2} \times 7.9 \\
&= \frac{(2275 + 1935.94)}{76.56} \times 7.9 \\
&= 434.5
\end{aligned}
$$

This shows that we need around 435 subjects per group, a total of 870 to meet the criteria set. This does not quite agree with paper B, where the authors state that a total 914 subjects is required (this may be as a result of the authors using the continuity correction for comparing proportions – see Chapter 5).

7.5.3   One-sided and two-sided tests

In sample size calculations we sometimes see that *one-sided* significance has been assumed. A *one-sided test* works on the assumption (perhaps based on other evidence) that the intervention can have an effect in only one direction. We therefore need fewer data to test our hypothesis and thus a smaller sample. Although using one-sided tests will result in a smaller sample size requirement, this is a risky approach, and one that is likely to be frowned upon by statistical referees of research-funding applications and papers. In a trial of some new intervention it is wise to allow for the possibility that the new treatment could actually be worse than the best existing treatment. We do not usually have reliable enough information about the direction of any difference and it is strongly recommended that *two-sided* tests be used so that the study has sufficient power to detect either a better or worse outcome.

7.5.4   Sample size for a trial with continuous data outcomes

Calculation of sample size for a continuous outcome variable follows the same principle as for the categorical outcome, although some of the information required is different.

As with the categorical outcome, we need to make a decision about the size of difference that we wish to be able to detect (demonstrate as statistically significant). If we label the population means of the control and intervention groups μ_1 and μ_2 respectively we need to decide the difference $(\mu_1 - \mu_2)$ to be detected. Since the standard error is calculated from the standard deviation we also need to have an estimate of the standard deviation of the outcome variable. In summary we require:

- $\mu_1 - \mu_2$: The difference between the population means of the outcome variable in the control group and intervention group.

- σ: The standard deviation of both groups. Usually it will be necessary to obtain an estimate of this from other studies on similar populations (e.g. from the literature), or preparatory studies that have been carried out on the same population.

- The significance level required for the hypothesis test; e.g. 5 per cent.

- The level of power for the study; e.g. 80 per cent.

The formula for calculating the number of subjects per group for the continuous outcome is:

Number n required per group is

$$n = \frac{2\sigma^2}{(\mu_1 - \mu_2)^2} \times f(\alpha, \beta)$$

where μ_1 and μ_2 are the population mean values in the control and intervention groups respectively and σ is the standard deviation of both groups.

The $f(\alpha, \beta)$ term is once again determined from Table 7.5.1, using the appropriate values of hypothesis test significance level and power. You will now have a chance to work through this formula in the following exercise. In this exercise, we shall look at the effect on sample size of trying to detect various size differences $(\mu_1 - \mu_2)$ for continuous variables.

 Self-Assessment Exercise 7.5.1

1. In paper B, Table 3 (not shown) gives data on a number of continuous variables. The 'balance range' was an important outcome for which the baseline mean was 13.3 cm with a standard deviation of 4.5 cm. Calculate the sample size for detecting a 1.5-cm improvement in the balance range, with a significance level of 5 per cent and power of 80 per cent.

2. Comment on what you find in respect of the actual study size.

3. What is the effect on sample size of halving the balance range difference you wish to detect to 0.75 cm?

Answers in Section 7.7

7.5.5   Estimation of sample size is not a precise science

We have now looked at sample size calculation for cohort, case-control and intervention studies. This calculation involves the estimation of at least one of the parameters involved: a judgement will always have to be made about the size of the effect that you wish to detect and often the prevalence, mean or standard deviation has to be estimated from other studies. As a result, a calculated sample size should be seen as a guide and not as a precise or absolute value. In making a final decision about sample size it is wise to err on the side of caution.

Finally, do not forget to make realistic allowances for non-response in recruiting the sample and for dropouts from the follow-up phase of the trial.

Summary

- Sample size calculation is a vital part of the planning of a trial and is carried out to reduce the chances of making type I and type II errors in any given situation.

- It is wise to obtain advice from a statistician on the correct approach to calculating sample size for a given study.

- It is recommended that the alpha values (significance level of hypothesis test) associated with two-sided tests be used for sample size calculation.

- A decision is always required about the size of effect to be detected and this in turn will depend on a judgement about what size of effect is important to demonstrate.

- Sample size calculation provides a guide for study design and should not be seen as a very precise exercise. If in doubt, err on the side of caution!

- Make realistic allowances for non-response and dropouts.

7.6 Further aspects of intervention study design and analysis

7.6.1 Introduction

A number of more complex features of intervention study design and analysis have been introduced in paper B (falls prevention trial) and we will now take a look at the most important aspects of these in some more detail. In your further reading of this paper do not be concerned at this stage that you are unfamiliar with a number of methods and statistical procedures described, including factorial design, analysis of variance, Cox proportional hazards and Kaplan–Meier curves. We will work through and explain these at various points in this and subsequent chapters, beginning here with factorial design.

7.6.2 Factorial design

We saw in the falls prevention study that, instead of simply comparing two groups (intervention and control) as in the nicotine inhaler study, there were a total of eight groups, some with combinations of interventions and one with none. The allocations are set out in Table 7.6.1.

Table 7.6.1 Summary of intervention allocation in the falls prevention study (paper B)

Intervention type			Number of subjects allocated	Number of interventions
Exercise programme	**Home hazard removal**	**Vision test and referral**		
Yes	No	No	135	One intervention
No	Yes	No	136	
No	No	Yes	139	
Yes	Yes	No	135	Two interventions
Yes	No	Yes	136	
No	Yes	Yes	137	
Yes	Yes	Yes	135	All three interventions
No	No	No	137	No intervention
Total			1090	

This design allows comparisons to be made in the following way:

- First of all, note that each type of intervention is experienced by half of the total sample. Thus, half the sample $(135 + 135 + 136 + 135)$ had the exercise programme and half did not, so it is possible to compare exercise with no exercise in the whole sample. This is the basis of the sample size calculation and what is meant by the **main effect** two-group comparison.

- Of course only 135 subjects have the exercise programme alone: all the other subjects with exercise also have one or more other interventions. The factorial design, together with the way it is analysed (**an**alysis **of** **va**riance, or 'ANOVA'), allows the main effects (single intervention effects) and the effects in combination (**interactions**) to be identified. ANOVA will be introduced in Chapter 11.

- Overall, the design also allows comparisons to be made of:

  - single intervention versus another single intervention;

  - single intervention versus no intervention;

  - two interventions together versus a single intervention, or no intervention;

  - three interventions together versus two interventions together, a single intervention, or no intervention.

7.6.3   Analysis and interpretation

We will now take a look at how the falls prevention study was analysed. You will find that some aspects of this are familiar, but some are new. Two familiar elements of the analysis include (a) checking whether the randomisation has balanced variables across interventions and control groups (characteristics of participants at baseline: Tables 2 and 3, reproduced in Table 7.6.2), and (b) analysis by intention to treat.

Checking the success of randomisation

It may seem that Table 7.6.2 presents the baseline characteristics in an unfamiliar way. Since there are eight groups, rather than listing the mean and standard deviation (SD) (or per cent) values for each group, the range across the groups is given (column 2). Thus, for age, the lowest group mean was 75.4 years and the highest 76.5 years, with the other six groups distributed in between these values. This suggests that randomisation had balanced the groups quite well by age, but what about the other variables? Look, for example, at the balance of males and females in row 2 of the upper table (Table 2 from paper B).

Compliance with interventions

It is important to take a close look at compliance with interventions, as this will help us in interpreting the results. Also, since **intention to treat** analysis has been used, comparisons are made according to the group that subjects were randomised to, not according to whether they complied with the intervention offered in that group. Please now read the excerpt below on intervention compliance, from the results section of paper B. Exercise 7.6.1 explores the level of compliance and considers the implications for the analysis.

Table 7.6.2 Baseline values in the intervention and control groups (Tables 2 and 3 from paper B)

Table 2 Characteristics of participants at baseline

Characteristic	All participants (n = 1090)	Range across intervention groups (n = 1090)*	Reassessed participants (n = 442)†
Mean (SD) age (years)	76.1 (5.0)	75.4–76.5 (4.7–5.5)	75.9 (4.9)
No (%) of women	652 (59.8)	77–93 (55.4–68.4)	261 (59.0)
No (%) of participants living alone	586 (53.8)	68–83 (50.0–61.0)	230 (52.0)
No (%) of participants who had a fall in past month	69 (6.3)	5–11 (3.7–8.1)	31 (7.0)
Mean (SD) score for activities of daily living‡	5.3 (1.1)	5.2–5.4 (0.92–1.2)	5.3 (1.1)
Mean (SD) No of medications	3.4 (2.6)	3.1–3.6 (2.4–2.9)	3.3 (2.6)

SD=standard deviation.

*Highest and lowest recorded among the eight groups. Measures for the remaining groups fall within the range.

†Participants randomly selected for reassessment at end of follow up.

‡Score for instrumental activities of daily living, plus bathing.

Table 3 Targeted risk factor measures at baseline. Values are means (standard deviation)

Measure	All participants (n = 1090)	Range across intervention groups (n = 1090)*	Reassessed participants (n = 442)†
Quadriceps strength in stronger leg (kg)	22.6 (10.5)	21.3–24.0 (9.6–11.8)	23.2 (10.7)
Postural sway on foam pad (log)	2.8 (0.35)	2.7–2.8 (0.32–0.40)	2.7 (0.37)
Maximal balance range (cm)	13.3 (4.5)	13.0–13.7 (4.2–5.0)	13.5 (4.7)
Coordinated stability (sum of errors)	12.4 (8.4)	11.4–13.0 (7.6–9.2)	11.6 (8.0)
Timed 'up and go'(s)	11.7 (5.3)	10.9–12.3 (3.6–6.2)	11.6 (5.6)
High contrast acuity in best eye (logMAR)	0.08 (0.19)	0.05–0.11 (0.18–0.21)	0.06 (0.19)
Low contrast acuity in best eye (logMAR)	0.38 (0.19)	0.34–0.42 (0.17–0.20)	0.38 (0.19)
Dot pattern (No of patterns identified)	5.8 (3.2)	5.5–6.1 (3.1–3.4)	6.0 (3.1)
Field of view in best eye (No of correct identifications)	25.2 (3.0)	24.8–25.5 (1.9–4.5)	25.4 (2.7)
Home Hazards (No identified)	9.3 (4.8)	8.3–10.1 (4.3–5.4)	9.6 (4.7)

Source: Reproduced from Day *et al.*, p. 32.

Intervention compliance

Of the 541 participants receiving the exercise intervention, 401 started a class. The mean number of sessions attended was 10 (SD 3.8) and 328 participants attended more than 50% of their sessions. The mean number of additional home exercise sessions was nine a month. Of the 543 participants receiving the home hazard management intervention, 478 participants were advised to have modifications in their homes; 363 of these participants received help to do these modifications, which included hand rails fitted (275 participants), modifications to floor coverings (72), contrast edging fitted to steps (72) and maintenance to steps or ramps (66).

Of the 547 participants receiving the vision intervention, 287 were recommended for referral, of whom 186 had either recently visited or were about to visit their eye care practitioner. Of the remaining 101 participants, 97 took up the referral, resulting in 26 having some form of treatment – new or modified prescription glasses (20) or surgery (6).

Self-Assessment Exercise 7.6.1

1. Briefly summarise the information given on compliance.

2. Comment on compliance with each of the three interventions.

Answers in Section 7.7

Reassessment of risk factors during follow-up

Not all of the study subjects were reassessed for risk factors at 18 months. Exercise 7.6.2 explores this further, including implications for the interpretation of results.

Self-Assessment Exercise 7.6.2

According to the information from excerpts on assessment (Section 7.4.1) and Table 7.6.2 (Section 7.6.3, Tables 2 and 3 from paper B):

1. How many (what percentage) of the subjects were reassessed at 18 months?

2. Why did the investigators not reassess all subjects?

3. How did they select those that were reassessed?

4. What information is available to judge how representative the reassessed individuals were of all study subjects?

5. How representative do you think these individuals were?

Answers in Section 7.7

Analysis of main effects of the intervention

The main results of the study are shown in Table 7.6.3 (Table 4 from paper B) below. You may have seen from paper B that the effect estimates, expressed as rate ratios, have been obtained by Cox proportional hazards regression. Cox regression is the method of choice when using outcome data that include time until the event occurs, as is the case in this study. This is known as survival analysis, and will be studied in Chapter 8. For now, we can treat the results of Cox regression as if these were ORs from logistic regression (which we would use for a categorical outcome such as falls). A number of other techniques used in the analysis of this study will be covered later in the book. Figure 2 in paper B (not reproduced here) shows the outcomes over time graphically in what are known as Kaplan–Meier curves and these are also covered in Chapter 8. Analysis of variance (ANOVA), which is used to test main effects and interactions in a factorial design, is introduced in Chapter 11, together with paired t-tests and the Fisher's exact test.

Table 7.6.3 Effect on falls outcome, single and combined interventions (Table 4 from paper B)

Intervention	No (%) having at least one fall	Rate ratio		% estimated reduction in annual fall rate (95% CI)	No needed to treat to prevent 1 fall
		Estimate (95% CI)	P value		
No intervention*	87/137 (63.5)	1.00 (Reference)			
Exercise	76/135 (56.3)	0.82 (0.70 to 0.97)	0.02	6.9 (1.1 to 12.8)	14
Vision	84/139 (60.4)	0.89 (0.75 to 1.04)	0.13	4.4 (−1.5 to 10.2)	23
Home hazard management	78/136 (57.4)	0.92 (0.78 to 1.08)	0.29	3.1 (−2.0 to 9.7)	32
Exercise plus vision	66/136 (48.5)	0.73 (0.58 to 0.91)	0.01	11.1 (2.2 to 18.5)	9
Exercise plus home hazard management	72/135 (53.3)	0.76 (0.60 to 0.95)	0.02	9.9 (2.4 to 17.9)	10
Vision plus home hazard management	78/137 (56.9)	0.81 (0.65 to 1.02)	0.07	7.4 (−0.9 to 15.2)	14
Exercise plus vision plus home hazard management	65/135 (48.1)	0.67 (0.51 to 0.88)	0.004	14.0 (3.7 to 22.6)	7

* No intervention until after the study had ended.
Source: Reproduced from Day *et al.*, p. 133.

First, look at Table 7.6.3. You will be familiar with the interpretation of rate ratios (relative risk), 95 per cent CIs and the p-value. The **number needed to treat** (NNT) (last column) is an important new concept and describes the number of subjects that need to be 'treated' (given the intervention) to prevent one event (in this case, a fall). It is calculated as 1/difference between proportions experiencing events in the intervention and comparison groups (or 100/difference if this is calculated from percentages). We will now look at interpretation of the main effect results and one example of NNT in Exercise 7.6.3.

Self-Assessment Exercise 7.6.3

From the information in Table 7.6.3 (Table 4 from paper B), above:

1. Interpret the rate ratios, 95 per cent CI and p-values for receiving (a) exercise and (b) vision interventions.

2. Now interpret the rate ratio, 95 per cent CI and p-value for receiving exercise and vision interventions in combination. How does this compare with the results for the interventions on their own?

3. The number needed to treat for all three interventions in combination is seven. See whether you can work out how this was derived. What does a NNT of seven for these interventions mean?

Answers in Section 7.7

7.6.4   Departure from the ideal blinded RCT design

In the foregoing sections we have emphasised two important themes in respect of the design and application of intervention studies:

- The strength of the 'ideal' RCT as a research design arises from the randomisation, controlled comparison, the use of placebo, and application of blinding.

- For many interventions, however, it is not possible to adhere to all aspects of this 'ideal' design. We have already discussed a number of interventions where blinding was not possible.

Table 7.6.4 summarises opportunities (or lack of them) for randomisation, use of placebo controls and blinding for a range of intervention types, from drug/vaccine trials, through to more complex preventive and health-care interventions.

Table 7.6.4   Methodological opportunities and constraints in trials of various types of intervention

Intervention	Randomisation	Control/placebo	Blinding
Drug or vaccine	Possible	Possible, often with placebo control	Blinding of all groups usually possible.
Surgical operation	Possible	Control operation, but placebo not possible	Not possible for surgical team, or for patient in some circumstances. Some blinding of assessment should be done if possible.

Medical treatment extending beyond medication alone, e.g. health education advice, management by a multidisciplinary team, etc.	Possible	Control treatment, but placebo not possible	Usually not possible. Some blinding of assessment should be done if possible.
Health promotion initiative at group level, e.g. whole (GP) practice	Can randomise clusters (groups, e.g. general practices) if a sufficient number are available	Control groups, but comparability may be difficult to achieve and maintain	Not possible. Some blinding of assessment should be done if possible.
Health promotion initiative at community, city or regional level	Not possible	Control area, but comparability will be difficult to achieve and maintain	Not possible. Blinding of assessment also very difficult with such a broadly applied intervention.

7.6.5   Cluster randomisation

Reasons for selecting cluster randomised design

In the two intervention studies discussed so far, individual people have been randomised. For some interventions it is more appropriate to randomise groups of people, such as schools or general practices. These groups are known as *clusters*, a term we have already encountered in sampling.

Group (cluster) randomisation is more suitable for interventions that involve, as part of their delivery, components that are not directed solely at individuals but at groups of service users – for example, health information posters in general practice or school-based health promotion activities. Although these may be adjuncts to interventions directed at individuals on a one-to-one basis, the group-based component means that randomisation of individual subjects within the practice or school would not be appropriate. When control subjects are exposed to influences intended to be solely for intervention subjects, this is known as *contamination*. This may operate in rather subtle ways. For example, even if a practice-based intervention is applied to individuals, it may be very difficult to prevent information exchange between intervention and control subjects, particularly for interventions that cannot be blinded and involve information and advice. An additional factor with a non-blinded intervention in settings such as general practice is that it may be difficult for the health-care staff to ensure even-handed treatment of intervention and control patients in the same practice. For all of these reasons it may be better to randomise the whole practice (or other type of cluster), rather than individuals within that cluster.

Most aspects of cluster randomisation trials are similar to individual-based randomisation studies, but there are some key features that do differ. As an example we will look briefly at a study of the effectiveness of exercise advice and prescription ('green prescription') for 40–59-year-olds habitually doing little physical activity, set in general practice in New Zealand (paper C). The abstract for this study is reproduced below.

Abstract

Objective: To assess the long term effectiveness of the 'green prescription' programme, a clinician based initiative in general practice that provides counselling on physical activity.

Design: Cluster randomised controlled trial. Practices were randomised before systematic screening and recruitment of patients.

Setting: 42 rural and urban general practices in one region of New Zealand.

Subjects: All sedentary 40–79 year old patients visiting their general practitioner during the study's recruitment period.

Intervention: General practitioners were prompted by the patient to give oral and written advice on physical activity during usual consultations. Exercise specialists continued support by telephone and post. Control patients received usual care.

Main outcome measures: Change in physical activity, quality of life (as measured by the 'short form 36' (SF-36) questionnaire), cardiovascular risk (Framingham and D'Agostino equations) and blood pressure over a 12 month period.

Results: 74% (117/159) of general practitioners and 66% (878/1322) of screened eligible patients participated in the study. The follow up rate was 85% (750/878). Mean total energy expenditure increased by 9.4 kcal/kg/week ($p = 0.001$) and leisure exercise by 2.7 kcal/kg/week ($p = 0.02$) or 34 minutes/week more in the intervention group than in the control group ($p = 0.04$). The proportion of the intervention group undertaking 2.5 hours/week of leisure exercise increased by 9.72% ($p = 0.003$) more than in the control group (number needed to treat = 10.3). SF-36 measures of self rated 'general health,' 'role physical,' 'vitality,' and 'bodily pain' improved significantly more in the intervention group ($p < 0.05$). A trend towards decreasing blood pressure became apparent but no significant difference in four year risk of coronary heart disease.

Conclusion: Counselling patients in general practice on exercise is effective in increasing physical activity and improving quality of life over 12 months.

Please now read the following excerpt from paper C describing the 'green prescription' used as the intervention in this cluster-randomised trial.

The 'green prescription' intervention

- Primary care clinicians are offered four hours of training in how to use motivational interviewing techniques to give advice on physical activity and the green prescription.

- Patients who have been identified as 'less active' through screening at the reception desk and who agree to participate receive a prompt card, stating their stage of change, from the researcher, to give to the general practitioner during consultation.

- In the consultation, the primary care professional discusses increasing physical activity and decides on appropriate goals with the patient. These goals, usually home based physical activity or walking, are written on a standard green prescription and given to the patient.

- A copy of the green prescription is faxed to the local sports foundation with the patient's consent. Relevant details such as age, weight and particular health conditions are often included.

- Exercise specialists from the sports foundation make at least three telephone calls (lasting 10–20 minutes) to the patients over the next three months to encourage and support them. Motivational interviewing techniques are used. Specific advice about exercise or community groups is provided if appropriate.

- Quarterly newsletters from the sports foundations about physical activity initiatives in the community and motivational material are sent to participants. Other mailed materials, such as specific exercise programmes, are sent to interested participants.

- The staff of the general practice are encouraged to provide feedback to the participant on subsequent visits to the practice.

 Self-Assessment Exercise 7.6.4

1. Why do you think the authors chose a cluster design rather than individual based randomisation?

2. What management do you think the control clusters would have received?

Answers in Section 7.7

Sample size

The calculation of sample size for a cluster trial is similar in most respects to that you have carried out for an individual-based two-group comparison. The new element is that we need to take account of the fact that subjects within a cluster are more alike (for example, socio-economically or in respect of influences of the practice) than subjects from different clusters.

An adjustment is therefore made by using an estimated value for ***intra-class correlation***. Please now read the following excerpt on sample size calculation from paper C, which describes how coefficients based on estimates from previous studies were used for the four main outcomes:

Sample size calculation

A sample size of 800 patients from 40 practices ($\alpha = 0.05$, power $= 90\%$) was required to detect differences in change between the intervention and control groups of one hour of moderate physical activity per week, 4.5 mm Hg systolic blood pressure, 10% relative risk of cardiovascular events and six points of SF-36 'vitality.' We assumed an attrition rate of 25%. To account for the effect of clustering, we adjusted the sample size calculations by using intraclass correlation coefficients of 0.05, 0.016, 0.0036 and 0.05 for physical activity, blood pressure, cardiovascular risk and 'vitality,' respectively, based on estimates from previous studies.[9–11]

We will not take the use of intra-class correlation for sample size further in this book and, at this stage, it is sufficient that you are aware of the need to allow for the greater similarity of individuals within clusters. As previously, we recommend that advice from a statistician be sought for all but the most straightforward sample size calculations.

Analysis

The analysis of cluster-randomised trials has much in common with the methods we have already studied. The main difference is that we should again take account of the greater similarity of people within clusters. Table 7.6.5 (Table 2 from paper C) is reproduced below and shows the main results: we can see that the analysis is carried out initially for all subjects, ignoring clustering (columns 2 and 3). In column 4 the differences between groups are shown as the 'difference between groups' (intervention minus control), allowing for clustering in practices. The statistical techniques used included mixed and random effects regression modelling. We will not discuss these methods further here, but you can interpret the regression coefficients (column 4) in the same way as you have done previously with multiple linear regression (these are all continues outcomes).

7.6.6 The community randomised trial

We began this chapter by looking at a pharmacological (drug-based) approach to helping people reduce and stop smoking using a nicotine replacement inhaler. A double-blinded, placebo-controlled, randomised trial was both feasible and appropriate. What approach would be appropriate, however, if we wanted to study the effectiveness of measures to prevent young people from taking up smoking?

We know that adoption of smoking by young people is influenced by a range of family, peer group, school and wider societal factors. Interventions to address these cannot realistically be delivered within tightly defined groups. In this last example of a randomised trial, we will look at a study designed to test community approaches to preventing adolescent tobacco use (paper D). The units of randomisation are small communities in Oregon, USA. Comparison was made between a school-based intervention only (control communities) and school plus community intervention (intervention communities). The community intervention was carried out by a paid community coordinator and included:

- media advocacy;

- anti-tobacco activities designed to be engaging and persuasive for young people;

- family communication about tobacco use;

- reducing youth access to tobacco in stores.

In this section we will study only the principal design issues involved in a randomised community trial. Please now read the abstract and excerpt from the methods section (design) from paper D, reproduced below. The following exercise will help you identify the key design points.

Table 7.6.5 Mean changes (95 per cent CIs) in physical activity, cardiovascular and quality-of-life outcomes in the control and intervention groups at 12 months (Table 2 from paper C)

No adjustment for clustering within practices

Adjustment for clustering within practices

Measure	Intervention* (n = 451)	Control*	Difference between groups† (n = 878)	P value
Primary outcomes:				
Total energy expenditure (kcal/kg/week)	9.76 (5.85 to 13.68)	0.37 (−3.39 to 4.14)	9.38 (3.96 to 14.81) (975 kcal/week)	0.001‡
Leisure physical activity (kcal/kg/week)	4.32 (3.26 to 5.38)	1.29 (0.11 to 2.47)	2.67 (0.48 to 4.86) (247 kcal/week)	0.02§
Leisure exercise (minutes/week)	54.6 (41.4 to 68.4)	16.8 (6.0 to 32.4)	33.6 (2.4 to 64.2)	0.04§
Systolic blood pressure (mm Hg)	−2.58 (−4.02 to −1.13)	−1.21 (−2.57 to 0.15)	−1.31 (−3.51 to 0.89)	0.2
Diastolic blood pressure (mm Hg)	−2.62 (−3.62 to −1.61)	−0.81 (−1.77 to 0.16)	−1.40 (−3.35 to 0.56)	0.2
4 year risk of coronary heart disease (%)	0.42 (0.23 to 0.60)	0.52 (0.32 to 0.72)	−0.10 (−0.43 to 0.23)	0.6
SF-36 quality of life scores:				
Physical functioning	3.16 (1.61 to 4.71)	1.63 (−0.04 to 3.31)	1.23 (−1.35 to 3.81)	0.3
Role physical	10.53 (6.8 to 14.3)	4.16 (0.63 to 7.68)	7.24 (0.16 to 14.31)	0.045§
Bodily pain	6.51 (4.28 to 8.74)	2.50 (0.15 to 4.86)	4.01 (0.78 to 7.24)	0.02§
General health	5.95 (4.43 to 7.47)	1.60 (0.22 to 2.99)	4.51 (2.07 to 6.95)	0.000‡
Vitality	5.36 (3.76 to 6.96)	3.06 (1.44 to 4.68)	2.30 (0.03 to 4.57)	0.047§
Social functioning	3.02 (0.68 to 5.36)	2.85 (0.57 to 5.13)	0.36 (−3.53 to 4.26)	0.9
Role emotional	5.32 (1.43 to 9.21)	5.70 (2.07 to 9.32)	−0.38 (−5.70 to 4.94)	0.9
Mental health	2.61 (1.17 to 4.04)	1.63 (0.28 to 2.98)	0.98 (−0.99 to 2.95)	0.3
Other variables:				
Body mass index (kg/m²)	−0.11 (−0.25 to 0.02)	−0.05 (−0.18 to 0.07)	−0.06 (−0.24 to 0.12)	0.5
Cholesteral concentration (mmol/l)	−0.019 (−0.08 to 0.05)	0.01 (−0.05 to 0.06)	−0.02 (−0.12 to 0.09)	0.7

*Unadjusted for clustering.
†Adjusted for clustering by medical practice.
‡Significant at 0.01 level.
§Significant at 0.05 level.

Abstract

Objective: Experimental evaluation of comprehensive community wide programme to prevent adolescent tobacco use.

Design: Eight pairs of small Oregon communities (population 1700 to 13 500) were randomly assigned to receive a school based prevention programme or the school based programme plus a community programme. Effects were assessed through five annual surveys (time 1–5) of seventh and ninth grade (ages 12–15 years) students.

Intervention: The community programme included: (a) media advocacy, (b) youth anti-tobacco activities, (c) family communications about tobacco use and (d) reduction of youth access to tobacco.

Main outcome measure: The prevalence of self-reported smoking and smokeless tobacco use in the week before assessment.

Results: The community programme had significant effects on the prevalence of weekly cigarette use at times 2 and 5 and the effect approached significance at time 4. An effect on the slope of prevalence across time points was evident only when time 2 data points were eliminated from the analysis. The intervention affected the prevalence of smokeless tobacco among grade 9 boys at time 2. There were also significant effects on the slope of alcohol use among ninth graders and the quadratic slope of marijuana for all students.

Conclusion: The results suggest that comprehensive community wide interventions can improve on the preventive effect of school based tobacco prevention programmes and that effective tobacco prevention may prevent other substance use.

Design

The design of the current study is shown in fig 1. It was a randomised controlled trial in which small Oregon communities were assigned to one of two conditions (see below). The population of these communities ranged from 1700 to 13 500. The principal economic activities are tourism, logging, fishing and farming. Communities were selected such that the possibility of contamination between communities was minimised. The communities share no common high schools and are at least 20 miles apart. In order to participate, school districts agreed to implement the school based intervention and to permit the in-school assessment sequence shown in fig 1.

Pairs of communities were matched on community socioeconomic status and population. One member of each pair was assigned at random (via the flip of a coin) to receive a school based tobacco and other substance use prevention programme (school based only (SBO) condition) in grades 6 through to 12. The other member received a community intervention programme in addition to the school based programme (CP condition). Communities in the two conditions did not differ statistically in size, per capita income, median household income, the percent of people below the poverty level, the proportion of minority students, the number of high school students per grade, or the proportion of high school graduates in the population.

Implementation of the design was carried out in three phases to allow refinement and streamlining of intervention procedures and to minimise demands on project personnel.

Self-Assessment Exercise 7.6.5

According to the information in the abstract and the excerpt on methods from paper D:

1. How many communities were involved?

2. How large (population size) were the communities?

3. What factors helped to minimise 'contamination' between communities?

4. How did the investigators try to minimise the effect of confounding factors in the comparison between control and intervention communities?

5. What evidence was there that they had succeeded in the objective described in (4) above?

Answers in Section 7.7

7.6.7   Non-randomised intervention study designs

Some studies do not carry out a randomised, controlled comparison of an intervention, but find other ways to provide a group with which to compare an intervention. This may be done for practical or ethical reasons. For example, a group (e.g. a practice or hospital sample) might be taken for comparison, but not as part of a randomised allocation. These types of comparison studies are sometimes termed *quasi-experimental* because there is a comparison group, but it is not subject to random allocation as in all of the examples so far in this chapter.

The main limitation of these study designs is that confounding factors are unlikely to be as well balanced as when randomisation is used. In order to address this and make the comparison as valid as possible, an attempt is sometimes made to 'match' study groups according to social, demographic or other characteristics. Adjustment for imbalance in confounding factors would normally be required by multiple regression, as described in Section 7.3.1.

Alternatively, a *before and after comparison* may be made. In this design subjects serve as their own controls: their status with respect to the variable of interest is measured before and after the intervention. This leads to *paired* data: for each subject we have a data value before intervention and a data value after intervention.

7.6.8   Paired comparisons

Here is a scenario for a study involving the generation of paired data:

In a study of the effect of education on patients' management of asthma, a group of asthma patients attended a series of talks about asthma and its treatment. The intention was that this would result in greater understanding about their disease and the way their medication works and that they would consequently make better use of their prescribed drugs and suffer less from asthma symptoms. To evaluate how much the patients had learned they took a short test on asthma and its treatment before the series of talks and a similar test at the end of the course and their scores were recorded.

In this example the two test scores for each patient are paired continuous outcome data (Table 7.6.6).

Table 7.6.6 Test scores of asthma patients before and after attending a series of talks about asthma and its treatment

| Subject | Test scores | | Difference (A–B) |
	Before talks (B)	After talks (A)	
1	51	55	4
2	43	49	6
3	48	52	4
4	19	32	13
5	57	62	5
6	39	44	5
7	37	40	3
8	46	46	0
9	43	39	−4
10	43	52	9
11	53	50	−3
12	58	61	3
13	49	54	5
Mean	**45.08**	**48.92**	**3.85**

We can see that this gives us a series of differences (A–B) for each person. The mean of these differences is 3.85, which is of course the difference between the mean of the after scores (A) and the mean of the before scores (B). When, in analysing paired data, we wish to carry out a hypothesis test, we need to use a test which is based on the distribution of these differences. These are called ***paired tests***. In this example we have continuous data (the scores), so we use a ***paired t-test*** (in contrast to the independent sample *t*-test we have already used). We will cover this and other paired tests in Chapter 11.

Paired data also arise if we ***match*** individuals in the control and intervention groups. The matching is with respect to factors that are likely to affect the outcome, such as age, sex, area of residence, etc. We have seen the use of this technique in case-control studies and you have already encountered the hypothesis test used for matched case-control studies, known as ***McNemar's test***. Here is an exercise to help you understand when it is appropriate to use a paired comparison.

Self-Assessment Exercise 7.6.6

Which of the following should use a paired approach to analysis?

(a) Thirty male volunteers take a psychological test to determine reasoning. Before the test 15 volunteers drink two glasses of whisky. The test scores are determined.

(b) Twenty male volunteers take two psychological tests to determine reasoning. Each volunteer has no alcohol before the first test, but drinks two glasses of whisky before the second test. Test scores are determined.

Answers in Section 7.7

7.6.9 The cross-over trial

This is a special form of RCT, which allows subjects to operate as their own controls. This design has been used most commonly for testing drugs. The structure is summarised in Figure 7.6.1.

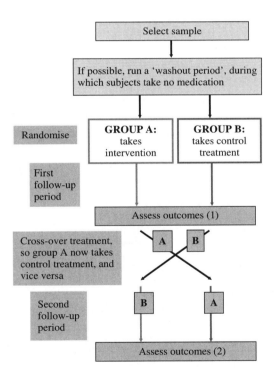

Figure 7.6.1 Schematic overview of a cross-over trial

During the course of the trial, each subject crosses over from receiving one treatment to receiving the other. This design is most suitable for treatments that bring rapid relief of symptoms in chronic diseases, where the long-term condition of the subjects remains fairly stable.

There are a number of advantages and disadvantages of this study design. One of the principal attractions of the cross-over trial is that subjects operate as their own controls, thus reducing the random error which has to be dealt with in the analysis. This means that the study can be done with much smaller numbers and is therefore cheaper and easier.

A crossover trial results in data in the form of matched pairs: there are two measurements for each subject, one for each treatment. These are clearly paired. Thus, we can analyse a cross-over trial by methods for paired data, such as the paired t-test for a continuous outcome. However, there is a bit more to the analysis of the cross-over trial. We need to take into account the order in which each subject received the two treatments and the possibility of the effect of one treatment carrying over to the next period in which the subject is receiving the alternative treatment. These methods are beyond the scope of this book.

Summary

- The elements of RCT design that contribute to its scientific strength become more difficult to apply with more complex preventative, health-care and community-based interventions.

- Cluster randomisation is appropriate for interventions that include components that can, or are intended to, impact on groups and where there is a high chance of so-called contamination (controls are exposed to influences intended only for the intervention group).

- Community-based trials, which may also be randomised, are appropriate where the intervention(s) address social determinants of behaviour and health, which are most effectively addressed through action at the level of communities.

- Quasi-experimental studies may be used when randomisation is not practical, but they require greater attention to the effects of confounding.

- It is important to be aware of what is lost by deviating from the 'pure' RCT design, and to preserve as much as possible. However, overzealous adherence to ideal RCT design where this is inappropriate may well result in an artificial intervention and/or an atypical study sample, and ultimately compromise the usefulness of the results and the extent to which these can be generalised.

- Paired data are generated in situations where subjects act as their own controls (the same people are assessed before and after an intervention), or when subjects are fairly closely matched. Paired data should be analysed by paired hypothesis tests.

- The cross-over trial is a special type of RCT which uses subjects as their own controls and thereby reduces random error and the sample size required. This strength has to be balanced against the problem of 'carry-over' and order effects, so it can only be used for certain types of intervention.

7.7 Answers to self-assessment exercises

Section 7.1

Exercise 7.1.1

If the research team had carried out an observational study (e.g. case-control or cohort), they would have to base their exposure assessment on measurement of existing patterns of nicotine inhaler use among people in a study sample. This was a relatively new product and may therefore not be used extensively, presenting practical difficulties for achieving the required sample size. Furthermore, people who were using the inhaler already would be unlikely to be typical of all 'smokers unable or unwilling to quit', so the research team would need to go to great lengths to try to characterise the features of users and non-users and adjust for these. It is unlikely they could avoid the bias resulting from this. By this approach, it would not be possible to blind the subjects or research team to whether or not subjects were using an inhaler, thus introducing another source of bias.

Thus, in order to gain more effective control of who used the inhaler and to minimise other sources of bias, it was very appropriate to carry out an intervention study.

Exercise 7.1.2

1. Objectives:

   - To determine the effectiveness of an oral nicotine inhaler in achieving long-term reduction in smoking.

   - To determine safety of nicotine inhaler use among people who are still smoking.

2. The population was people (male and female), aged 18 and over, living in (and around, depending on the readership of newspapers) Basle and Lausanne, Switzerland, who were smokers 'unable or unwilling to give up, but interested in reducing their smoking'. When we look at the eligibility criteria you will see that this was further defined, and we will consider this further in Exercise 7.2.1.

3. The sample was selected by using newspaper advertisements, asking for healthy smokers 'unable or unwilling to give up, but interested in reducing their smoking'. These were therefore volunteers. The question of whether this sample is representative of the population is considered further in Exercise 7.2.1 but, even if demographic characteristics are similar between sample and population, one must always ask whether volunteers differ in other ways that are relevant to the study; for example, having a higher level of motivation, or being prepared to try something new.

4. The intervention was an inhaler containing nicotine and menthol. The control was a placebo inhaler, containing only menthol. The use of placebos is considered further in Section 7.2.

Section 7.2

Exercise 7.2.1

1. The criteria that determined whether or not a person took part were as follows:

Criteria of eligibility to be included	Criteria for exclusion
• Aged 18 and over • Both sexes • Smoke 15 or more cigarettes per day • Have a CO concentration in exhaled air of $\geq 10\,ppm$ • Have smoked regularly for 3 or more years • Have failed in at least one serious attempt to quit smoking in the last 12 months • Want to reduce smoking as much as possible with the help of the nicotine inhaler • Are prepared to adhere to the protocol • [Willing to provide informed consent]	• Current use of nicotine replacement therapy or any other behavioural or pharmacological smoking cessation or reduction programme • Use of other nicotine-containing products • Have any condition that might interfere with the study

It is very important that these criteria are clearly defined prior to the selection process, and described in the report so that others can see exactly who was included in the sample and who was excluded. The criteria specified do seem to be clear and easily understandable – although the last exclusion criterion does seem rather vague and is not further defined or discussed.

2. The selection process was not random as volunteers were sought through newspaper adverts. It is also useful to refer to the study flow diagram in paper A (this is reproduced in Section 7.3.3 of this chapter). Diagrams such as this are an extremely useful way of summarising the recruitment, selection, randomisation and follow-up process: you can see at a glance how many people got though each stage. At present we are only concerned with the initial stages. Of 1115 people answering the advert, less than 50 per cent (468) had telephone screening, of whom 407 were invited to a baseline visit. The paper does not explain why only 468 out of 1115 were screened, nor does it indicate how representative those who progressed into the study were of all those responding to the advert. Of the 407 invited to baseline visit, only seven did not meet the 'admission' criteria (of course, many more were deemed ineligible at earlier stages of the process) and 400 were 'eligible and randomised'.

3. How representative is the sample of the Swiss population? As there is no sampling frame (list of names with identifying characteristics), we have no way of knowing whether the sample was representative of the Basle and Lausanne populations of 18 years or older smokers unable or unwilling to give up. Based on the process review in (no. 2) above, there are some questions about why less than 50 per cent of those answering the advert progressed past the telephone screening and we have no further information to judge how representative the sample is of the populations of the two cites. We would need additional information to assess whether findings on the response of these smokers to the nicotine inhaler is likely to be typical of how people throughout Switzerland would respond.

Exercise 7.2.2

1. The nicotine inhaler (which also contained 1 mg of menthol), termed the ***active treatment***, was compared with a placebo inhaler that contained only menthol. In all respects, the placebo appeared identical to the nicotine inhaler.

2. The general principle for deciding what the appropriate comparison 'treatment' should be is as follows. The control (comparison) group must be offered the best existing treatment in routine use. If there is no known effective treatment, then the controls can be given no active treatment (which, if practical, may be as placebo). In the case of this nicotine study, although it is well established that nicotine replacement can help smokers reduce or quit, it seems that 'successful abstinence is usually obtained in smokers with low to moderate nicotine dependence' (p. 329 of paper A). Heavily dependent smokers have the highest relapse rates, and are at highest risk of smoking-related disease, and smoking reduction should seen as a useful (possibly intermediate) goal. As the inhaler is a relatively new product, it is implied (as this is not explicitly discussed) that it is not unethical to compare the new inhaler with no active treatment in this group of smokers.

   This is a different situation from, say, testing the effect of a new surgical procedure that is thought might improve on an existing procedure. So long as there is evidence that the existing procedure has some beneficial effect, it would be unacceptable to compare the new operation with no operation at all. No ethical committee would allow a study to proceed that did not address this matter appropriately.

Exercise 7.2.3

1. The main outcome, or measure of success (the 'primary efficacy measure') was defined as 'self-reported reduction of daily cigarette smoking by at least 50 per cent compared with baseline from week six to month four.'

2. This outcome was validated by 'decreased breath carbon monoxide (CO) concentrations at week six and months three and four'. The authors do not appear to state how large a reduction in CO (or to what concentration) is required for validation.

3. The other key outcome was smoking cessation, defined as not smoking from week 6 and a breath CO concentration of < 10 ppm at all subsequent visits.

Exercise 7.2.4

1. Blinding in the nicotine inhaler study:

Group	Blinding applied
1. Subjects	Placebo should have ensured blinding, but it is likely that smokers who are highly nicotine dependent would notice that the active inhaler is having some effect on their craving, and vice versa for those with the placebo inhaler. By giving ***informed consent***, all subjects would know they are being randomised to receive either active or inactive inhalers.
2. Research team	The research team would not know the allocation until completion of the study, but could probably pick up some signals in the follow-up assessments, based on comments by subjects. Counselling was

(Continued)

Group	Blinding applied
	provided at each visit, although it is not clear by whom: this is one point at which – if subjects suspected which inhaler type they had and talked about it – some bias could have been introduced.
3. Health-care staff	The most important staff are the independent pharmacists who dispensed the inhalers and they should have remained blind. Other health-care staff could become involved, such as GPs. Although this was a healthy group of subjects (despite being smokers!), no doubt they sought care for the usual ailments and in doing so they might mention their involvement in the study, what they felt about the type of inhaler they had been randomised to use and the advice from the GP could have been influenced by this.

2. Reasons why blinding is important for these three groups:

Group	Reasons
1. Subjects	• Could affect compliance if they felt they may be missing out on effective treatment. • May influence reporting of outcomes and side effects.
2. Research team	• May influence objectivity of data collection on outcomes and side effects.
3. Health-care staff	• Knowledge of allocation may influence modifications to treatment for related or other health problems, with management potentially differing between treatment and control subjects.

3. Examples of interventions which cannot be blinded:

- A surgical procedure, the nature of which is clearly obvious to those carrying it out and caring for the patient post-operatively; such procedures may well be apparent to the patient, at least post-operatively.

- Counselling or other similar support and indeed the verbal advice/support component which relates to any treatment.

- Health education advice and materials.

It is possible that some of these could be blinded to the research team, or some members of it. The technique of blinding some people involved in the assessment of outcomes is very important. Thus, in an unblinded study, the outcome should, if possible, be assessed by people or techniques that are not influenced by the open nature of the study. Using self-administered questionnaires (for the subjects themselves to fill in) will also help. Although this will not remove *bias* introduced by the subjects' knowledge of their own treatment, the *instrument* is likely to be more objective than an interviewer (who is very likely to find out the allocation during the course of the interview). Measurements, such as breath CO, are also very useful, as these are less likely to be affected by knowledge of the allocation.

Section 7.3

Exercise 7.3.1

1. 2×2 table with numbers and percentages:

	Placebo	Active	Total
Men	104 (52%)	86 (43%)	190
Women	96 (48%)	114 (57%)	210
Total	200	200	400

2. The appropriate test is the chi-squared test.

3. The result of this hypothesis test is as follows: chi-squared $= 2.89$ (df $= 1$) $0.1 > p > 0.05$. This is not statistically significant at the 0.05 level (thus, it is unclear what the authors mean by 'the only significant difference was that there were more women in the active treatment group' (first paragraph of results section, p. 330). Hypothesis tests can be applied to all the variables compared in Table 1 to establish whether any are unlikely to have arisen by chance. One should be wary of acting on such testing too rigidly for the following reasons. First, if (as in some studies) the baseline characteristics table has a large number of variables, applying hypothesis tests without adjustment for multiple comparisons could throw up significant results at the 0.05 level by chance – a type I error (adjustment of p-values for multiple hypothesis testing is discussed further in Chapter 11, Section 11.4.3). Secondly, we should always remember that the great strength of randomisation is that it balances confounders that we know about, as well as those we do not know about and/or have not measured. While some variables we may have measured and displayed in a baseline characteristics table could differ between intervention and control groups, this could be 'balanced' by variation (in the opposite direction) among other influential variables we do not know about. Overenthusiastic adjustment for a few confounders we have measured and found to differ between groups may therefore actually disrupt what is, unknown to us, an overall well-balanced allocation. If in doubt, seek advice.

Exercise 7.3.2

1. Overall, inhaler use decreased over time (as expected) from 60 per cent at 6 weeks down to 10 per cent at 18 months.

2. Table 7.3.2 provides information on subjects in both groups who used the inhaler every day. The number of subjects using inhalers and the number of inhalers (cartridges) used per day decreased in both groups from the same starting levels. The rate of decrease in numbers of subjects using inhalers appears to have been greater in the placebo group, but the number of inhalers used per day by these subjects was very similar.

Exercise 7.3.3

1. For primary efficacy measure at 24 months (Table 7.3.3)

    (a) 2×2 table for sustained reduction at 24 months. Note (from the percentages in Table 7.3.3), the total numbers are those that were randomised to each treatment ($n = 200$ per group), consistent with the **intention to treat** analysis.

	Intervention	Control	Total
Reduced	19	6	25
Did not reduce	181	194	375
Total	200	200	400

    (b) The Fisher's exact test would normally be used if one or more of the cells in the table has an expected value of less than 5. The smallest expected value in this case is in the reduced/control cell, and is $200 \times 25/400 = 12.5$. Thus, although use of the Fisher's exact test is not strictly necessary (the chi-squared test with continuity correction could have been used), it may be that the authors were erring on the side of caution, or wished to use the same test for all comparisons, some of which have smaller numbers.

    (c) The OR is 3.39, with a 95 per cent CI of 1.39–8.29. Hence, in the study (paper A), those using the nicotine inhaler are around 3.4 times more likely to have a sustained reduction in smoking at 24 months and we can be 95 per cent sure that the true effect (in the population) lies between 1.4 and 8.3 times. This interval does not include 1 (unity), which is the value for no effect. This is consistent with a significant p-value result reported for the hypothesis test.

2. An appropriate hypothesis test for comparing mean values of breath CO, a continuous variable, would be the independent samples t-test, so long as the assumptions are met. If the distributions were very skewed (if you look at the means, standard deviations and ranges in Table 2, there is evidence of positive skewing), you could transform the data and use the t-test, or use a non-parametric test such as the Mann–Whitney U test. Transformation of data and so-called non-parametric tests, such as the Mann–Whitney U test, are described in Chapter 11.

Exercise 7.3.4

1. This seems reasonable. Although we have identified and discussed some concerns, (for example whether the groups were really blind to whether or not their inhaler contained nicotine), the validation of reported smoking reductions with breath CO does add weight to the findings. It is always possible that subjects deliberately reduced their smoking for several days prior to their scheduled visit and CO test, but it seems unlikely that the nicotine group would be so much more aware of this that they would do so more consistently than the control group. We might however point out that the numbers of subjects with sustained reduction at 24 months was somewhat disappointing (19 intervention, 6 control), given that the point prevalence for reduction (around 25 per cent) and quitting (about 10 per cent) at that stage was not very impressive and was

virtually the same in the intervention and control groups (differences non-significant, Table 3 of paper A).

2. This is quite difficult to answer. It is not helped by knowing so little about how representative this sample is of all 'healthy smokers in Basle and Lausanne who are unable or unwilling to give up, but are interested in reducing'. Then we are faced with the question, if the intervention works in these smokers, would it work as well in other parts of Switzerland, and in other countries? Perhaps the first step would be to look for other evidence, but one might reasonably assume that the response of adult smokers in Basle and Lausanne to this inhaler is probably quite typical of how other people living in Western Europe (at least) would respond.

Section 7.4

Exercise 7.4.1

1. Eligibility for inclusion and exclusion criteria.

Eligibility for inclusion	Exclusion
• City of Whitehorse, Melbourne • 70 years and over • Living in own home or leasing similar accommodation and allowed to make modifications	• Did not expect to remain in the area for 2 years (except for short absences) • Participated in regular to moderate physical activity with a balance improvement component in the previous 2 months • Could not walk 10–20 metres without rest, help, or having angina • Severe respiratory or cardiac disease • Psychiatric illness prohibiting participation • Dysphasia (difficulty with speech) • Recent home modifications • Education and language adjusted score of > 4 on the short portable mental status questionnaire • Did not have approval of their general practitioner

2. The sample was drawn from the electoral roll and Figure 1 provides numbers progressing through each stage. Response is difficult to judge as (the authors point out) they do not know how many of the total group contacted would have been eligible. Details are given in the text (recruitment) of how the study group compared with the general population (based on national census and health survey). Towards the end of p. 133 in paper B, the authors comment on the applicability of the findings saying that these would be most relevant to 'older adults living at home with similar characteristics – namely Australian born, aged 70–84 and rating their health as good to excellent'.

3. The intervention and control 'treatments' are as follows:

Intervention groups	Control
Offered as single interventions or in various combinations: • Strength and balance exercise programme, 1 hour/week for 15 weeks plus home exercises • Home hazard identification and removal • Vision assessment and referral for treatment as required	• No intervention (deferred until the end of the study)

4. All of these interventions either are, or could be, made available through routine services. So, depending on which turned out to be most effective, there is no reason why the interventions could not be made widely available, subject (of course) to costs. One aspect that may be quite challenging to reproduce is the coordination of the interventions, particularly if it is shown that two or more interventions should be combined.

5. The comparison groups are of two types in this study:

   • Other types of interventions (and combinations of interventions), none of which have been shown to be more effective than others used in the study, either singly or in combination.

   • No intervention at all, although in effect these are deferred until the end of the study, which lasted 18 months. The introduction section does state that there is evidence that a number of interventions (including those in the study) are effective, so it may be considered surprising that the ethics committee approved this 'no intervention' control group. We would need to know more about the case made to the committee to judge this further.

6. Blinding to the intervention:

Group	Blinding
Subjects	It was not possible to blind the subjects. Although we do not know exactly how aware they were of other options, it should be assumed that they would have a good general idea from the informed consent. The main outcome was self-reported by the subjects, although followed up by a blinded research assistant.
Research team	The team would be aware of the allocation, but some blinding was designed into the study. The assessor who carried out the initial home visits was blind to the allocation, as was the assessor who carried out risk factor assessments on a proportion of subjects ($n = 442$) at 18 months. Follow-up of self-reported falls and of subjects not returning the record card at the end of each month was carried out over the telephone by a blinded research assistant.
Health-care staff	Staff delivering the interventions could not have been blinded to the allocation. GPs (and presumably other primary care staff) were informed of the study (approval was sought from the GP) and probably would know the allocation. Whether this knowledge would have affected their management in respect of falls is not known. This type of uncertainty is inevitable in an unblinded study, but there is really little alternative.

Section 7.5

Exercise 7.5.1

1. $(\mu_1 - \mu_2) = 1.5$; $\sigma = 4.5$; $f(\alpha, \beta) = 7.9$. Hence $n = 142$ per group, total 284, before allowing for non-response, dropouts, etc.

2. The total study sample size is more than adequate to detect this difference.

3. Decreasing the treatment effect to 0.75 cm results in a sample size requirement of 569 per group: halving the effect leads to a fourfold increase in sample size.

Section 7.6

Exercise 7.6.1. Compliance with interventions (paper B)

1. Summary of compliance:

Group	Allocated	Initiated	Compliance
Exercise	541	401	401 (74%) out of 541 started sessions, and 328 (82%) of the 401 attended > 50% sessions. Mean (SD) number of sessions = 10 (3.8)
Home hazard	543	478	363 (76%) of the 478 advised received help to do modifications.
Vision	547	287	186 of 287 (65%) had recently visited or were about to visit for eye care; 97 of 101 others (96%) took up referral.

Some additional information is to be found in the discussion section; for example, with exercise (described as having achieved 'relatively poor compliance'), sessions were intended to be daily, but in fact were performed twice weekly on average.

2. Commentary:

- Exercise: around three-quarters started the sessions, and 328 (61 per cent) of the total allocated attended 50 per cent of the sessions. Put another way, 40 per cent either did not attend any (26 per cent) or attended less than half of the sessions (14 per cent).

- Home hazard: around three-quarters of those thought to need modifications had the work done.

- Vision: almost all of those needing a new referral took up this advice.

Overall, given the types of intervention and the fact that these were people living independently at home (as opposed to in an institutional setting), compliance was fairly good. However, the 'intention to treat' analysis has to 'absorb' the fact that around 40 per cent of the exercise groups did no exercise sessions or did less than half of the sessions and one-quarter of those recommended to make changes in the home hazard group did not do so. Although virtually all of those needing attention to their vision took up this advice, the intervention only applied to 97 people

(18 per cent of the total allocated), as all others were either not in need of eye care or had already arranged this.

Exercise 7.6.2 Reassessment at 18 months

1. 442 out of 1090 (40.6 per cent) were reassessed at 18 months. Figure 7.4.1 (Figure 1 from paper B) shows the numbers in each of the intervention groups who were reassessed (from which you can calculate percentages).

2. The reasons given are (a) resources were not available to reassess the whole group and (b) this assessment was of secondary importance to the study's main goal (this being falls, which were measured by a calendar completed by all subjects continuing in the study).

3. They were randomly selected by an assessor blind to the intervention group.

4. The percentage of each group reassessed can be determined from Figure 7.4.1. The baseline characteristics are shown in Table 7.6.2 (Tables 2 and 3 from paper B).

5. Comparison of reassessed subject characteristics (column 4 in Table 7.6.2 (Table 2 and 3 from paper B)) with those for all participants (column 1) shows that the reassessed individuals were similar in all respects studied.

Exercise 7.6.3

1. (a) Exercise: 18 per cent reduction in risk (95 per cent CI, 3 percent to 30 per cent reduction), p = 0.02, which is significant; (b) vision: 11 per cent reduction in risk (95 per cent CI, 4 per cent increase to 25 per cent reduction), p = 0.13, which is non-significant and consistent with a 95 per cent CI that includes 1.

2. Exercise and vision in combination: 27 per cent reduction (95 per cent CI, 9 per cent to 42 per cent reduction), p = 0.01. This shows, more or less, that the effect of the two interventions in combination is roughly that of the individual effects added together (additive). This implies there is no **interaction**, whereby the effect of one (or both) is enhanced by the presence of the other. This is reported in the first paragraph of the discussion.

3. The NNT has been calculated by the per cent estimated reduction in the annual fall rate, which for the three interventions combined is 14 per cent (or 0.14 as a proportion). The NNT therefore is 100/14 (or equivalently 1/0.14)= 7. This means that seven people need to receive the intervention for 1 year in order to prevent one fall over the same time period. Note that this is based on the central estimate of 14 per cent and does not take account of the 95 per cent CI (which you could do).

In interpreting the effectiveness of the interventions, it is important to remember that intention to treat analysis was used, and compliance was not perfect. Hence, a NNT of 7, which allows for the level of compliance with interventions, may be considered as quite favourable.

Exercise 7.6.4

1. Although the intervention was initiated on an individual basis (mainly delivered by the GP through the consultation), there was some wider involvement of practice staff (encouraged to give feedback). If within-practice individual randomisation had been used, there would have been a risk of contamination between intervention and control subjects (see discussion section,

p. 798 of paper C). In addition, GPs (and other staff) would have found it extremely difficult to manage intervention and control patients strictly to protocol and to avoid bias.

2. Control clusters received 'usual care', as described in the Abstract (no further information is given on details of this, but they were offered the intervention at the end of the study).

Exercise 7.6.5

1. There were 16 communities (8 intervention, 8 control).

2. Populations ranged from 1700 to 13 500.

3. The communities shared no common high schools and were at least 20 miles apart.

4. Pairs of communities were matched on socio-economic status and population and randomisation was carried out within each pair.

5. It was reported that communities 'in the two conditions' (this means intervention and controls) did not differ statistically in respect of a range of demographic, social and economic factors, implying that a good balance had been achieved.

Exercise 7.6.6

(a) No, as these are two independent groups (whisky versus none).

(b) Yes, since these are the same volunteers before and after.

8

Life tables, survival analysis and Cox regression

Introduction and learning objectives

Introduction

In the work we have done so far on cohort studies and trials we have used incidence rates as the measure for outcomes, that is, the number of people dying (mortality) or becoming ill (morbidity) in a given time period. The simplest concept was **cumulative incidence**:

$$\frac{\text{Number of new cases arising in the specified time period}}{\text{Number of people at risk during specified time period}}$$

We also saw that a more useful measure was **incidence density** for which we used person-time (months, years, etc.) in the denominator.

With **survival analysis** we introduce a new but intuitively simple and important dimension. This is the time that people in the study survive until dying (mortality), falling ill (morbidity), or any other event of interest. Apart from that, what we are covering in this chapter builds on concepts we have already covered.

We will start by looking at the use of the Kaplan–Meier method (**Kaplan–Meier survival curves**) to study survival in cohort studies and trials, where we are following up specific groups of people over time. We will then discuss **Cox proportionate hazards regression**. This sounds complicated, but is in fact another form of regression analysis–used for the purposes we have already covered in previous chapters (adjustment for confounding, prediction, etc.)–but in this new situation where we have the added ingredient of 'time until the event of interest'. Finally, we will introduce the purpose and method of **current life tables** which allow the calculation of life expectancy for a population using age-specific death rates.

Quantitative Methods for Health Research   Nigel Bruce, Daniel Pope and Debbi Stanistreet
© 2008 John Wiley & Sons, Ltd

Learning objectives

By the end of this chapter, you should be able to do the following:

- Describe how survival analysis differs from comparisons of cumulative incidence or incidence density.

- Describe the circumstances when it is appropriate to use Kaplan–Meier survival curves and interpret examples of these, including using the curve to determine median survival and the proportion of a population surviving to a given time.

- Describe the use of the log-rank test for hypothesis testing with survival data and interpret the results of the test.

- Describe the circumstances when it is appropriate to use Cox proportional hazards regression, determine that the assumption of proportional hazards has been met, and interpret results from such an analysis.

- Describe the purposes and principles of current life table analysis.

Resource papers

Two papers have been selected for this chapter. The first (paper A) investigates the risk of coronary heart disease (CHD) and stroke associated with passive smoking in the British Regional Heart Study, a cohort study which we introduced in Chapter 5. The second (paper B) is a RCT comparing early with delayed palliative (symptom relieving) radiotherapy for advanced lung cancer.

Paper A

Whincup, P. H. *et al.* (2004). Passive smoking and risk of coronary heart disease and stroke: prospective study with cotinine measurement. *Br Med J* **329**, 200–205.

Paper B

Falk, S. J. *et al.* (2002). Immediate versus delayed palliative thoracic radiotherapy in patients with unresectable locally advanced non-small cell lung cancer and minimal thoracic symptoms: randomised controlled trial. *Br Med J* **325**, 465–472.

8.1 Survival analysis

8.1.1 Introduction

In this section we will focus on methods for analysing data, typically derived from cohort studies or trials, which uses information on time until the event of interest for each person in the study. This is called *survival analysis*.

Thus, if we are looking at death as the 'event of interest', the analysis uses information on whether or not a person died within the study period, but also on how long the person survived from the time he or she entered the study.

We can apply survival analysis to many situations as well as survival time until death. For example, in a study of the duration of breastfeeding we may record the length of time to completion of weaning. Completion of weaning is the ***terminal event*** or ***end point***. We refer to any 'time to event' situation by the common terminology of ***survival time***. Thus, the event of interest could be recovery from disease, relapse, leaving intensive care, introduction of bottle-feeding, conception following fertility treatment or any other discrete event. When we refer to 'survival time' we mean 'time to the event of interest', whatever that event may be.

8.1.2 Why do we need survival analysis?

In the analysis of cohort studies and trials, we are usually interested in one or more of the following questions:

- Describing the survival experience of a group of individuals; for example, what proportion of cancer patients are alive, or free of recurrent disease, 5 years after diagnosis and treatment?

- Comparing the survival experience of two or more groups of individuals; for example, is there a difference between the proportions of individuals taking treatments A and B who are still alive after 5 years? Or, alternatively, what are the average survival times for treatments A and B?

- Predicting the length of survival for an individual given a number of characteristics or prognostic factors; for example, what is the predicted time to recurrence of gallstones after dissolution given age, sex, history of previous gallstones and other clinical information?

We already know some methods of estimating and comparing proportions and means by ***confidence intervals (CIs)*** and ***hypothesis tests***. We have also seen how a ***regression model*** can be used for prediction. But the methods we have already met cannot usually be used to answer our questions about 'survival'. This is because survival data differ from the types of data we have studied so far in two important respects:

- Survival times are hardly ever normally distributed – but instead are usually quite markedly skewed, as illustrated in Figure 8.1.1 (these data, for which the mean is 67.8 and the median 61.0, have been generated for this example and are presented in more detail in Table 8.1.1, below);

- only some of the individuals studied actually experience the event of interest during the study period. The rest have what are known as ***censored*** observations. This is a critical element of survival analysis and is now discussed.

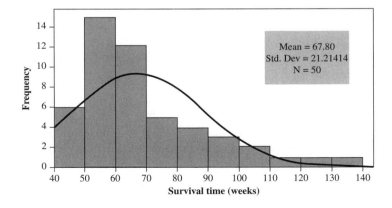

Figure 8.1.1 Survival data are usually positively skewed

8.1.3 Censoring

In a study of survival we may observe a survival time of 5 years for each of two individuals. If one person died 5 years after entering the study and the other was still alive when the study ended 5 years after joining it, then these are clearly two different types of information. The fact that a person remained alive for the full 5 years is important and we need a way of dealing with this difference in the analysis. This is called *censoring*. In this example the time for the second person is censored; that is, the period of observation ended before the event (death) occurred.

Censoring also occurs if individuals become lost to follow-up, or withdraw from the study, and we do not know whether or not they have died. We still need to be able to represent the fact that for the period they were under observation they did not experience the event of interest. These examples are termed *right censored* as they occur after (to the right on graphs of survival over time) recruitment and follow-up started. If there is a delay between base-line assessment and the start of follow-up surveillance, people lost at that stage are termed *left-censored*.

In a set of survival data it is usual to indicate in some way which of the survival times are censored. Commonly, this is done by using an indicator variable (that is, a variable that can have the value 0 or 1 for each individual) called a *censoring indicator*. This indicator has the value 0 for each individual with a censored survival time and the value 1 for those whose survival times are not censored. There is an example of this in Section 8.1.4.

In the following sections we will first look at a graphical display of survival data (*Kaplan–Meier survival curve*)–remember we always picture the data first–and then go on to consider an hypothesis test used to compare the survival of two or more groups (*log-rank test*) and lastly the predictive model used for survival data (*Cox regression*).

Summary – survival data

- We use survival analysis when we have data showing the times to occurrence of an event.

- Survival data are usually positively skewed, often highly skewed.

- Usually some observations are censored and this information needs to be taken into account in the analysis.

- Censoring arises when an individual has not experienced the event of interest by the end of the study (e.g. is still alive), or the event had not occurred when the individual was last observed, but records stop before the end of the study (e.g. lost to follow-up).

We will now start to look at how survival analysis is applied in practice through the example of the cohort study investigation of passive smoking and heart disease (paper A). Please now read the following excerpts which cover (i) the abstract and (ii) the introduction and methods (apart from the statistical methods, as we need to cover more on survival analysis first).

Abstract

Objective To examine the associations between a biomarker of overall passive exposure to tobacco smoke (serum cotinine concentration) and risk of coronary heart disease and stroke.

Design Prospective population based study in general practice (the British Regional Heart Study).

Participants 4729 men in 18 towns who provided baseline blood samples (for cotinine assay) and a detailed smoking history in 1978–80.

Main outcome measure Major coronary heart disease and stroke events (fatal and non-fatal) during 20 years of follow up.

Results 2105 men who said they did not smoke and who had cotinine concentrations < 14.1 ng/ml were divided into four equal sized groups on the basis of cotinine concentrations. Relative hazards (95% confidence intervals) for coronary heart disease in the second (0.8–1.4 ng/ml), third (1.5–2.7 ng/ml), and fourth (2.8–14.0 ng/ml) quarters of cotinine concentration compared with the first (≤ 0.7 ng/ml) were 1.45 (1.01 to 2.08), 1.49 (1.03 to 2.14), and 1.57 (1.08 to 2.28), respectively, after adjustment for established risk factors for coronary heart disease. Hazard ratios (for cotinine 0.8–14.0 $v \leq 0.7$ ng/ml) were particularly increased during the first (3.73, 1.32 to 10.58) and second five year follow up periods (1.95, 1.09 to 3.48) compared with later periods. There was no consistent association between cotinine concentration and risk of stroke.

Conclusion Studies based on reports of smoking in a partner alone seem to underestimate the risks of exposure to passive smoking. Further prospective studies relating biomarkers of passive smoking to risk of coronary heart disease are needed.

Introduction

Active cigarette smoking is a well established major preventable risk factor for coronary heart disease (CHD).[1] Many studies have reported that passive smoking is also associated with increased risk of CHD.[2 3] Generally such studies have compared the risks of non-smokers who do or do not live with cigarette smokers,[4—9] though a few have also considered occupational exposure.[10—12] Meta-analyses of case-control and cohort studies examining the effect of living with a cigarette smoker on risk among non-smokers have generally shown an overall increase in risk of about one quarter, after adjustment for potential confounding factors[2 3] and with little evidence of publication bias. Passive smoking may also be related to risk of stroke.[13] Although living with someone who smokes is an important component of exposure to passive smoking, it accounts for less than half of the variation in cotinine concentration among nonsmokers[14] and does not take account of additional exposure in workplaces and in public places (particularly pubs and restaurants).[15] Biomarkers of passive exposure to smoking, particularly cotinine (a nicotine metabolite), can provide a

(Continued)

summary measure of exposure from all these sources.[16] Although cotinine concentration in non-smokers has been related to prevalent CHD,[17] there are no published reports of the prospective associations between serum cotinine concentration and risk of CHD and stroke in non-smokers. We have examined these associations in the British Regional Heart Study, a prospective study of cardiovascular disease in middle aged men, using retained baseline samples for retrospective measurement of cotinine.

Methods

The British Regional Heart Study is a prospective study of cardiovascular disease in 7735 men aged 40–59 years selected from the age and sex registers of one general practice in each of 24 towns in England, Wales, and Scotland (78% response rate).[18]

Baseline assessment

In 1978–80, research nurses administered a questionnaire on present and previous smoking habits (cigarettes, cigar, pipe), alcohol intake, physical activity, and medical history (including angina, myocardial infarction, stroke, and diabetes diagnosed by a doctor). Participants also completed a questionnaire on chest pain (Rose, World Health Organization). Two seated blood pressure measurements were taken with a London School of Hygiene and Tropical Medicine sphygmomanometer; the mean was adjusted for observer variation within each town. Non-fasting total serum cholesterol concentration was measured with a modified Liebermann-Burchard method on a Technicon SMA 12/60 analyser. High density lipoprotein (HDL) cholesterol was measured by the same procedure after precipitation with magnesium phosphotungstate. Serum samples were placed in long term storage at $-20\,^{\circ}C$ in the last 18 study towns. In 2001–2, these were thawed and cotinine concentration was measured with a gas-liquid chromatography method (detection limit 0.1 ng/ml).[19]

Follow up

All men were followed up for all cause mortality and cardiovascular morbidity. We collected information on deaths through the established 'flagging' procedures provided by the NHS central registers. We obtained information on non-fatal CHD events and strokes from general practitioners' reports, supplemented by reviewing patients' records every two years throughout follow up. Major CHD events included deaths with coronary heart disease as the underlying cause, including sudden death of presumed cardiac origin (international classification of diseases, ninth revision (ICD-9), codes 410–414) and non-fatal myocardial infarction, diagnosed in accordance with standard WHO criteria.[18] Stroke events included deaths with cerebrovascular disease as the underlying cause (ICD-9 codes 430–438) and non-fatal stroke diagnosed in accordance with WHO criteria.[18] The analyses presented are based on all first major CHD or stroke events during the follow up period to December 2000, with an average follow up of 18.5 years for men who had no myocardial infarction or stroke (range 0.2–20.0 years).

Definition of baseline smoking status

Men were classified as 'current non-smokers' at baseline if they reported that they did not smoke cigarettes, cigars, or a pipe and had a serum cotinine concentration < 14.1 ng/ml.[20] Among these men, 'lifelong non-smokers' were those who reported never having smoked cigarettes, cigars, or a pipe. For comparison purposes, 'light active smokers' were men who reported smoking 1–9 cigarettes a day, irrespective of cotinine concentration.

Other definitions
Pre-existing CHD included one or more of angina or possible myocardial infarction, or both, on the WHO Rose questionnaire; electrocardiographic evidence of definite or possible myocardial infarction or ischaemia; or participant's recall of myocardial infarction or angina diagnosed by a doctor. Study towns were considered to be in the south if they were to the south or east of a line joining the River Severn and the Wash. Physical activity and alcohol intake were categorised as in earlier reports.[21][22]

 Self-Assessment Exercise 8.1.1

1. You should be familiar with the methods of this cohort study. To make sure you are clear about the subjects being studied in this report, make brief notes on who was included.

2. What outcomes were studied?

3. How was passive smoking exposure determined? Comment on the likely validity of this assessment.

4. Can you see why survival analysis would be appropriate to this investigation? Does the research team have information on 'time to the events of interest'?

Answers in Section 8.4

8.1.4   Kaplan–Meier survival curves

One of the most important methods in dealing with survival data from one or more groups is the graphical display, known as the ***Kaplan-Meier*** survival curve. To compare two or more groups, we show each group's survival curve on the same graph. We can then use the graph (or more accurately the calculations which produced it) to estimate the proportion of the population of such people who would survive a given length of time in the same circumstances.

Summary statistics such as the ***median survival time***, or the proportion of individuals alive at a specified time (say, 1 month, or 1 year), can be read directly from the Kaplan–Meier graph (we will look at how to do this shortly). CIs should be calculated for these summary statistics. If there are no censored values we can use standard methods for calculating CIs: a 95 per cent CI for a population proportion is given by:

$$p \pm 1.96\sqrt{\frac{p(1-p)}{n}}$$

where p is the proportion observed in the sample and n is the sample size. Generally, however, we need to use a modified formula to allow for the censoring (see for example Gardner and Altman, 1989).

We will not go into the detail of how to calculate the Kaplan–Meier survival curve here, which in any case is easily done on a computer. Essentially, however, for each unit of survival time we estimate the proportion of the sample surviving for that period of those who have not experienced the outcome event during the immediately preceding time period. This results in the survival curve being presented as a *step function*; that is, the proportion surviving remains unchanged between events, even if there are some intermediate censored observations. The times of these censored observations are usually indicated by tick marks on the curve to show when they occurred. The median survival time is the time corresponding to a survival probability of 0.5. Therefore, if the curve does not fall below 0.5, we cannot estimate the median. The following example will help you to understand these key elements of the Kaplan–Meier method.

Example

Table 8.1.1 shows times (in months) before recurrence for two groups of cancer patients in a trial comparing a new treatment against the existing standard treatment. These data are not real but are typical of such a trial. In this example, we are interested in *recurrence-free* survival–that is the time that each person remains well, without recurrence of the cancer.

Table 8.1.1   Survival times and censoring information for intervention and control groups

Intervention (new treatment)			Control (standard treatment)		
Subject ID	Survival (months)	Censoring indicator*	Subject ID	Survival (months)	Censoring indicator*
1	3.00	1	26	2.00	1
2	6.00	1	27	3.00	0
3	6.00	1	28	4.00	1
4	6.00	0	29	5.00	1
5	7.00	1	30	5.00	1
6	9.00	0	31	6.00	1
7	10.00	1	32	7.00	0
8	10.00	0	33	8.00	1
9	11.00	0	34	8.00	1
10	13.00	1	35	9.00	1
11	16.00	1	36	11.00	1
12	17.00	0	37	11.00	1
13	19.00	0	38	12.00	0
14	20.00	0	39	13.00	1
15	22.00	1	40	15.00	1
16	23.00	1	41	17.00	0
17	25.00	0	42	19.00	1
18	32.00	0	43	21.00	1
19	32.00	1	44	21.00	1
20	34.00	0	45	23.00	1
21	35.00	0	46	25.00	0
22	36.00	1	47	26.00	1
23	42.00	0	48	29.00	1
24	45.00	0	49	31.00	0
25	51.00	0	50	33.00	1

* Censoring indicator: 0 = censored; 1 = event (recurrence of cancer).

In the table, the ***censoring indicator*** shows whether the times are censored or not. A code of 0 means that the time observation is censored and a code of 1 means that the event (recurrence) has occurred. The Kaplan–Meier survival curves for the two groups are displayed in Figure 8.1.2 (calculated with SPSS) and show that the treatment group has a higher recurrence-free survival rate than the control group.

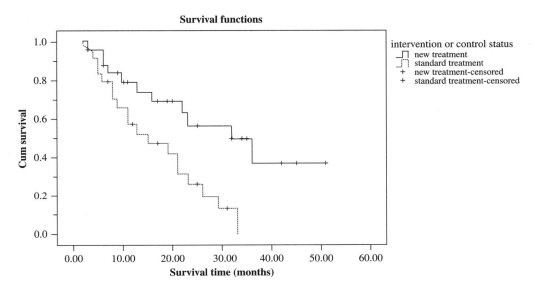

Figure 8.1.2   Kaplan–Meier survival curves for cancer trial example

In Figure 8.1.2 the cumulative survival (y-axis) gives the probability of 'surviving' (not having a recurrence of the cancer) at any given time after treatment. The median survival is given by a probability of 0.5, but any other probability can be read off the graph. Similarly, the probability of surviving until a specified time can be determined: for example, the probability of controls surviving to 10 months is (approximately) 0.65. Check that you can read this off the graph. The following exercise will help consolidate your understanding of this technique.

 Self-Assessment Exercise 8.1.2

1. In the example above (Table 8.1.1), how many of (a) the intervention (new treatment) and (b) control groups were censored? What are the possible reasons for this difference?

2. Use Figure 8.1.2 to estimate the median recurrence-free times for the two groups.

3. What proportions of (a) controls and (b) those treated with the new treatment are estimated to survive to 30 months?

Answers in Section 8.4

As fewer and fewer subjects remain at risk, the interpretation of the survival curves may become misleading because the tail of the curves become unstable due to the small numbers at risk. The curves have a tendency to flatten out as events become less frequent, but this will not be very meaningful unless there are a large number of subjects still at risk.

Also, as occurs for the control group in this example, if the last event occurred after the last censored time the curve will plunge to zero (see Figure 8.1.2). However, this does not necessarily mean that no one in that group will survive past that point. In fact, although the censored subjects had not experienced the events when last studied, we do not know what happened to them subsequently.

8.1.5   The log-rank test

This hypothesis test is used to compare survival in two (or more) groups, such as in the cancer trial we have been discussing. The test uses all of the available survival information, not just information at one point as when comparing the median survival times or the proportions surviving at a given time. This test is available in standard computer programmes and our discussion of this test is confined to looking at how it utilises all of the available information.

The **log-rank test** is a form of chi-squared test and as it is **non-parametric**, it does not require assumptions to be made about the distribution of survival times (non-parametric hypothesis testing will be described in more detail in Chapter 11). This test, in effect, compares the total number of events in each group with the number of events expected if there was no treatment effect. Hence, the null hypothesis (H_0) is that there is no difference in survival between the two groups.

 Statistics reference section

The principle of the test is to divide the survival time scale into intervals, according to the distinct observed times of death (or other event), but ignoring censored times. First, the survival times for all events are ranked in ascending order, combining data from both groups. For the purpose of this discussion, we will call the people on the new treatment group A and those on the control treatment group B. Then, for each time period, we calculate the contribution from each group to the overall expected deaths for each group. These contributions to expected events at each time period are then summed to yield the total number of expected events for group A (notation is E_A). The total expected for group B (E_B) is also calculated, though this is simply the total number of observed events$-E_A$. This is how the log-rank test uses all of the available survival information.

The notation for the number of observed events in group A is O_A and for group B the notation is O_B. The log-rank test statistic has one degree of freedom and is calculated as:

$$X^2 = \frac{(O_A - E_A)^2}{E_A} + \frac{(O_B - E_B)^2}{E_B}$$

As noted above, the log-rank test can also be used to compare the survival of more than two groups.

 Reference section ends

8.1.6 Interpretation of the Kaplan–Meier survival curve

We have now covered enough on survival methods to start looking at what has been done in the passive smoking study, though we will have to skip the description of Cox regression until we have looked at this in Section 8.2.

Please now read the following excerpts (text, table and figures) from paper A and complete Exercise 8.1.3.

Statistical methods

We used Cox proportional hazards models, stratified by town of residence, to examine the independent contribution of serum cotinine concentration to the risks of CHD and stroke. These produced relative hazards, adjusted for age and other risk factors, for each quarter of the distribution of serum cotinine concentration compared with the lowest. We carried out overall tests of the association, fitting the continuous relation between log cotinine concentration and risk of CHD. Relative hazard estimates for each five year interval were calculated by fitting interaction terms with time (using three binary factors to separate the effects in the second, third, and fourth intervals from those in the first). Kaplan–Meier curves were used to display the differences in incidence of major CHD by cotinine exposure group; differences were assessed using the log rank test. All P values were two sided.

We fitted age, body mass index, height, systolic blood pressure, diastolic blood pressure, serum total cholesterol, high density lipoprotein cholesterol, white cell count, lung function (forced expiratory volume in one second (FEV_1)), and triglycerides as continuous variables. Physical activity was fitted as a factor with four levels (none, occasional, light, moderate or more), alcohol intake with three levels (none/occasional, light/moderate, heavy), and social class with seven levels (six registrar general categories and Armed Forces). History of cigarette smoking, pre-existing CHD, and diabetes were fitted as dichotomous variables.

Results

In the last 18 towns of the study, 5661 men took part (78% response rate). For 4729 of these we had detailed histories on smoking and blood samples for cotinine analysis. These men resembled the whole study population in reported smoking habits and risks of CHD and stroke. A total of 2158 men reported that they were current non-smokers, of whom 2105 (97.5%) had serum cotinine concentrations < 14.1 ng/ml. Of these, 945 men were classified as lifelong non-smokers, the remaining 1160 as former smokers. The cotinine distributions of these two groups (fig 1)* were skewed, with a slightly higher geometric mean cotinine among former smokers than among lifelong nonsmokers (1.49 v 1.18 ng/ml). Few men in either group had cotinine concentrations close to the 14.1 ng/ml cut off.

(Continued)

Serum cotinine and cardiovascular risk factors—Among current non-smokers, cotinine concentrations were not consistently related to age, total cholesterol concentration, physical activity score, or prevalent CHD but showed graded positive associations with mean body mass index, systolic and diastolic blood pressure, high density lipoprotein cholesterol, white cell count, and triglycerides (weakly) and positive associations with the prevalence of former smoking, heavy drinking, and manual occupation (table 1).* Cotinine concentrations were inversely associated with FEV_1, prevalence of low alcohol intake, and residence in southern England. These associations were generally little affected when we excluded former smokers. Light active smokers had lower mean body mass index, diastolic blood pressure, and FEV_1 and a higher mean white cell count than men who did not smoke.

_____

* Figure 1 is reproduced in Figure 8.1.3 and Table 1 is reproduced in Table 8.1.2 (below).

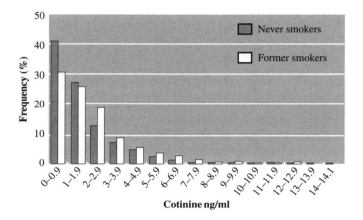

Figure 8.1.3 Distribution of serum cotinine concentrations among current non-smokers; lifelong non-smokers and former smokers are shown separately (Figure 1 from paper A)

 Self-Assessment Exercise 8.1.3

1. Why are geometric means quoted for the comparison of cotinine levels in ex-smokers and never smokers?

2. Why do you think ex-smokers may have had higher cotinine levels than lifelong never smokers? (see text and Figure 8.1.3).

3. What type of graph is Figure 8.1.4?

Table 8.1.2 Means (SDs) and numbers (percentages) of cardiovascular risk factors by cotinine concentration: non-smokers and light active cigarette smokers (Table 1 from paper A)

	Passive smoke exposure (ng/ml cotinine)					Active smokers (1–9/day)	P value for trend*
	≤0.7	0.8–1.4	1.5–2.7	2.8–14.0			
Mean cotinine (ng/ml)	0.5	1.1	2.0	4.9		138.4	–
No of men	575	508	506	516		192	–
Age (years)	50.5 (5.7)	49.9 (5.7)	50.2 (5.8)	50.5 (6.1)		50.7 (5.7)	0.96
BMI (kg/m²)	25.5 (2.9)	25.4 (3.1)	26.3 (3.1)	26.5 (3.4)		25.0 (3.4)	<0.001
Height (cm)	174.0 (6.6)	173.5 (6.6)	173.5 (6.6)	172.4 (6.5)		172.8 (6.1)	0.03
Systolic blood pressure (mm Hg)	144 (22)	145 (21)	147 (20)	151 (22)		144 (22)	<0.001
Diastolic blood pressure (mm Hg)	82 (14)	83 (13)	85 (14)	87 (15)		83 (14)	<0.001
Total cholesterol (mmol/l)	6.3 (1.0)	6.3 (1.0)	6.3 (1.0)	6.3 (1.0)		6.3 (1.0)	0.50
HDL cholesterol (mmol/l)	1.14 (0.25)	1.16 (0.27)	1.14 (0.26)	1.20 (0.26)		1.15 (0.25)	<0.001
White cell count (10⁹/l)	6.4 (1.4)	6.5 (1.4)	6.6 (2.3)	6.7 (1.4)		7.2 (1.6)	0.02
FEV₁ (ml)	357 (68)	355 (72)	346 (74)	329 (80)		329 (78)	<0.001
Triglycerides† (mmol/l)	1.65	1.61	1.77	1.78		1.74	0.04
Evidence of CHD	134 (23)	126 (25)	117 (23)	142 (28)		48 (25)	0.19
Diabetes (diagnosed by doctor)	8 (1)	8 (2)	7 (1)	5 (1)		4 (2)	–
Physical activity: none or occasional	182 (32)	169 (33)	163 (32)	208 (40)		70 (36)	0.25
Alcohol intake: never or occasional	261 (45)	189 (37)	145 (29)	104 (20)		52 (27)	<0.001
Alcohol intake: heavy (> 6 drinks/day)	10 (2)	22 (4)	38 (8)	85 (16)		22 (11)	<0.001
Former smoker	267 (46)	259 (51)	309 (61)	325 (63)		–	<0.001
Manual workers	246 (43)	258 (51)	287 (57)	346 (67)		120 (63)	<0.001
Live in south	303 (53)	196 (39)	158 (31)	113 (22)		64 (33)	<0.001‡

* Across passive smoking groups only. Adjusted for age and town.

† Geometric means as log transformed (use of transformed data and geometric means for skewed data are discussed fully in Chapter 11, and also explored in Exercise 8.1.3, below).

‡ Adjusted for age only.

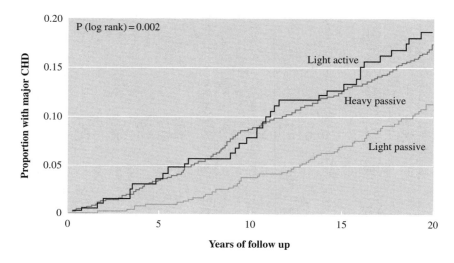

Figure 8.1.4 Proportion of men with major CHD by years of follow-up in each smoking group. 'Light passive' refers to lowest quarter of cotinine concentration among non-smokers (0–0.7 ng/ml), 'heavy passive' to upper three-quarters of cotinine concentration combined (0.8–14.0 ng/ml), and 'light active' to men smoking 1–9 cigarettes a day (Figure 2 from paper A).

4. What is the probability of having a CHD event after 10 years for (a) light passive and (b) heavy passive smoking? Can you determine the median probability of a CHD event?

5. Interpret the result of the log-rank test (result top left of Figure 8.1.4).

6. Why do the curves in Figure 8.1.4 start at a probability of 0.0, whereas those in our cancer trial example (Figure 8.1.2) started at a probability of 1.00?

Answers in Section 8.4

8.1.7 Survival analysis in a RCT

Paper A reports survival analysis of a cohort study. The other common application of survival analysis is for intervention studies. We will now briefly review paper B, a RCT of palliative radiotherapy[1] in lung cancer, to see how this is done in practice. Please now read the abstract, review Figures 8.1.5 and 8.1.6 and complete Exercise 8.1.4.

---

[1] 'Palliative radiotherapy' means treatment of cancer with radiation to ameliorate symptoms of pain and discomfort in cases of the disease that are advanced and for which cure is not expected. Further explanation of technical terms in the excerpts is given in the answers to Exercise 8.1.4.

Abstract

Objective To determine whether patients with locally advanced non-small cell lung cancer unsuitable for resection or radical radiotherapy, and with minimal thoracic symptoms, should be given palliative thoracic radiotherapy immediately or as needed to treat symptoms.

Design Multicentre randomised controlled trial.

Setting 23 centres in the United Kingdom, Ireland, and South Africa.

Participants 230 patients with previously untreated, non-small cell lung cancer that is locally too advanced for resection or radical radiotherapy with curative intent, with minimal thoracic symptoms, and with no indication for immediate thoracic radiotherapy.

Interventions All patients were given supportive treatment and were randomised to receive palliative thoracic radiotherapy either immediately or delayed until needed to treat symptoms. The recommended regimens were 17 Gy in two fractions one week apart or 10 Gy as a single dose.

Main outcome measures Primary—patients alive and without moderate or severe cough, chest pain, haemoptysis, or dyspnoea six months from randomisation, as recorded by clinicians. Secondary—quality of life, adverse events, survival.

Results From December 1992 to May 1999, 230 patients were randomised. 104/115 of the patients in the immediate treatment group received thoracic radiotherapy (90 received one of the recommended regimens). In the delayed treatment group, 48/115 (42%) patients received thoracic radiotherapy (29 received one of the recommended regimens); 64 (56%) died without receiving thoracic radiotherapy; the remaining three (3%) were alive at the end of the study without having received the treatment. For patients who received thoracic radiotherapy, the median time to start was 15 days in the immediate treatment group and 125 days in the delayed treatment group. The primary outcome measure was achieved in 28% of the immediate treatment group and 26% of patients from the delayed treatment group (27/97 and 27/103, respectively; absolute difference 1.6%, 95% confidence interval -10.7% to 13.9%). No evidence of a difference was observed between the two treatment groups in terms of activity level, anxiety, depression, and psychological distress, as recorded by the patients. Adverse events were more common in the immediate treatment group. Neither group had a survival advantage (hazard ratio 0.95, 0.73 to 1.24; P = 0.71). Median survival was 8.3 months and 7.9 months, and the survival rates were 31% and 29% at 12 months, for the immediate and delayed treatment groups, respectively.

Conclusion In minimally symptomatic patients with locally advanced non-small cell lung cancer, no persuasive evidence was found to indicate that giving immediate palliative thoracic radiotherapy improves symptom control, quality of life, or survival when compared with delaying until symptoms require treatment.

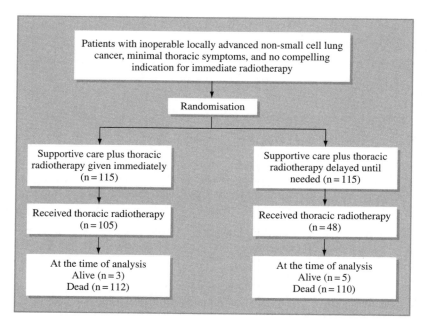

Figure 8.1.5   Trial profile (Figure 1 from paper B)

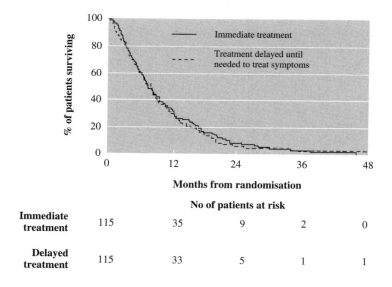

Figure 8.1.6   Percentage of patients surviving after date of randomisation (Figure 2 from paper B)

Self-Assessment Exercise 8.1.4

1. List the criteria that defined the patients included in this study.

2. What were the (a) primary and (b) secondary events (outcomes) of interest?

3. From the Kaplan–Meier curve (Figure 8.1.6), what was the (a) median 'survival time' and (b) the probability of surviving to 12 months for the two groups? (single estimates are sufficient as the curves do not differ appreciably). Do your answers agree with the figures for the two groups provided in the abstract?

4. The hazard ratio (see abstract) is reported as 0.95, with a 95 per cent CI 0.73–1.24 ($p = 0.71$). Although you have not yet been introduced to hazard ratios (we do that next in Section 8.2), you can regard this, for now, just like a relative risk. Have a go at interpreting this result.

Answers in Section 8.4

Summary : survival analysis

- We use survival analysis when we have data with times to occurrence of an event.

- These data require special treatment because;

  (i) survival times are usually positively skewed, often highly so;

  (ii) some observations are censored.

- We first picture the data as a Kaplan–Meier survival curve.

- Median survival and the proportion surviving at a given time can be read off the Kaplan–Meier survival curve. Although these are useful measures, they do not utilise all of the available data for comparison purposes.

- We use the log-rank test to test the hypothesis of no difference in survival between two or more groups; this test uses all of the available survival data.

8.2 Cox regression

8.2.1 Introduction

We have seen that the log-rank test can be used to compare the survival of two or more groups. Often, however, we want to explore the effect of several variables on survival; for example, to compare the effects of two different treatments while allowing for the confounding effects of age and previous history. Indeed, you will have seen from the statistical methods section of paper A (British Regional Heart Study) that the research team intended to adjust for a large number of confounding variables. Thus, we want to be able to model how the risk of the event depends on a number of *explanatory variables*. As with the examples of multiple linear and logistic regression we saw earlier in Chapters 5 and 6, these explanatory variables may be a mixture of continuous variables (such as age) and categorical variables (such as smoking status).

Cox regression is the method of choice for modelling the relationship between the risk of the event occurring and a number of explanatory variables. It is also called *proportional hazards regression*–we will see why shortly. It is analogous to the multiple and logistic regression models we have met previously, but it is a regression model that takes into account time until the event occurs.

8.2.2   The hazard function

In survival analysis, the risk of an event occurring is called the *hazard*. This risk can vary with time, and the risk of individuals experiencing the event at time t given that they have survived up to that time is denoted by $h(t)$ and is called the *hazard function*. The fact is that the hazard function is generally unknown, as we cannot mathematically describe how the risk of the event is related to time. Cox regression deals with this by making an important assumption about the hazard, thereby allowing us to model how a *ratio of hazards* in the two groups of people being studied is related to the explanatory variables. We will look now at this assumption, and then briefly at the Cox regression model to help illustrate what it has in common with methods you are already familiar with.

8.2.3   Assumption of proportional hazards

In Cox regression, for any possible explanatory variable such as treatment, we assume that if it affects the hazard, it does so by the same ratio at all times. Thus, although the hazard (risk of dying) on treatment A may vary over time, and similarly for B, it is assumed that the ratio of the hazards is the same at all times. So, if being on treatment B rather than A doubles the risk of dying at 1 week, it is assumed that it also doubles the risk of dying at 2 months, at 1 year, and so on.

8.2.4   The Cox regression model

Taking this example, we can write mathematically the statement (in Section 8.2.3) that the hazard ratio is 2 at all times as:

$$\frac{h_1(t)}{h_0(t)} = 2 \qquad \text{for all times } t$$

where $h_0(t)$ is the hazard function for group A and $h_1(t)$ the hazard function for group B. The hazards are therefore in constant proportion. This is why the method is called *proportional hazards regression*. In practice, and more generally, we want to be able to include several explanatory variables. Then $h_0(t)$ is the hazard function for individuals having values of zero for all the explanatory variables, and we write $h(t)$ for the hazard function of an individual with other values of the predictors. We are assuming that $h(t)/h_0(t)$ depends only on the predictors, and not on time t, as it is constant over time.

$h(t)/h_0(t)$ is called the **hazard ratio**. It is the relative risk of an endpoint occurring at any given time and $h_0(t)$ is called the **baseline hazard function**. The **Cox regression model** generates the log hazard ratio:

$$\log\left(\frac{h(t)}{h_o(t)}\right) = \beta_1 x_1 + \beta_2 x_2 + \cdots + \beta_k x_k$$

Where β_1 is the regression coefficient for the first explanatory variable x_1 and so on.

You can see the similarity between the Cox regression model and the multiple logistic regression model we studied earlier. Cox regression can be carried out in standard statistical software.

8.2.5 Checking the assumption of proportional hazards

It is important that, before fitting the Cox regression model to survival data, we check whether the assumption of **proportional hazards** is reasonable for the data. The Kaplan–Meier survival curves can be used for this purpose; the curves for each group should remain (at least approximately) proportional to each other and certainly not cross. We will look at this again in subsequent exercises. Another way of checking this assumption is to include an **interaction term** in the Cox regression model: this will identify whether or not there is a statistically significant change over time in the risk associated with a given explanatory variable (e.g. treatment).

8.2.6 Interpreting the Cox regression model

Interpretation of the Cox regression model is similar to that for logistic regression. The hazard ratios are found by exponentiating the estimated regression coefficients $b_1, b_2, \ldots$ (that is, we raise the natural log e to the power of b, written as e^b). A hazard ratio:

- Greater than 1 indicates an increased hazard relative to the baseline hazard.
- Less than 1 indicates a reduced hazard relative to the baseline hazard.
- Equal to 1 indicates that the hazard is equal to the baseline hazard.

Example

In another cancer drug trial (not the study reported in paper B), 37 patients were randomised to the treatment group and 32 patients to the control group. Their survival times (until death, in this case) are measured in months and some observations are censored. The main question of interest is whether survival is related to treatment, but survival time is thought to be related to the age and sex of the patient as well. As shown above, the Cox regression model is:

$$\log\left(\frac{h(t)}{h_o(t)}\right) = \beta_1 x_1 + \beta_2 x_2 + \beta_3 x_3$$

where the explanatory variables are:

> Group $x_1 = 0$ for controls; 1 for treatment
> Sex $x_2 = 0$ for males; 1 for females
> Age x_3 in years

The results of the Cox regression are similar to the output from logistic regression, and look like this (Table 8.2.1):

Table 8.2.1   Results of Cox regression for the cancer trial example (see text)

	Explanatory variable	Regression coefficient b_i	Hazard ratio e^{bi}	95% CI	p-value
1	Group	−1.896	0.1052	0.086–0.262	<0.0001
2	Sex	−0.09135	0.9127	0.732–1.366	0.4342
3	Age	0.1196	1.127	1.103–1.152	0.002

Interpretation

1. The death hazard in the treatment group is 0.1052 times (95 per cent CI: 0.086–0.262) that in the control group, reducing the risk by almost 90 per cent at any given time. The 95 per cent CI does not include 1.0 (no effect)–indeed, the upper limit is still well below 1.0 at 0.262 equivalent to a 74 per cent reduction in risk. As expected, this is a highly significant result ($p < 0.0001$).

2. The death hazard for females does not significantly differ from that for males (the CI includes 1.0, the p-value is large): the sex of the patient does not affect survival.

3. Each 1-year increase in age results in the death hazard increasing by a factor of 1.127, with a 95 per cent CI that does not include 1.0 and a p-value of 0.002: age has a significant effect on survival.

Important note

It is important to note that a 5-year increase in age multiplies the death hazard by $1.127^5 = 1.818$. This calculation is $1.127 \times 1.127 \times 1.127 \times 1.127 \times 1.127$; this is *not* the same as 5×1.127, which would give a factor of 5.635–very different! We saw in Chapter 6 that this also applies to the interpretation of odds ratios from logistic regression which, as you will recall, are also derived by exponentiating the beta coefficient.

8.2.7 Prediction

We have seen that one of the functions of regression is **prediction**. The quantity $(b_1 x_1 + b_2 x_2 + \ldots + b_k x_k)$ is known as the **risk score** or **prognostic index** and can be used to predict the survival of new cases by substituting their particular set of explanatory variable values into the equation.

8.2.8 Application of Cox regression

We have now covered enough on Cox regression to look at how this method was used in the analysis of paper A. Please now read the following excerpt from the results of paper A and review Table 8.2.2 (Table 3 from paper A).

Results (continued)

Serum cotinine concentration and CHD risk—We examined the association between quarters of the cotinine distribution and CHD hazard ratios among all 2105 current non-smokers using the complete follow up period (table 2). The risks in the upper three cotinine groups were markedly higher than the risk in the lowest group, with a relative hazard of 1.61 in the highest group in the simplest model (adjusted for town and age), a hazard estimate similar to that of light active smokers. The association between cotinine concentration and CHD seemed graded and was not markedly affected by adjustment for other cardiovascular risk factors. The results of analyses restricted to lifelong nonsmokers were similar, though the confidence intervals were wider. Exclusion of men with pre-existing CHD had no effect on these findings (data not presented). When we examined the overall association between cotinine concentration and CHD, we found that a doubling of cotinine concentration was associated with a hazard increase of 16% (95% confidence interval 6% to 27%).

Influence of follow up period—In a Kaplan–Meier plot showing the cumulative proportions of men with major CHD over time among three groups (light passive (lowest cotinine quarter), heavy passive (upper three cotinine quarters), and light active (1–9 cigarettes/day)) we found that the heavy passive and light active groups diverged rapidly from the light passive group during the first years of follow up but remained almost parallel during later years (fig 2). The corresponding hazard ratios for cotinine and risk of CHD in separate five year follow up periods were highest in the early years of follow up and declined with increasing duration of follow up (table 3). These patterns were little affected by adjustment for cardiovascular risk factors, and again the hazard ratios for the heavier passive smoking groups were comparable with those of light active smokers. Restriction of these analyses to lifelong non-smokers or to men with no evidence of pre-existing CHD had no material effect on the results.

Serum cotinine exposure and stroke—There was no strong association between cotinine concentration and stroke among non-smokers, either before or after adjustment for major cardiovascular risk factors (table 4). Analyses based on lifelong non-smokers showed similar results. For stroke, there was no strong evidence that hazard ratios changed over time (data not presented).

Table 8.2.2 Cotinine group and risk of coronary heart disease (CHD): hazard ratios (95 per cent CIs) for specific 5-year follow-up periods (Table 3 from paper A)

	Follow up period (years)			
	0–4	5–9	10–14	15–20
Passive smokers*†				
Adjustment 1	3.45 (1.36 to 8.80)	1.90 (1.09 to 3.31)	1.27 (0.72 to 2.22)	1.09 (0.66 to 1.82)
Adjustment 2	3.14 (1.23 to 8.04)	1.93 (1.09 to 3.42)	1.10 (0.63 to 1.95)	1.00 (0.60 to 1.67)
Adjustment 3	3.73 (1.32 to 10.58)	1.95 (1.09 to 3.48)	1.13 (0.63 to 2.04)	1.04 (0.62 to 1.76)
Low active smokers†‡				
Adjustment 1	3.44 (1.07 to 11.02)	1.50 (0.63 to 3.55)	1.59 (0.70 to 3.62)	1.41 (0.66 to 3.03)
Adjustment 2	2.99 (0.90 to 9.97)	1.58 (0.66 to 3.80)	1.43 (0.61 to 3.38)	1.47 (0.68 to 3.15)
Adjustment 3	3.32 (0.87 to 12.64)	1.66 (0.66 to 4.18)	1.71 (0.71 to 4.10)	1.34 (1.23 to 1.47)

* Hazard ratios for CHD events for passive smokers with cotinine above 0.7 versus passive smokers with cotinine below 0.7.

† For CHD: adjustment 1 stratified by town and adjusted for age; adjustment 2 additionally adjusted for systolic blood pressure, diastolic blood pressure, total cholesterol, HDL cholesterol, FEV_1, height, and pre-existing CHD; adjustment 3 additionally adjusted for BMI, triglycerides, white cell count, diabetes, physical activity (none, occasional, light, moderate or more), alcohol intake (none/occasional, light/moderate, heavy), and social class (I, II, III non-manual, III manual, IV, V, and Armed Forces).

‡ Hazard ratios for CHD events for low active smokers (1–9 cigarettes/day) versus passive smokers with cotinine below 0.7.

 Self-Assessment Exercise 8.2.1

1. Can you explain why Cox regression, rather than logistic regression, has been used for the analysis of this study?

2. What assumption should be satisfied before applying Cox regression? Was this requirement met? You should refer to Figure 8.1.4 (Figure 2 from paper A), reproduced in Section 8.1.6.

3. In Table 8.2.2 (Table 3 from paper A), the result for passive smokers observed with adjustment model 2, for the follow-up period 10–14 years, was 1.10 (0.63–1.95). Interpret this result, noting which confounding factors had been included in the model.

4. Why do you think the hazard ratio is highest for the first 5-year follow-up period and declines thereafter?

Answers in Section 8.4

Summary: Cox regression

• The Cox regression model allows investigation of the simultaneous effect of several explanatory variables on survival.

- As with other multivariate regression methods, this allows adjustment for confounding and obtains estimates of the independent effects of variables we are interested in.

- We must be able to assume that hazards are proportional over time. Examination of survival curves allows assessment of whether the difference in hazards is (approximately) proportional at all times, a key test being that the curves do not cross.

- The result of Cox regression is a relative hazard for the event, and is calculated by exponentiating the regression coefficient for each explanatory variable in the same way as for logistic regression.

8.3 Current life tables

8.3.1 Introduction

The life table is a method for studying the survival pattern of a population or group of people. There are essentially two ways in which the method can be used:

- **The current life table**: this is a particular way of expressing age-specific death rates experienced by a given population, at a specified period of time. The method has been extensively used by the life insurance industry to assess the risk of death of a prospective client, given age, sex, and various demographic and lifestyle factors for which age-specific death rates are available.

- **The cohort life table**: This application allows us to look at and compare the survival of specific group(s) (cohorts) of people followed up over time as in a cohort study or trial. It can be used as an alternative to the Kaplan–Meier survival curve. However, since it is generally less useful than the Kaplan–Meier method for this type of analysis (mainly because time intervals are constant rather than determined by the timing of events), we will not consider it further. See, for example, Kirkwood 1988 for further discussion of this technique.

8.3.2 Current life tables

It is helpful to think of the *current life table* as a way of illustrating the survival of an arbitrary number (say, 100 000) of people (which would be newborns if we wish to study life expectancy from birth), if the age-specific death rates we currently experience applied to these people. The figure of 100 000 is known as the *radix*, and is chosen on the basis of convenience. Although this is clearly a fictional device, the method provides a useful means of describing mortality and in comparing populations. For example, if we wish to compare life expectancy of newborn infants in two or more areas of a country, this would be an appropriate method. Life tables provide a measure of life expectancy, for example from birth or across a specified age range, by summarising the impacts of age-specific mortality rates across all relevant ages.

8.3.3   Overview of method

Table 8.3.1 shows the structure and elements that make up a life table, with data entered just for year 1 (an explanation of how this is obtained follows). The columns in the life table can provide the following kinds of information:

- the average life expectancy from birth;
- the average life expectancy at a given age, say, 25;
- how many people would still be left alive at a specific age, say, 65;
- the probability of dying between specified ages, say, from age 5 to 10;
- the probability of surviving between specified ages, say, from age 20 to 65.

The top row of Table 8.3.1 gives an explanation of what each column contains, while the second row shows the conventional notation for each of these values. Only a few rows are shown here, but in a *full life table* such as this there would be a row for every year of life (see also Section 8.3.4 below on abridged life tables). Please note that the notation for *expectation of life*, e^o_x, has nothing to do with natural log to base e, nor is it raised to any power–this is just the conventional way it is written.

Table 8.3.1   Structure of a full life table

Age: for explanations here, each age is termed age_x	Number surviving at age_x	Number of deaths between age_x and age_{x+1}	Probability of surviving from age_x to age_{x+1}	Probability of dying between age_x and age_{x+1}	Expectation of life at age_x
X	l_x	d_x	p_x	q_x	e^o_x
0	**100 000** *(radix)*	647.06	0.9935294	0.0064706	
1	99 352.94				
2					
Etc.					
Etc.					
99					
100					

We will now briefly describe look at how the life table is calculated. The starting point is the *age-specific mortality rate* for age x. We use this to calculate q_x, the risk of dying between that age and the next year of age $(x + 1)$, as follows:

$$q_x = \frac{\text{mortality rate (for age x)}}{1 + 0.5 \,(\text{mortality rate for age x})}$$

So, we start off with $x = 0$, that is the first year of life. The mortality rate for this age group is the *infant mortality rate* (IMR). As the majority of deaths in the first year of life occur before 6 months, it is usual to make some adjustment for this, and the denominator for the formula for q_x becomes $1 + 0.7$ (IMR)–we will use this for the current example. If we know the risk of dying for that year (q_x), then we can work out the number of people who die in that year (d_x). Let us take a typical IMR for a developed country, 6.5 deaths per 1000 live births, which is 0.0065 expressed as a proportion. For the first year, then, we have:

- The infant mortality rate (IMR) (rate for age 0) $= 0.0065$.

- Hence q_x (the probability of dying between birth and age 1 year) $= 0.0065/[1+0.7\,(0.0065)] = 0.0064706$.

- Hence d_x (the number of deaths between birth and 1 year) $= 100\,000$ (the arbitrary *radix*) $\times 0.0064706 = 647.06$.

- Hence l_x (the numbers surviving to year 1) $= 100\,000 - 647.06 = 99352.94$

- And p_x (the probability of surviving from birth to 1 year) $= 1 - q_x = 0.9935$.

And so on. For the next year ($x+1$), we start again with the age-specific rate for age 1 (the second year of life) and calculate d_{x+1}, and so on.

The ***expectation of life*** ($e^o{}_x$) is calculated when the table is complete, using the total number of person years still to be lived by people starting from year x. This might be between specific years (say, from 20 to 65, in which case year $x = 20$), or if we are interested in full life expectancy, from birth to the oldest age survived (in which case year $x = 0$). To obtain life expectancy, we add up all the values in the l_x column from l_{x+1} onwards, divide by l_x and add 0.5.

8.3.4 Abridged life tables

A full life table (as in Table 8.3.1) has the information entered for each year. In practice, however, age-specific death rates for each year of life may not be available and an ***abridged life table*** may be used. These would typically have data for 5-year intervals, although the first 5 years of life may be included separately, as in the example below (Table 8.3.2). An additional column (interval) is

Table 8.3.2 Structure of an abridged life table

Age: for explanations here, each age is termed age_x	Interval (years)	Number surviving at age_x	Number of deaths between age_x and age_{x+1}	Probability of surviving from age_x to age_{x+1}	Probability of dying between age_x and age_{x+1}	Expectation of life at age_x
X	n	$_n l_x$	$_n d_x$	$_n p_x$	$_n q_x$	$e^o{}_x$
0	1	100000				
1	1					
2	1					
3	1					
4	1					
5	5					
10	5					
15	5					
Etc.	Etc.					

included to show the size of the unequal intervals. The notation is also slightly different, with the n included for columns 3–6 to indicate the interval (in years) referred to.

The main points from this brief introduction to life tables are summarised below.

Summary: current life tables

- The current life table is a means of summarising death (or other) rates in a given population at a specific time.

- The calculation of a life table is based on age-specific (mortality) rates. A full life table includes every year; an abridged one has larger intervals.

- Since death rates for a specific time period are used, the life table does not indicate the true mortality experience of a cohort of people over time, as the death rates those people actually experience as they age will change over time (as social circumstances and health services improve, or maybe deteriorate).

- Information about each age (or age group in an abridged table) is preserved and available for comparison.

- The information from life tables can be compared across populations as age-specific rates are used.

- Life tables can be calculated in standard statistical packages.

8.4 Answers to self-assessment exercises

Section 8.1

Exercise 8.1.1

1. The subjects were a subsample of men from the British Regional Heart Study, a prospective investigation of men aged 40–59 at recruitment drawn from 24 towns in Great Britain. The subsample for this analysis ($n = 4729$) was drawn from the last 18 towns, which included serum samples (that could be subsequently analysed for cotinine). From the men in these towns, self-reported non-smokers ($n = 2158$: this number provided in later excerpt – see Section 8.1.6) were selected, but only those with a serum cotinine of <14.1 ng/ml ($n = 2105$) were included in the analysis.

2. Outcomes studied were (a) major CHD events (deaths and non-fatal myocardial infarction), and (b) strokes (deaths and non-fatal strokes).

3. By serum cotinine levels. Cotinine is a metabolite of nicotine, and is a 'sensitive and specific' indicator of exposure to tobacco smoke (the definition and interpretation of the terms *sensitivity* and *specificity* are covered in Chapter 10). While it is a good indicator of recent history of exposure to tobacco smoke, the single baseline measurement will become a progressively less accurate measure over time as the men's exposure to tobacco changes.

4. The research team does have information on time between the baseline survey (recruitment) and the event; hence the 'survival' time. In these circumstances, survival analysis is an appropriate method.

Exercise 8.1.2

1. A total of 14 intervention group observations and six control group observations were censored. Possible reasons for this difference include: (i) the better survival among intervention subjects mean that these people are more likely to reach the end of their follow-up period without experiencing the outcome event (recurrence) and (ii) there may be more losses to follow-up among intervention subjects.

2. On the Kaplan–Meier curve (see annotated figure below), we have run a horizontal line across the graph from probability $= 0.5$. Where this line intersects the curves for (a) control and (b) intervention groups, we run a vertical line down to the x-axis (survival time). This gives values of approximately 15 (control) and 32 (intervention). These are confirmed when calculated in SPSS: median (with 95 per cent CI) on control treatment $= 15$ (3.9, 26.1); on new treatment, median $= 32$ (16.4, 47.6).

3. We can run a vertical line up from 30 months and see where this intersects with the two curves (and then run horizontal lines across to the y-axis, the survival probability). This is approximately at 0.13 (13 per cent) for the control group and 0.55 (55 per cent) for the intervention group.

Exercise 8.1.3

1. Geometric means are used because the distribution of cotinine levels is markedly right skewed, and this is normalised by log transformation. The use of transformation for skewed data and the interpretation of geometric means are discussed fully in Chapter 11.

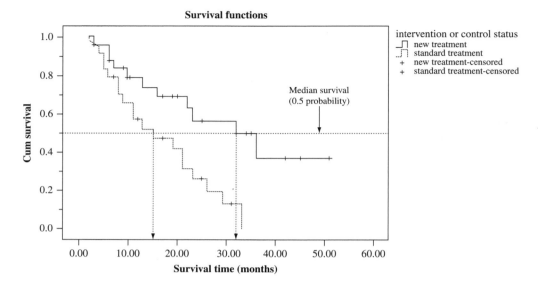

2. Self-reported ex-smokers could have higher cotinine levels if they are still smoking some cigarettes, although, according to the interim surveys at 5 and 12 years, almost all (99 per cent) continued to report they were non-smokers. Alternatively (or in addition), ex-smokers may be more likely than never smokers to associate socially and at work with current smokers.

3. Figure 8.1.4 is a Kaplan–Meier curve.

4. The probability of having a CHD event after 10 years for (a) light passive is approximately 0.04 (4 per cent); (b) for heavy passive smoking, it is approximately 0.085 (8.5 per cent). It is not possible to read median probability of a CHD event from this Kaplan–Meier curve, as the probability does not exceed 0.5: indeed, the probability of a CHD event after 20 years among the highest exposure group is just under 0.2.

5. The result of the log-rank test (result top left of Figure 8.1.4) is $p = 0.002$, a very significant finding. This indicates that we can reject the null hypothesis of no difference in survival between the groups studied (light passive, heavy passive, light active). Since the last two curves are close and cross several times, it is the difference between light passive and the other groups that is important.

6. The curves in Figure 8.1.4 start at a probability of 0.0 because this study looks at the probability of having an event, not avoiding it (i.e. survival without recurrence), as in the cancer trial example. At the start of follow-up, none of the men have had a new event; hence, the probability is 0.0.

Exercise 8.1.4

1. The criteria that defined the patients included in this study were:

- recruited from 23 centres in the UK, Ireland and South Africa;

- unresectable (not possible to remove surgically) non-small cell lung cancer;

- no, or only minimal, thoracic (chest) symptoms;

- no compelling indication for immediate radiotherapy;

- performance status of any WHO grade;

- non-metastatic or metastatic disease (that is, patients whose cancer had spread outside the lungs (metastatic), and those whose cancer had not spread (non-metastatic) were included);

- not suitable for radical radiotherapy with curative intent.

2. *Primary outcome*: patients alive and without moderate to severe cough, chest pain, haemoptysis (coughing blood), or dyspnoea (shortness of breath) 6 months after randomisation, as recorded by clinicians. *Secondary outcomes*: quality of life, adverse events, survival.

3. The Kaplan–Meier graph is for survival (not dying), one of the secondary outcomes. The graph is presented as percentage of patients surviving, where 100 per cent is equivalent to a probability of 1.0. As a result of the very high death rate (low survival), the probability of survival drops below 50 per cent during the course of the study, and it is therefore possible to read the median survival from the graph (unlike in paper A). The results in the abstract are (a) medians 8.3 and 7.9 for immediate and delayed, respectively, and (b) 31 and 29 per cent surviving at 12 months, respectively. These results are consistent with those you would read off the Kaplan–Meier curves.

4. A hazard ratio for survival of 0.95 with a 95 per cent CI 0.73–1.24 (p = 0.71) implies that subjects receiving the immediate radiotherapy had a 5 per cent lower risk of dying, but since the 95 per cent CI includes 1.0 there is no strong evidence that this finding is anything other than chance. The p-value of 0.71 is consistent with this conclusion. We therefore cannot reject the null hypothesis of no survival advantage.

Section 8.2

Exercise 8.2.1

1. Time to event data was available and Cox regression makes the most of this information. Logistic regression could have been used for incidence density (CHD events/person years), but this would not have been the most efficient use of the data. Cox regression is now commonly used in the analysis of prospective studies for this reason.

2. The Kaplan–Meier curves in Figure 8.1.4 do not cross (at least not those for light and heavy passive, which are the curves of principal interest for this analysis). However, we do know from the curves and particularly from the analysis of 5-year follow-up periods in Table 8.2.2, that the hazards do not remain proportional over the 20 years. Carrying out the Cox regression separately for each 5-year period, however, overcomes any concern about the assumption not being met across the whole 20-year period.

3. Interpretation: there is a 10 per cent increase in the relative hazard (risk of CHD if exposed to passive smoking with cotinine above 0.7 ng/ml compared to less than 0.7 ng/ml), but the 95 per cent CI is quite wide and includes 1.00, so this is a non-significant result. Adjustment 2, in addition to stratification for town and adjustment for age, included systolic blood pressure, diastolic blood pressure, total cholesterol, high-density lipoprotein cholesterol, FEV_1 (a measure of lung function), height, and pre-existing CHD.

4. Some comment on this is to be found in the paper, in the Discussion section. This considers the effect of relying on a single baseline measure of cotinine to characterise passive smoking exposure for (up to) the next 20 years. With changing smoking patterns (for example, spouses of subjects giving up, and growing restrictions on smoking at work, in public transport and in public places) and generally greater awareness of the dangers of passive smoking, it is likely that many of these men will have experienced considerable changes to their passive smoking exposure over the follow-up period.

9

Systematic reviews and meta-analysis

Introduction and learning objectives

A literature search on any particular research question may yield several, if not many, published studies which in one way or another may contribute to answering the question. No two studies will report identical results. The methods and outcome measures may differ. Not infrequently, we find that studies appear to contradict each other. What are we to make of all this information? Does a large number of studies help us to arrive at a definitive answer, or do more studies lead to more confusion and lack of clarity? And what about all the unpublished studies investigating the same question?

As we will see over the course of this chapter, reviews of all available evidence on a particular question can be extremely useful. However, in order to assess the validity of the various studies, integrate appropriate information, and arrive at an overall result, we need a rigorous, systematic approach. That is, we need to carry out a *systematic review* of all the evidence, both published and unpublished.

> A *systematic review* is a review of the methods and results of all individual studies designed to answer the same research question and that conform to set criteria.

As part of this process we may want to obtain a quantitative summary (for example, of a treatment effect or an exposure risk) across comparable studies. This may be (most commonly) through combining the results of the individual studies, or by analysing the raw data from the studies if they are available. The statistical methods required to carry out such analyses are known as *meta-analysis*.

> *Meta-analysis* is the statistical analysis of the data/results from studies included in a systematic review to produce an overall, pooled result.

Quantitative Methods for Health Research   Nigel Bruce, Daniel Pope and Debbi Stanistreet
© 2008 John Wiley & Sons, Ltd

Meta-analysis is commonly used to combine data from a number of randomised, controlled trials (RCTs) of therapies or interventions. However, the techniques may also be used for observational epidemiological studies of risk factors.

The results of any one study may have too much random error to show any clear effect. That is, the study may not be powerful enough to demonstrate significant differences (type II error). In combining data from several studies, we increase the sample size and so increase power and obtain more precise estimates.

Systematic reviews and associated meta-analyses are playing an increasingly important role in both research and practice. In this chapter we will explore the rationale for carrying out systematic reviews and the methods for selecting, reviewing and analysing the results, and look at some practical applications of the reviews. We will then explore the principles and practicalities of carrying out a meta-analysis based on the results of a systematic review. This will incorporate assessment of the suitability of studies to be included in a meta-analysis, methods of statistically pooling results from the selected studies and approaches to investigating the effects of study quality on the results. Finally we will introduce the Cochrane Collaboration, one of most important contemporary initiatives in the field of systematic reviews.

Learning objectives

By the end of this chapter, you should be able to:

- Describe the purpose of systematic reviews, and the contribution these can make to earlier introduction of effective practice.

- Describe the main steps in carrying out a systematic review, including how to minimise selection bias and assess the methodological quality of selected studies.

- Describe the most commonly used approaches to reporting the results of systematic reviews of RCTs and observational studies.

- Describe what is meant by publication bias and the commonly used techniques for determining whether publication bias is present and the implications for a meta-analysis.

- Describe what is meant by statistical heterogeneity between studies selected for a meta-analysis and the commonly used methods for determining the presence and extent of heterogeneity.

- Describe the two main statistical approaches to combining results from studies in a meta-analysis, namely fixed effect and random effects models, and the implications of heterogeneity for the choice of method.

- Interpret the results of a meta-analysis as illustrated in a forest plot.

- Describe what is meant by sensitivity analysis and how this may be used to investigate the impact of differing methodological quality of studies on the results of a meta-analysis.

- Describe those aspects of methodology requiring special attention where a systematic review and meta-analysis of observational study designs is being carried out, rather than a review of randomised trials.

Resource paper

One resource paper has been selected for this chapter; it reviews a range of interventions aimed at reducing the incidence of diarrhoea in developing countries.

Paper A

Fewtrell, L., Kaufmann, R. B., Kay, D. *et al.* (2005). Water, sanitation and hygiene interventions to reduce diarrhoea in less developed countries: a systematic review and meta-analysis. *Lancet Infect Dis* **5**, 42–52.

Please now read the abstract from paper A, reproduced below.

Abstract

Many studies have reported the results of interventions to reduce illness through improvements in drinking water, sanitation facilities, and hygiene practices in less developed countries. There has, however, been no formal systematic review and meta-analysis comparing the evidence of the relative effectiveness of these interventions. We developed a comprehensive search strategy designed to identify all peer-reviewed articles, in any language, that presented water, sanitation, or hygiene interventions. We examined only those articles with specific measurement of diarrhoea morbidity as a health outcome in non-outbreak conditions. We screened the titles and, where necessary, the abstracts of 2120 publications. 46 studies were judged to contain relevant evidence and were reviewed in detail. Data were extracted from these studies and pooled by meta-analysis to provide summary estimates of the effectiveness of each type of intervention. All of the interventions studied were found to reduce significantly the risks of diarrhoeal illness. Most of the interventions had a similar degree of impact on diarrhoeal illness, with the relative risk estimates from the overall meta-analyses ranging between 0.63 and 0.75. The results generally agree with those from previous reviews, but water quality interventions (point-of-use water treatment) were found to be more effective than previously thought, and multiple interventions (consisting of combined water, sanitation, and hygiene measures) were not more effective than interventions with a single focus. There is some evidence of publication bias in the findings from the hygiene and water treatment interventions.

9.1 The why and how of systematic reviews

9.1.1 Why is it important that reviews be systematic?

Conducting a systematic review involves a great deal of work, although it is generally quicker and less costly than carrying out a new study. Clearly, it is important to establish why all of this activity is so important.

An example of the importance of synthesising results from studies in a meta-analysis can be illustrated by studying the relationship over time between accruing evidence from meta-analyses with the recommendations made by experts in review articles and textbooks. In a now classic study of thrombolytic drugs (drugs used to break down blood clots in heart attack patients) and recommendations for their routine implementation into current therapy, Antman *et al.* (1992) showed that such drugs were only first recommended for routine use in 1987, some 14 years after a statistically significant ($p < 0.01$) beneficial effect would have been identified if meta-analysis had been done at that time. The results from this study are illustrated in Figure 9.1.1.

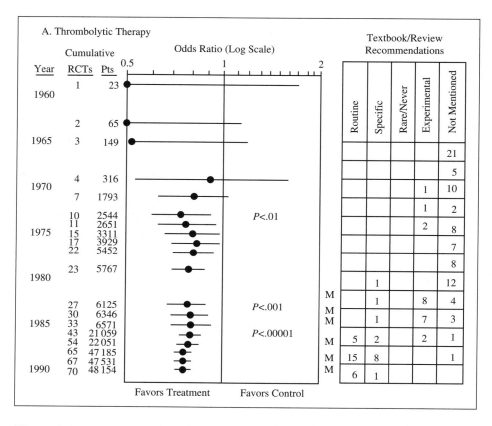

Figure 9.1.1 Recommendations to use thrombolytic therapy lagged well behind the evidence that would have been available from a systematic review and meta-analysis (from Antman *et al.*, 1992)

Figure 9.1.1 is a graphical display of a ***cumulative meta-analysis*** of 70 RCTs of thrombolytic therapy. In the centre box, odds ratios (ORs) (blobs) and confidence intervals (CIs) (the lines through the blobs) are displayed, showing the pooled results of all studies up to a particular point in time. For example, at the top is an estimated OR of 0.5 (the OR is likely to have been less than 0.5 but scale has been truncated for the figure) and a wide CI (only the right half is shown), which is the result of a single, pre-1960, trial with 23 patients. The wide CI includes 1, corresponding to no treatment effect, and reflects the lack of precision in this small trial. Between 1960 and 1965 a second study of 42 patients was completed. So the second line shows the pooled estimate from the two trials, with a total of 65 patients, and so on. With each additional study more data are included in the meta-analysis, so the sample size increases and the CI for the pooled OR becomes narrower, reflecting increased statistical precision and hence certainty of the estimate.

By 1990, 70 trials had been completed with a total of 48 154 patients. The estimated OR and CI from all the trials clearly show the benefit of the treatment, although the evidence of this benefit was in fact available in the 1970s, if a systematic review had been carried out at that time. However, thrombolytic therapy was not recommended for routine treatment until some years after the available evidence actually confirmed the efficacy of the treatment. In fact, the entry in the second edition of the *Oxford Textbook of Medicine* (1987), more than 10 years after pooled results showed a statistically significant effect, stated:

> *The clinical benefits of thrombolysis whether expressed as improved patient survival or preservation of left ventricular function, remain to be established.*

Interestingly, this was published 2 years after a systematic review of the relevant RCTs had shown that the treatment reduced the risk of premature death after myocardial infarction (Yusuf *et al.*, 1985). Antman concluded:

> *Because reviewers have not used scientific methods, advice on some life-saving therapies has been delayed for more than a decade, while other treatments have been recommended long after controlled research has shown them to be harmful.*

9.1.2 Method of systematic review – overview

We require systematic methods in order to establish whether research findings are consistent and generalisable. The process of carrying out a systematic review comprises the following steps:

1. Decide on the objectives of the review.

2. Define criteria for including/excluding studies in the review.

3. Find/locate studies.

4. Select studies according to the eligibility criteria.

5. Assess the methodological quality of the studies.

6. Extract data.

7. Describe and compile the results.

8. Report the results of the review.

We will now work through each of these steps to explain the process in more detail.

9.1.3   Deciding on the objectives of the review

As we saw previously, with any study design, it is very important to state clearly the research question and study objectives prior to carrying out the study, and this is just as relevant to a systematic review. If the objectives are not explicitly stated, there is a risk that a reviewer will use the results to support a hypothesis that was not intended. For example, if after analysis of the results of individual studies, one or more are found to give unexpected or contrary findings in respect of the postulated objectives, there might be a temptation to revise the objectives of the review or to exclude some of the studies.

For this reason the review objectives should clearly state who the study participants are, what interventions are to be investigated (or what risk factors are to be measured for observational study designs), what outcomes are to be assessed and the settings of studies for the review. In addition, the criteria that will be used for inclusion/ exclusion of subjects in the study should be clearly defined.

Please now read the following excerpt from the introduction of paper A.

Introduction

Diarrhoeal disease is one of the leading causes of morbidity and mortality in less developed countries, especially among children aged under 5 years.[1,2] Since the seminal reviews of Esrey and colleagues in 1985, 1986, and 1991,[3-5] additional studies have been published on various water, hygiene, and sanitation related interventions aimed at population health improvements. The original reviews,[3-5] and a study by Blum and Feachem,[6] have led to a better understanding of methodological issues in this area. The reviews by Esrey and colleagues[3-5] included studies that measured differences in health outcomes between groups that had different water or sanitation conditions. Since these original reviews, many studies have reported additional results of interventions to reduce illness through improvements in drinking water, sanitation facilities, and hygiene practices in the less developed world. There has, however, been no formal systematic review and meta-analysis comparing the relative evidence on the effectiveness of these interventions. We present a systematic review of all published studies and, where appropriate, meta-analysis of studies that reported interventions (planned or occurring as natural experiments) in water quality, water supply, hygiene, and sanitation in less developed countries. Less developed countries are defined here as any country not within a class A region under the WHO comparative risk assessment (class A countries have very low child and adult mortality).

 Self-Assessment Exercise 9.1.1

According to the abstract (in the introduction of the chapter) and introduction of paper A above:

1) What were the stated objectives of this systematic review?

2) Was the context of the study clearly described (in terms of population, setting, intervention and outcome)?

3) From the introduction, what types of studies were stated as eligible for the review?

Answers in Section 9.5

9.1.4 Defining criteria for inclusion and exclusion of studies

When we looked at intervention studies (Chapter 7), we saw the importance of clearly stating the subject inclusion and exclusion criteria. In a similar way, for a systematic review, it is important to specify the criteria studies need to meet before being eligible for inclusion. Failure to do this can result in bias in terms of which studies are selected. The inclusion criteria should relate to the required study populations, treatments (which may be interventions or risk factors in observational studies), study outcomes, length of follow-up and aspects of methodological quality. We will see later in the chapter how the methodological quality of studies can be assessed and how we can measure the influence that differing quality of studies can have on results of meta-analyses. The particular issues relating to reviews of observational studies are discussed in Section 9.3.

Please now read the following excerpt relating to the initial selection criteria of paper A, taken from the methods section.

Methods

Initial selection criteria and data extraction
Two selection criteria were used to identify articles: (1) description of specific water, sanitation, or hygiene interventions, or some combination of such interventions; and (2) diarrhoea morbidity reported as the health outcome, measured under endemic (non-outbreak) conditions. In addition, only published studies were used, to maintain quality (via peer review) and transparency. . . .

No study was excluded from the review or meta-analysis on the basis of quality criteria alone.

 Self-Assessment Exercise 9.1.2

What were the main selection criteria used to identify relevant articles for the review?

Answers in Section 9.5

9.1.5 Identifying relevant studies

Publication bias

When carrying out a systematic review it is important to include relevant unpublished studies, as well as published, peer-reviewed studies. Thus a simple literature search using electronic databases is not sufficient. One of the most important reasons for this is that studies reporting statistically significant results are more likely to be published than those with non-significant results. This selective publication, or ***publication bias***, means that we may reach over-optimistic or misleading conclusions if we include only published studies in our systematic review. This is particularly the case with small studies: we have seen that any study might occasionally produce a significant effect when no such effect really exists (type 1 error), but since small studies are more difficult to publish than large ones, there is a tendency for those with significant results to be offered (and accepted) for publication more frequently than small studies without 'interesting' results.

Statistical significance does not guarantee the quality, validity or clinical significance of the research and good studies which have conclusively demonstrated a lack of treatment effect or lack of association may never be published. Since 2005, in accordance with the International Committee of Medical Journal Editors (ICMJE), prior entry of clinical trials in a public registry is a condition for publication of results in ICMJE journals (including *The New England Journal of Medicine*, *Journal of the American Medical Association* and *The Lancet*, among others). For UK clinical trials, the ICMJE recommends a website for public registration: www.controlled-trials.com, a UK site developed and maintained by Current Controlled Trials Ltd, part of the Current Science Group of biomedical publishing companies. In the future such registries will make it easier to identify studies for a systematic review in order to reduce the risk of publication bias.

Publication bias is minimised by a comprehensive search strategy including unpublished work and foreign language journals. However, it should be noted that the inclusion of data from unpublished studies can itself introduce bias. The studies that can be located might be an unrepresentative sample of all unpublished studies, and in general unpublished trials may have a poorer methodological quality than those that are published.

As we shall see in Section 9.2 when we consider how to conduct a meta-analysis, it is possible to investigate both graphically (by a funnel plot) and quantitatively (by statistical methods) whether the selection of studies for a systematic review is likely to have been subject to publication bias.

 Self-Assessment Exercise 9.1.3

Refer to the previous excerpt from paper A (Section 9.1.4) that described the initial selection criteria and data extraction.

1. What reasons did the authors give for only including published studies in their review?

2. Do you think that these reasons were sufficient justification for excluding unpublished studies from their review?

Answers in Section 9.5

Searching the literature

The next important step in ensuring that a review is systematic is to state what the search strategy will be prior to identifying relevant studies. The Cochrane website (www.cochrane.org – the

Cochrane initiative is described further in Section 9.4) contains detailed information about how to develop a search strategy. In this section we will briefly look at the main approaches to carrying out a thorough literature search.

The sources chosen to search for studies will be influenced by the type of study to be included in the review, that is, whether these are to be clinical trials, observational studies, qualitative studies, etc., but generally the first step is to search the main health-related electronic databases. If the review relates to clinical trials, the *Cochrane Controlled Trials Register (CCTR)* (see also Section 9.4) is the best single source of trials published in peer-reviewed journals: the database currently contains over 270 000 published trials. To ensure the literature is up to date, however, searches of *Medline* and *EMBASE (Excerpta Medical Database)* should also be carried out. This would also be the starting point for systematic reviews of observational studies. The main attributes of Medline and EMBASE are shown in Table 9.1.1.

Table 9.1.1 Summary of the main attributes of the two main electronic journal databases for quantitative studies of health outcomes (Medline and EMBASE)

Medline	EMBASE
• approximately 10 million references	• approximately 8 million references
• Uses specific indexing (MeSH)	• Uses specific indexing (EMTREE)
• 1966 to present	• 1974 to present
• Available through CD-ROMS and on the Internet	• Available through CD-ROMS and on the Internet
• 52% from the USA	• 33% from the USA

It is advisable to search both Medline and EMBASE because the overlap between the databases is only approximately 34 per cent. In addition, just over half the references on Medline are published in the USA compared to only a third of references on EMBASE, which has better coverage of European journals.

The next step is to supplement the literature search by utilising additional electronic databases of published health-related research. The most common of these databases are listed in the box below.

Examples of additional electronic databases of published studies in health fields

- Allied and Alternative Medicine (AMED)

- Biological abstracts (BIOSIS)

- CAB Health

- Cumulative Index to Nursing and Allied Health Literature (CINAHL)

(Continued)

- Derwent Drug File

- Psychological abstracts (PsychInfo)

- Science Citation Index/Current contents

- PASCAL (original journal articles – including foreign language)

- Latin American and Caribbean Health Sciences Information System (LILACS).

After searching the electronic databases of published studies, it is also advisable to search the so-called *grey literature* for additional studies that have not been published in peer-reviewed journals. For example, a proportion of trials and observational studies will only be published as meeting/conference abstracts. The main grey literature electronic databases are listed in the box below.

Principal electronic databases of grey literature

- British Library 'inside' database

- System for Information on Grey Literature in Europe (SIGLE)

- Patents database

- Indexes to conference proceedings (including the British Library Index to Conference Proceedings)

- PASCAL (conference proceedings, dissertations, patents, reports, etc.).

To complete the search checks should be made to ensure that the review has captured all relevant studies by checking the reference lists of published papers and reports, by hand searching the reference lists of key journals and by contacting experts in the field to identify any research they have conducted or know about that has not yet been published.

We will now look at the search strategy used for paper A, described in the following excerpt:

Methods

Search strategy

Database searches of the Cochrane Library, Embase, LILACS, Medline, and Pascal Biomed were done with keyword searches that paired aspects of 'water', 'sanitation', and 'hygiene' with 'diarrhoea', and, separately, with 'intervention'. The Cochrane Central Register of Controlled Trials was particularly useful for identifying intervention studies; Embase and Medline provided very good coverage of English language papers; and LILACS and Pascal

Biomed provided coverage of foreign language, Latin American, and Caribbean papers. Searches were limited to articles published before June 26, 2003 (when the search was done), and to articles about human beings. The reviews by Esrey and colleagues[3–5] were used as an additional source to identify early studies, and author-based searches were used to identify subsequent work by the primary investigators, with additional information. All titles and abstracts (if available) from each of the searches were examined and then the relevant articles were obtained for review. Bibliographies of those articles were examined for additional references. No restrictions were put on study design, location, or language of publication.

Self-Assessment Exercise 9.1.4

1. List the databases and sources used for the search.

2. Do you feel these were sufficiently comprehensive?

Answers in Section 9.5

9.1.6 Assessment of methodological quality

What is methodological quality?

The concept of *methodological quality* is hard to define but typically it is used to describe the design, procedures and conduct of a study, how the analysis has been carried out, the relevance of the study to policy and practice, and/or the quality of the reporting. For example, ideally, we might set the following inclusion criteria for a systematic review of clinical trials:

- placebo controls (if possible);

- evidence of effective randomisation;

- blinding used, ideally at least double blinding; that is, of study participants and research staff assessing the outcome;

- near complete follow-up of subjects;

- analysis by intention-to-treat.

Complete information is not always available however, even in published journal articles, and it is sometimes necessary to define the methodological quality of studies in terms of only basic criteria. Alternatively, it may be necessary to contact the authors to obtain the missing information.

Why measure methodological quality?

Even after we have excluded studies with poor methodological quality, it is likely that the remaining studies will still be of variable quality. It has been demonstrated empirically that studies with poor quality can distort the results from systematic reviews and meta-analyses. For example, a study of 250 trials from 33 meta-analyses of a range of interventions relating to pregnancy and childbirth found that non-random treatment allocation and lack of double blinding of controlled intervention trials were associated with larger treatment effects. The main findings of this study are presented in Table 9.1.2, comparing the effect estimates of trials defined as having inadequate/unclear methodology with those from trials defined as having adequate methodology (an OR ratio of less than 1 indicates an exaggerated treatment effect).

Table 9.1.2 Summary of the results of a study investigating methodological aspects of RCTs in relation to the size of treatment effect (adapted from Shulz *et al.*, 1995 in Egger *et al.*, 2003).

Methodological quality item	Ratio of OR*	95% CI	Interpretation
Treatment hidden from subjects			
- adequate	1.0	(reference group)	
- unclear	0.67	0.60 – 0.75	Exaggerated effects
- inadequate	0.59	0.48 – 0.73	Exaggerated effects
Randomisation method			
- adequate	1.0	(reference group)	
- inadequate/ unclear	0.95	0.81 – 1.12	Similar effects
Double blinding			
- yes	1.0	(reference group)	
- no	0.83	0.71 – 0.96	Exaggerated effects

* Comparison of ORs of studies with inadequate methodology and studies with adequate methodology.

The authors did not find that the randomisation method or exclusions after randomisation influenced the treatment effect. If the treatment was not adequately hidden (blinded) from study subject, however, there appeared to be an exaggerated treatment effect of 41 per cent (95% CI: 27 to 52 per cent). In addition, a lack of double blinding was associated with an exaggeration of treatment effect by 17 per cent (95% CI: 4 to 29 per cent). These results highlight the importance of assessing the methodological quality of studies included in a systematic review, especially if the results are to be included in a meta-analysis.

How should we measure methodological quality?

We saw previously that poor quality could be among the criteria for excluding studies from a review. Given the somewhat subjective nature of the decision process as to whether studies meet minimum inclusion criteria in relation to quality, it is good practice for two reviewers independently to check the eligibility of candidate studies, with disagreements being resolved through discussion with a third reviewer.

Methodological quality can be quantified by scoring the quality of studies on a pre-existing scale, such as that developed for randomised trials by Jadad *et al.* (1996). This scale has five items: two relate to blinding, two to randomisation, and one to the description of withdrawals/dropouts. When using the Jadad scale, each of the five items receives a 'yes' or a 'no', resulting in an overall/composite quality score that can range from 0 to 5; higher scores reflect better methodological quality.

An example of a quality scale for assessing the quality of observational studies to be included in a systematic review is the Newcastle-Ottawa Scale (NOS) (Wells *et al.*, 2000). We will look more closely at systematic reviews of observational studies in Section 9.3 of this chapter. Although assessment of quality is a very important step, recent evidence suggests that the use of quality scales might be problematic. Comparisons of assessments of the quality of trials using different composite scales have found that the perception of the quality of a clinical trial, and hence (potentially) whether or not it is included in the review, varies according to which scale is used. The conclusions of a meta-analysis can therefore be affected by the choice of quality scale.

An alternative to using a quality score is to measure individual components of methodological quality. These can then be examined quantitatively for their influence on the results from a meta-analysis. An example of this was seen in Table 9.1.2, where the authors identified that inadequately hiding the treatment from subjects and not using double blinding were associated with exaggerated treatment effects. As we will see in Section 9.2, this can be investigated by performing a *sensitivity analysis*. Let's now look at the assessment of quality in paper A, described in the following excerpt:

Methods
The quality of each study was examined on the basis of a set of methodological criteria for such studies previously suggested by Blum and Feachem.[6] No study was excluded from the review or meta-analysis on the basis of quality criteria alone. If possible, issues of study quality were examined in the meta-analysis as a source of possible heterogeneity between results. Poor quality studies, for the purposes of this review, were defined as those that had any of the following design flaws: inadequate or inadequately described control groups, no clear measurement or control for confounders, no specific definition of diarrhoea or the particular diarrhoeal health outcome used, or a health indicator recall period (ie, the maximum time between illness occurrence and the reporting of the illness) of more than 2 weeks. Studies without these flaws were categorised as being of good quality. Fewtrell and Colford[8] have outlined further details on issues of study quality.

 Self-Assessment Exercise 9.1.5

1. How were 'poor-quality' studies defined?

2. How did the authors deal with studies of poor quality?

Answers in Section 9.5

9.1.7 Extracting data and describing the results

We have now come to the stage of extracting data from articles selected for the systematic review to report in a narrative summary of the main results.

The process of data extraction should be carried out with as much care as was taken for assessing the methodological quality of studies. Again, it is important that two independent observers extract the data to ensure that errors are minimised. Data extraction requires that a (data extraction) form be used for all the studies selected for the review, and this should be carefully designed, piloted and revised if required. Typically information required for randomised trials will comprise (i) the reference, (ii) the setting and sample of people being studied, (iii) the intervention or treatment and how this is measured, (iv) the health outcome and how this is measured and (v) a measure of the size of effect (e.g. OR or relative risk) with associated CIs.

The descriptive presentation of results from a systematic review normally involves three stages. First, it is important to state clearly the numbers of studies included and rejected from the review. Second, the results of the articles included in the systematic review are tabulated presenting a summary of the main attributes of the studies. The third stage is to outline descriptively the main results of the review. The emphasis on presenting the results from a systematic review is placed on a descriptive narrative summary of the findings. As we shall see in the next section, the value of a systematic review in providing a quantitative summary of results is through the pooling of data in the form of a meta-analysis.

Please now read the excerpt below and review Table 9.1.3 (Table 1 from paper A), reproduced from the results section of paper A. The table and text relate to one objective of the systematic review (hygiene interventions) and show how the results of the review are presented as a descriptive summary of the studies. At this stage, ignore the information given at the bottom of Table 9.1.3, as this refers to the meta-analysis – we will return to this information in Section 9.2.

Results

Hygiene
15 articles, representing 13 distinct studies, were identified that examined hygiene interventions. 11 of these studies presented data that could be used for meta-analysis (Table 1). . . . Hygiene interventions were typically of two types, those concentrating on health and hygiene education, and those that actively promoted handwashing (usually alongside education messages). The number of messages, the content of those messages, and the way in which they were delivered varied between studies. In general, education was aimed at the mothers, although the outcome was measured in children.

 Self-Assessment Exercise 9.1.6

1. From the text excerpt, how did the authors summarise the types of hygiene intervention?

2. Referring to Table 9.1.3, briefly describe how information from the systematic review relating to hygiene is presented.

Answers in Section 9.5

Table 9.1.3 Studies of hygiene interventions and health effects (Table 1 from paper A)

Reference	Intervention	Country (location)	Study quality*	Health Outcome	Age Group	Measure	Estimate (95% CI)
Khan, 1982	Handwashing with soap	Bangladesh (unstated)	Good	Diarrhoea	All	RR†	0.62(0.35–1.12)‡
Torún, 1982	Hygiene education	Guatemala (rural)	Poor	Diarrhoea	0–72 months	RR†	0.81(0.75–0.87)‡
Sircar et al, 1987	Handwashing with soap	India (urban)	Good	Diarrhoea	0–60 months	RR†	1.13(0.79–1.62)
					> 5 years	RR†	1.08(0.86–1.37)
				Dysentery	0–60 months	RR†	0.67(0.42–1.09)
					> 5 years	RR†	0.59(0.37–0.93)
				Combined outcome	Combined ages	RR†	0.97(0.82–1.16)‡
Stanton et al, 1988 Stanton and Clemens, 1987	Hygiene education	Bangladesh (urban)	Good	Diarrhoea	0–72 months	IDR#	0.78(0.74–0.83)‡
Alam et al, 1989	Hygiene education (and increased water supply)	Bangladesh (rural)	Good	Diarrhoea	6–23 months	OR	0.27(0.11–0.66)‡
Han and Hlaing, 1989	Handwashing with soap	Burma Myanmar (urban)	Good	Diarrhoea	0–60 months	RR	0.70(0.54–0.92)
					0–24 months	RR	0.69(0.48–1.01)
					25–60 months	RR	0.67(0.45–0.98)
				Dysentery	0–60 months	RR	0.93(0.39–2.23)
					0–24 months	RR	0.59(0.22–1.55)
					25–60 months	RR	1.21(0.52–2.80)
				Combined outcome	0–60 months	RR†	0.75(0.60–0.94)‡

Table 9.1.3 (Continued)

Reference	Intervention	Country (location)	Study quality*	Health Outcome	Age Group	Measure	Estimate (95% CI)
Lee et al, 1991	Hygiene education	Thailand (unstated)	Good	Diarrhoea	0–60 months	RR†	0.43(0.32–0.56)‡
Wilson et al, 1991	Handwashing with soap	Indonesia (rural)	Good	Diarrhoea	<11years	RR†	0.21(0.08–0.53)‡
Haggerty et al, 1994	Hygiene education	Zaire (rural)	Poor	Diarrhoea	3–35 months	RR†	0.89(0.80–0.98)‡
Pinfold and Horan, 1996	Hygiene education	Thailand (rural)	Poor	Diarrhoea	0–60 months	RR†	0.61(0.37–1.00)‡
Shahid et al, 1996	Handwashing with soap	Bangladesh (periurban)	Good	Diarrhoea	All	IDR#	0.38(0.33–0.43)‡
					0–11 months	IDR#	0.39(0.29–0.54)
					12–23 months	IDR#	0.53(0.37–0.77)
					24–59 months	IDR#	0.44(0.34–0.59)
					5–9 years	IDR#	0.27(0.19–0.37)
					10–14 years	IDR#	0.28(0.16–0.49)
					> 15 years	IDR#	0.38(0.30–0.49)

Results of the meta-analyses: fixed-effect estimate of relative risk (RR) 0.75 (95% CI 0.72–0.78); heterogeneity p < 0.01; random-effects estimate of RR 0.63 (95% CI 0.52–0.77); Begg's test p = 0.19.

*For definition of quality see main text.

†Calculated.

‡Result used for the overall meta-analysis, which provided a pooled estimate of relative risk.

#IDR = Incidence Density Ratio (interpreted as RR but is the ratio of incidence density rates rather than incidence rates).

Summary

- A systematic review is a review of the methods and results of all individual studies designed to answer the same research question and that conform to a set of pre-agreed criteria.

- Systematic reviews can provide essential information for the early introduction of effective practice.

- It is important that reviews employ systematic methods in order to establish whether research findings are consistent and generalisable.

- The process of carrying out a systematic review comprises the following stages:

  (i) decide on the objectives of the review, which should be clear and explicit;

  (ii) define the inclusion and exclusion criteria, which should also be clear and explicit;

  (iii) identify relevant studies, by carrying out an effective and wide-ranging literature search that will minimise the likelihood of publication bias;

  (iv) assess the methodological quality of studies to be included in the review using independent assessors;

  (v) extract data using independent reviewers;

  (vi) present results from the review in the form of a descriptive summary of the selected studies in a table, with text commentary.

9.2 The methodology of meta-analysis

After investing a substantial amount of time and effort in conducting a careful and thorough systematic review the icing on the cake is to be able to combine the results from studies selected into the review quantitatively by a ***meta-analysis***. Meta-analysis is the name given to the statistical analysis of data from studies included in a systematic review.

The importance of this final step was illustrated in the previous example by Antman *et al.* (1992) in Section 9.1.1, where we saw that by conducting a meta-analysis demonstrated a statistically significant treatment effect for thrombolytic drugs would be demonstrated some 14 years prior to the drugs being used routinely.

9.2.1 Method of meta-analysis – overview

Essentially there are four main steps in carrying out a meta-analysis. These are:

- An assessment of publication bias using a funnel plot (or a statistical analogue of the funnel plot) to look for asymmetry.

- A statistical test for heterogeneity (difference) of the intervention effect between the selected studies.

- A pooled estimate (e.g. RR or OR) and 95% CI for the intervention effect after combining all the trials, the statistical approach used depending on whether or not statistical heterogeneity has been identified between the selected studies.

- An hypothesis test for whether the intervention effect is statistically significant or not.

We shall go on to discuss each of these steps in the remainder of this section.

9.2.2 The funnel plot

Graphical presentation

Funnel plots are used to identify whether a systematic review might have suffered from publication bias (or other bias) in the selection of studies for the review (see Section 9.1.5 for an overview of publication bias). If substantial publication bias is identified the results should not be pooled in a meta-analysis.

A funnel plot is a scatterplot showing the spread of results from studies selected for a review. Each point on the graph corresponds to one study and shows the relevant effect estimate (for example, an OR) and its precision (that is, how precisely it is estimated). The precision of the estimate is measured by its estimated standard error (SE), which depends on the variability in the study and the sample size: larger samples provide more precise estimates.

The examples illustrated in Figure 9.2.1(a) and (b), will clarify this and show why this type of graph is called a funnel plot. The plots show the estimated OR for each study on the x-axis, (with a vertical line through the value for no effect (OR = 1.0)), and its precision (1/SE) shown on a log scale on the y-axis. Moving up the scale (1/SE) on the y-axis, corresponds to a more precise estimate. In general larger studies will have smaller standard errors and hence provide more precise estimates with higher values on the y-axis. Ideally we are looking for a symmetrical

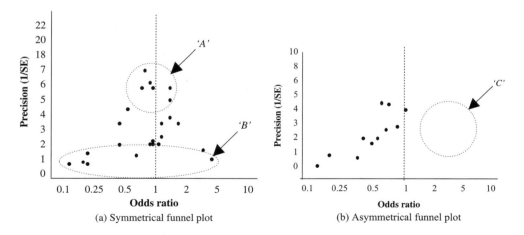

Figure 9.2.1 Funnel plots from 2 different systematic reviews

funnel plot illustrated in Figure 9.2.1(a). We will consider this first and then go on to look at an asymmetrical funnel plot illustrated in Figure 9.2.1(b), which is suggestive of publication bias.

In Figure 9.2.1(a), larger studies with greater precision (denoted by 'A') will have a narrow spread, whereas smaller studies (denoted by 'B') will scatter widely at the bottom of the graph due to the lack of power to estimate effects precisely. In the absence of bias, the plot will resemble a symmetrical inverted funnel because the large (precise) studies all have estimates fairly close to the true effect (OR a little below 1.0 in this example), while the less precise, smaller studies will have greater variability, but these should still be scattered symmetrically either side of the true effect. We can see that this is indeed the case, and there are more or less the same number of studies (whether large or small) scattered on either side of the true effect.

In Figure 9.2.1(b), we have an asymmetrical funnel plot because studies that have found against a beneficial treatment effect (that is, studies with an OR greater than 1.0 (denoted by the area of the plot labelled 'C') have not been included in the systematic review. We would expect a number of medium-sized and smaller studies to be in this area, to balance those on the side with ORs below 1.0. This is evidence of publication bias.

If the funnel plot is not symmetrical, as in Figure 9.2.1(b), we should not calculate an overall estimate from the combined studies. The asymmetry may be due to publication bias: for example, (i) studies demonstrating no effect or the 'opposite' effect have not been published and not been included in the review and/or (ii) small studies have not been published unless significant results or sizeable risks/ protective associations have been found and have not been included in the review. It should be noted that smaller studies are often conducted and analysed with less methodological rigour than larger studies. An asymmetrical funnel plot could therefore also be the result of exaggerated treatment effects of smaller studies of lower methodological quality.

Statistical methods for detecting funnel plot asymmetry

Statistical methods are commonly used to detect whether funnel plot asymmetry is present. This translates the graphical approach given by the funnel plot into a statistical model. The two main statistical approaches include a rank correlation method proposed by Begg and Mazumdar (1994) and a linear regression method proposed by Egger *et al.* (1997).

The rank correlation method examines the association between the effect estimates and their variances (or their standard errors), whereas the linear regression approach is equivalent to a weighted regression of effect estimate (for example, log OR) on its standard error, with weights inversely proportional to the study variance. Since both approaches look for an association between the study's treatment effect and its standard error, they can be seen as statistical analogues of funnel plots.

For both methods, evidence of possible publication bias (corresponding to an asymmetrical funnel plot) is indicated by a p-value of less than 0.05. However the sensitivity of both methods has been found to be low in meta-analyses based on less than 20 trials and this can result in evidence of publication bias being missed, a false-negative test result (type II error). For this reason a higher significance level (e.g. $p < 0.1$ or $p < 0.2$) is often taken to judge statistical significance. Of course, increasing the significance level causes a greater likelihood of detecting a false-positive result (type I error) – falsely identifying publication bias.

Please now read the following excerpt taken from the methods section of paper A, describing the approach used to carry out a meta-analysis. For now, concentrate on how the publication bias was assessed, and we will return to the issues of heterogeneity and random and fixed-effect models later in this section.

Methods

Meta-analysis

Risk estimates from the selected studies for each category of intervention were pooled in meta-analyses by use of STATA software (version 8; STATA Corporation, College Station, TX, USA). Random-effects models and fixed-effect models (which both use a form of inverse variance weighting) were generated for each analysis.[9] Random effects models were used to summarise the relative risk estimates if the test of heterogeneity for a group of study results was significant (defined conservatively as p < 0.20). In the absence of heterogeneity, fixed-effects models were used. Publication bias was explored through the use of Begg's test,[10] and a result with a p value less than 0.20 was defined, a priori, to indicate the possible presence of bias.

 Self-Assessment Exercise 9.2.1

1. What approach was used to ascertain whether publication bias might have occurred?

2. How do you think the authors' choice of a p-value of <0.2 would have affected their judgement of whether publication bias had occurred?

3. Refer back to Table 9.1.3 (Table 1 from paper A, in Section 9.1.7), and in particular the paragraph at the bottom of the table. Did the authors identify whether there was any publication bias in their review of hygiene interventions?

Answers in Section 9.5

9.2.3 Heterogeneity

By *heterogeneity* we mean 'not of the same type'. In the previous section on systematic reviews we discussed how studies with a similar design should be selected by set criteria. When deciding whether or not it is wise to carry out a meta-analysis, it is important (in addition to examining the funnel plot for symmetry) to assess the extent to which the actual results of the various studies differ. If these differ too much pooling the results is likely to be misleading since the studies might actually be measuring different effects. Thus, (statistical) *heterogeneity* of results across studies means that the estimates from individual studies have different magnitudes, or even different directions (e.g. some showing increased risk; others reduced risk).

Statistical heterogeneity may be caused by recognisable differences in treatment or subjects in a trial or by methodological differences, or it may be related to unknown or unrecorded trial characteristics. We can assess the heterogeneity of study estimates of effect by:

- Looking to see whether the 95% CIs for each of the studies included in a systematic review overlap. This can be ascertained by looking at individual study results on a *forest plot* (discussed in Section 9.2.5 – presentation of results).

- Carrying out a hypothesis test to assess whether there is evidence of statistically significant heterogeneity in the results of the studies. As we shall see, it is possible to use the **critical value** of the hypothesis test to quantify statistically the amount of heterogeneity between studies included in a meta-analysis.

The hypothesis test for assessing whether there is statistically significant heterogeneity between studies to be included in a meta-analysis is a version of the **chi-squared test** known as **Cochran's Q** (producing the **Q statistic**). The test examines whether the observed variability in effect sizes of included studies is within the range that can be expected if all the studies shared a common population effect size. Because the value of the Q statistic has a chi-squared distribution, results of meta-analyses frequently quote the value of the Q statistic from a test of heterogeneity as χ^2 (chi-squared).

A p-value for the Q statistic is frequently quoted as an indication of the extent of between-study variability. However, as with the statistical test for funnel plot asymmetry, the sensitivity of the Q statistic is low when only a few studies (e.g. $n < 20$) are included in the meta-analysis, so that the test could fail to detect even a moderate degree of heterogeneity. To compensate for this poor sensitivity, a higher significance level is usually taken (e.g. $p < 0.1$ or $p < 0.2$) for statistical significance. In most published meta-analyses the test for heterogeneity will be non-significant but this cannot be interpreted as direct evidence for **homogeneity** of all the results in the selected studies – we can never say that we accept the null hypothesis, but only that there is insufficient evidence to reject it.

It is, however, possible to quantify the amount of statistical heterogeneity between studies by using the Q statistic to calculate the *proportion of total variability between studies* explained by the heterogeneity, over that occurring by chance. This is done by calculating the I^2 *statistic* (calculated by the formula below):

$$I^2 = 100 \times \frac{Q - df}{Q}$$

In the formula, Q represents the Q statistic for the hypothesis test for heterogeneity and *df* (degrees of freedom) represents the number of studies minus 1 included in the meta-analysis. Negative values of the I^2 statistic (which will arise if the degrees of freedom are larger than the value of Q) are put to zero so that the I^2 statistic lies between 0 and 100 per cent. A value of 0 per cent indicates no observed heterogeneity and larger values show increasing heterogeneity. As a rule of thumb, low, moderate and high values of the I^2 statistic are assigned to 25, 50 and 75 per cent respectively to aid interpretation of the statistic.

To some extent we must decide for ourselves whether the differences between the studies described in the review are acceptable and of practical importance. The I^2 statistic will help us make this decision but we must also try to understand what methodological and other features of the studies have led to the observed heterogeneity. Not surprisingly there is often room for disagreement about whether results should be pooled.

Self-Assessment Exercise 9.2.2

1. Referring back to the previous excerpt describing the methods of meta-analysis of paper A (Section 9.2.2), how did the authors investigate whether there was statistical heterogeneity between the studies included in their meta-analysis?

2. Look again at the last paragraph of Table 9.1.3 (Table 1 of paper A) in Section 9.1.7. Did the authors identify significant heterogeneity between studies included in their meta-analysis of hygiene interventions?

Answers in Section 9.5

9.2.4   Calculating the pooled estimate

The quantitative summary of study results is generally considered the most important conclusion from a meta-analysis. The choice of method for calculating this pooled estimate will depend mainly on whether or not significant heterogeneity has been identified.

The fixed-effect model

If we are confident that the studies in our review are all providing similar estimates (that there is no significant heterogeneity between the studies), then we can calculate a common estimate from all the data. This is known as a *fixed-effect* meta-analysis. The summary measure used in a fixed-effect meta-analysis will depend on the outcome of interest, such as a RR, an OR or a difference in means.

The pooled estimate is essentially a summary measure of the results of the selected studies in the review. It is not simply an average, however, as different studies do not all provide information of equal value. It is therefore a *weighted* combination where the weight given to each study is related to the inverse of the variability within the study. This means that more account is taken of the more precise studies (larger sample sizes, more information) than the studies with low precision (smaller samples, less information).

There are a number of different methods for calculating a pooled estimate by a fixed-effect model. Specific details are not given here and are beyond the scope of this book, but methods you may commonly see referred to are the *Mantel–Haenszel*, *Peto* and *general inverse variance-weighted* methods.

The random-effects model

If we suspect that there is moderate or substantial heterogeneity between the studies an alternative approach is required to obtain a pooled effect estimate. This alternative is the *random-effects* meta-analysis. This approach assumes a different underlying effect for each study included in the meta-analysis and takes this into consideration as an additional source of variation. Effects are assumed to be randomly distributed, and the central point of this distribution is the focus of the combined effect estimate. In other words, the effects for the individual studies are assumed to vary around some overall average effect.

Under the random-effects model, individual effect sizes are assumed to have a normal distribution with mean and variance (this variance is denoted by the Greek letter τ^2, pronounced 'tor' – squared). This variance (τ^2) is taken into account when weighting each individual study, with the result that weights are smaller and more similar to each other than the weights in fixed-effect models that are based on the sample sizes of the individual studies. This means that random-effects meta-analyses will be more conservative (the CIs will be wider) than fixed-effect meta-analysis. It also means that random-effects models give relatively more weight to smaller studies than the fixed-effect model.

The most commonly used approach for conducting a random-effects meta-analysis is the method of *DerSimonian and Laird* (1986). Again specific details of this approach are beyond the scope of this book.

If we identify significant heterogeneity between studies selected for a meta-analysis we should always exercise caution before using random-effects models. Quite often the heterogeneity between studies is overlooked when using a random-effects model. In fact, rather than ignoring heterogeneity, we should look carefully at what the heterogeneity is and explore possible reasons as to why it has occured.

Please now read the following excerpt from the results section of paper A, describing the meta-analysis of hygiene interventions.

Results

Hygiene
Although the studies show a wide range of effectiveness, the summary meta-analysis suggests that hygiene interventions act to reduce diarrhoeal illness levels (random-effects model pooled estimate of relative risk 0.63, 95 per cent CI 0.52–0.77), although there is some evidence of publication bias (Begg's test p<0.20). Reanalysis of the data after exclusion of studies thought to be of poor quality resulted in a pooled estimate of the relative risk of 0.55 (95% CI 0.40–0.75).[12,20–22]

 Self-Assessment Exercise 9.2.3

1. Referring to the text excerpt above and the last paragraph of Table 1 of paper A (Section 9.1.7), what method of pooling the study results was used for the analysis of the hygiene interventions? Why was this approach adopted?

2. What did the authors' main meta-analysis for the hygiene interventions reveal?

Answers in Section 9.5

9.2.5   Presentation of results: forest plot

As we saw in Table 9.1.3 (Table 1 of paper A) for the hygiene interventions, the results of a meta-analysis can be displayed in tables showing the results for each individual study, the pooled summary estimate and CI, and the results of the tests for heterogeneity and publication bias.

The estimates and CIs for each study and the pooled results should also be illustrated pictorially in a ***forest plot***. Figure 9.2.2 (Figure 2 from paper A) is a forest plot illustrating the results of the meta-analysis of studies investigating the effect of household treatment water quality interventions on diarrhoea. We will now look in more detail at the information provided, and how this should be interpreted.

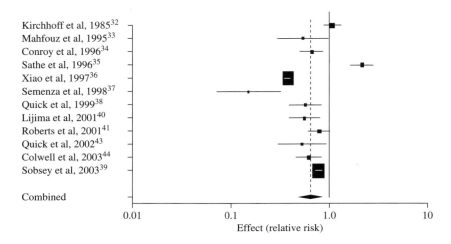

Figure 9.2.2   Random-effect meta-analysis of household treatment water quality interventions (Figure 2 from paper A)

Interpretation of a forest plot

The vertical solid line represents no difference between the two groups, as, for example, when the relative risk equals one. Each rectangle represents the results of one trial in terms of its effect estimate, the rectangle having an area which reflects the weighting given to each study. The horizontal line through each of the rectangles is the CI for each effect estimate (note that for the two largest studies by Xiao *et al.* and Sobsey *et al.*, the 95 per cent CI is shown within the borders of each study rectangle). Estimates to the left of the vertical solid line are indicative of a treatment or protective effect with (in this case), a relative risk (RR) of less than 1.0. Estimates to the right of the vertical line represent results that are associated with an increase in risk (RR > 1).

The final result illustrated with a diamond shape illustrates the combined result. The central points of the diamond indicate the pooled estimate and the lateral points the 95 per cent CI around that estimate. In the figure, the dashed vertical line aids location of the pooled estimate relative to the individual study estimates. The combined result generally has a narrow CI relative to any one study (although in a random-effects meta-analysis the confidence interval for the pooled estimate might be wider than for large individual studies that are not weighted in their contribution to the pooled estimate, as in Figure 9.2.2), indicating the increased power of the combined analysis and is usually placed at the bottom of the forest plot.

Figure 9.2.2 illustrates well the presentation of results for a random-effects model. We can see that the 95% CIs for the studies conducted by Sathe *et al.* (1996) and Semenza *et al.* (1998) do not overlap with the other studies included in the meta-analysis. This is visual confirmation that the results of studies included in this meta-analysis are heterogeneous. All of the studies, except the outlier conducted by Sathe *et al.* (1996), are consistent with a protective effect of the household treatment water quality interventions. The pooled result (diamond) indicates a statistically significant protective effect for the interventions.

9.2.6 Sensitivity analysis

A final stage in carrying out a meta-analysis is to investigate how sensitive the results of the meta-analysis are to the inclusion of studies of differing size, quality and other specified method-ological differences. This is known as *sensitivity analysis*. A sensitivity analysis can involve repeating the analysis on *subsets* of the original data as well as determining how any one study (or group of studies with similar attributes) might influence the overall summary statistics. One very large study might have a profound, and perhaps misleading (if the study has methodolog-ical problems), influence on the overall result. Sensitivity analysis can provide insight into the individual study factors that can affect the results and that will be important to consider in future studies.

We saw earlier how poor methodological quality can distort the findings of a meta-analysis (Table 9.1.2), and assessment of the influence of methodological quality on pooled estimates should be considered an integral part of the process. Sensitivity analysis can be conducted on separate aspects of study quality, as we saw in Table 9.1.2. It is also possible to carry out an analysis to study the effects of multiple aspects of quality on treatment effects, for example, by using a composite quality score, although the methods for this are beyond the scope of this book.

Let us now return to how methodological quality and the impact on the meta-analysis were assessed in the water and sanitation review. Please now read the following excerpt taken from the discussion section of paper A, which considers the quality of studies included in the review.

Discussion

In general, estimates calculated after the removal of poor quality studies from the meta-analyses indicated a stronger effect of the intervention. Although some of the studies identified in this review pre-dated the methodological critiques provided by Blum and Feachem[6] and Esrey and Habicht,[4] poorly done or poorly reported studies still make up a substantial part of the literature with 32% (12 of 38) of the identified studies classified as poor, with 50% (six of 12) of these being published after 1990. In addition to the studies classified as being of poor quality, data could not be extracted from 17% (eight from 46) of the studies identified. It seems clear that this research agenda would benefit from further guidance in terms of issues to be examined, reiteration of quality considerations, and guidelines in terms of reporting and presentation of results.

Self-Assessment Exercise 9.2.4

According to the excerpt from the discussion (above) and the previous excerpt describing the results of paper A (Section 9.2.4):

1. How did the authors address the possible influence of methodological quality on pooled estimates derived from meta-analyses?

2. Was there evidence that methodological quality had influenced the pooled estimates?

Answers in Section 9.5

9.2.7 Value of meta-analysis – an important historical example

The following example is taken from a 1998 paper on the treatment of critically injured patients and contains a salutary lesson on the value of meta-analysis (Cochrane Injuries Group Albumin Reviewers, 1998). This is a systematic review of randomised trials comparing the administration of albumin with no albumin in critically ill patients. Patients in the studies had one of three types of problem following severe injury: (i) hypovolaemia (reduced blood volume); (ii) burns, and (iii) hypoalbuminaemia (reduced blood albumin level). The outcome measure was mortality from all causes. Thirty-two trials met the criteria for inclusion in the review. Deaths occurred in 24 of the studies, and a meta-analysis of these studies was carried out. A funnel plot of the results of the included studies is shown in Figure 9.2.3, and Exercise 9.2.2 provides an opportunity to interpret this.

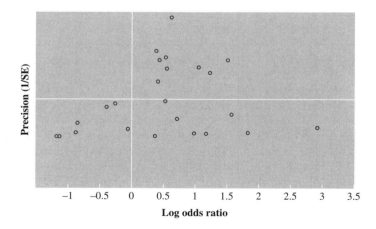

Figure 9.2.3 Funnel plot of the 24 trials in which deaths occurred (*Br Med J* (1998) **517**, 235–240)

Self-Assessment Exercise 9.2.5

Describe the appearance of the funnel plot in Figure 9.2.3. What are the likely implications of this pattern for publication bias?

Answers in Section 9.5

Figure 9.2.4 shows how the results of the meta-analysis are presented in a forest plot. The results from each trial are presented separately, grouped according to type of injury. For example, the first trial is by Lowe *et al.* (1977), and the results were as follows:

	Deaths	Survivals	Total
Albumin	3	54	57
Control	3	81	84
Total	6	135	141

The estimated relative risk (RR) of death for those given albumin compared with controls is

$$RR = \frac{3/57}{3/84} = 1.47$$

and the 95 per cent CI is (0.31, 7.05). This interval is very wide and includes 1, corresponding to no treatment effect.

We saw that, in a forest plot, the square shows the estimated treatment effect (i.e. the relative risk) for each trial, the horizontal line through the square is the 95 per cent CI, and the area of each square represents the amount of information (number of subjects) contributed by that trial to the pooled estimate. The solid diamonds are pooled estimates. There is one for each subgroup and an overall estimate for all types of injury, labelled 'total'. As we identified previously, the centre points of each diamond indicate the pooled estimate of the relative risk and the lateral points of the diamond show the 95% CI. The following exercise is based on this example and will help consolidate your understanding of meta-analysis including the interpretation of the forest plot.

 Self-Assessment Exercise 9.2.6

1. In the forest plot (Figure 9.2.4), do any of the 95 per cent CIs for individual studies not overlap? If so, which studies? What do you conclude from this?

2. The chi-squared statistics at the bottom of each section of the forest plot (below the 'subtotal' lines, and for the whole set of studies (below 'total') are derived from the Cochran's Q test for heterogeneity. P-values are not given, but the values (with the stated degrees of freedom) all have a p-value of > 0.1. What do you conclude from this? Are your conclusions consistent with those you arrived at from looking at the 95% CIs (question 1)?

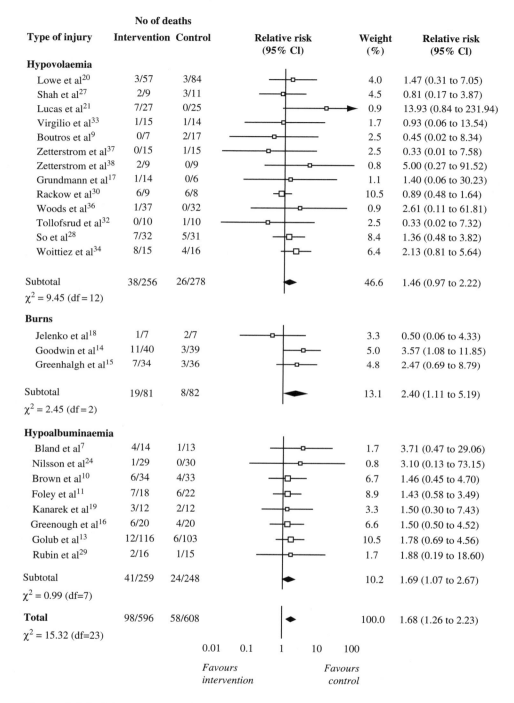

Figure 9.2.4 Meta-analysis of relative risk of death associated with intervention (albumin) compared with control (no albumin) in critically ill patients (*Br Med J* 1998; **517**, 235–240)

3. The amount of heterogeneity can be estimated with the I^2 statistic, which was described in Section 9.2.3. Calculate this statistic from the information on the test for overall heterogeneity (Q = 15.32, df=23), and interpret the result.

4. Given the findings so far, what type of statistical model should be used for meta-analysis?

5. Interpret the pooled estimates for (i) hypovolaemia, (ii) burns, and (iii) total. What do you conclude?

Answers in Section 9.5

Unfortunately a *sensitivity analysis* was not conducted as part of this meta-analysis, so it is not possible to investigate how different aspects of study quality might have influenced the pooled estimate.

Conclusion – albumin administration was increasing the risk of death

The clinical implications from this review bear some emphasis. The meta-analysis found that the administration of albumin in critically ill patients leads to a significant increase in mortality, not identified in any single previous study. It is likely that albumin had been given routinely to patients for some time prior to this meta-analysis and that earlier recognition of the harmful effects of albumin administration might have avoided unnecessary deaths.

Summary: meta-analysis

- A meta-analysis is the statistical analysis of the data from studies included in a systematic review.

- It is an efficient way of analysing and interpreting the results from many studies.

- The main steps and techniques of a meta-analysis are as follows:

  1. carry out and review a funnel plot and/or statistically assess whether there is funnel plot asymmetry;

  2. carry out and review tests of heterogeneity (Cochran's Q-statistic and I^2 statistic);

  3. if there is no significant heterogeneity, derive a pooled estimate and the 95% CI with a fixed-effect meta-analysis;

  4. if there is significant heterogeneity, derive a pooled estimate and 95% CI using a random-effects meta-analysis, but an attempt should be made to explain any heterogeneity);

  5. present the results in the conventional format, namely the forest plot;

  6. carry out a sensitivity analysis to investigate the effects of study quality and/or different characteristics of interventions or risk factors being studied.

(Continued)

- Meta-analyses help to formulate hypotheses for future work.

- Meta-analyses help to derive consensus for clinical treatments and other interventions.

9.3   Systematic reviews and meta-analyses of observational studies

9.3.1   Introduction

Traditionally systematic review and meta-analysis methodology has been concerned with RCTs of, typically, medical interventions. However of growing importance and becoming increasingly more common are systematic reviews and meta-analyses of observational studies. In fact, it has been suggested that as many as 40 per cent of published meta-analyses now concern systematic reviews of observational study designs (Egger *et al.*, 2003).

9.3.2   Why conduct a systematic review of observational studies?

As we have seen in previous chapters, there are many research questions for which randomised intervention studies would be inappropriate. For example, we saw how a cohort study design was utilised to investigate the protective effect of vigorous physical activity in relation to cancer (Chapter 5). We also saw how a case-control study design was adopted to investigate caffeine as a risk factor for spontaneous abortion (Chapter 6). Clearly, for both of these research questions, and for many others, trials would be at best difficult and in most cases impractical and / or unethical.

   For these other research questions and potential health interventions, systematic review and meta-analysis methods can offer the same benefits as we have seen for data derived from intervention studies, by summarising all of the available evidence and increasing the statistical power by pooling estimates from multiple studies. In principle, these methods can be applied to observational studies, but there are important issues arising from key differences in study design that we need to take into account.

9.3.3   Approach to meta-analysis of observational studies

Observational studies of risk factors and potential interventions often investigate relationships with relatively small underlying risks and will, not uncommonly, report conflicting results. It is therefore very desirable to combine the results of such studies statistically, using meta-analysis, with the intention of obtaining more precise and definitive answers. However extra care needs to be taken when combining the results of observational studies in this way due to methodological problems inherent in this type of study design.

   As we saw in earlier chapters, observational study designs are susceptible to both *bias* (particularly associated with case-control studies, although bias can also affect trials) and *confounding*, which exclusively affects non-randomised studies. Although good study design and appropriate analysis can reduce these problems in observational studies, we need to be aware that it is generally difficult to avoid them altogether. This is particularly the case with confounding, and even after careful design (e.g. matching) and thorough adjustment in analysis, there may well be some *residual confounding*.

   We should keep in mind that meta-analyses are carried out with the assumption that the studies being combined to produce the pooled effect estimate are free from bias and confounding and that any differences between the results of the studies are due to random variation (essentially sampling error, and the effects of differing sample sizes). Bias and confounding result in effect estimates that may deviate from the true underlying relationships beyond the effects of chance. Thus, a meta-analysis incorporating biased studies or studies suffering from residual confounding will lead to an incorrect effect estimate. Furthermore, if this pooled estimate is based on a reasonable number of studies of moderate size, it will appear to be precise with relatively narrow CIs. This precision may lead to unjustified confidence in the result, and in turn lead to misleading conclusions and potentially inappropriate decisions about health care or prevention policy. Reinforcement of a biased result in this way will be more likely if most or all of the studies on a given issue are biased in the same direction due to common difficulties in avoiding such bias; for example, if a similar set of confounders exists that are difficult to avoid and fully adjust for.

An example of this is given by Egger *et al.* (2003), who carried out a meta-analysis of cohort studies that had investigated the association between cigarette smoking and suicide. By pooling the studies they found a significant *dose-response* relationship between the number of cigarettes smoked and the risk of suicide (Table 9.3.1); the more cigarettes smoked the greater was the risk of suicide.

Table 9.3.1 Relationship between daily cigarette consumption and suicide: pooled relative risk based on four cohort studies (Egger *et al.*, 2003)

Cigarette consumption	Relative risk	95% CI
Non–smokers	1.00	
1–14 cigarettes	1.43	1.06–1.93
15–24 cigarettes	1.88	1.53–2.32
25 or more cigarettes	2.18	1.82–2.61

A causal relationship between smoking and suicide was considered improbable and it is likely that the social and mental states that make an individual susceptible to suicide are also related to smoking behaviour; such factors confound the relationship between smoking and suicide. The authors pointed out that, even though the cohort studies had adjusted for a number of known confounders, residual confounding of factors that cannot be precisely measured is likely to have occurred. This is unfortunately often the case for observational epidemiological studies of complex social and environmental issues.

This cautious introduction and the example from Eggar *et al.* might lead us to question whether we should ever carry out a meta-analysis of observational studies. However there are still important benefits in summarising the evidence from a systematic review with a pooled quantitative estimate of effect, so long as this is done carefully. We will now look in more detail at these requirements.

9.3.4   Method of systematic review of observational studies

The methods of conducting a systematic review of observational studies are in many respects the same as described for trials in Sections 9.1 and 9.2. The key differences in approach and emphasis are summarised in Table 9.3.2.

The most important additional considerations for a systematic review of observational studies relates to the assessment of methodological design issues, specifically in relation to bias and

Table 9.3.2   Stages of a systematic review: intervention studies versus observational studies

Review stage	Section described for intervention studies	Particular issues to consider when considering review for observational studies
1. Decide on the objectives of the review	Section 9.1.3	Same process.
2. Define inclusion/ exclusion criteria for studies	Section 9.1.4	Same process, but should detail types of observational studies to be included in the review (e.g. cohort, case-control, cross-sectional, etc.).
3. Search the literature (published/ unpublished)	Section 9.1.5	Same process. Cochrane Controlled Trials Register (CCTR) not relevant.
4. Assess methodological quality	Section 9.1.6	Some elements are the same (e.g. sampling, measurement, how well bias has been minimised etc.). In addition, it is important to assess how well and confounding has been dealt with at the design stage, or adjusted for in analysis. Composite quality assessment scales are available, tailored to individual observational designs (e.g. Newcastle-Ottawa Scale).
5. Extract data from studies for the review	Section 9.1.7	Same process. The data extraction sheet should include information about study design (and features of the design) together with details of all confounders measured, matched (if relevant) and adjusted for.
6. Describe/ present results from the review	Section 9.1.7	Same process. Summary table should be presented by study design (if more than one observational study design is included). Quality scores should be indicated according to scale used.

confounding. For this reason, it is necessary to provide detailed information about the types of study design selected for review. We must also consider methodological issues of quality relevant to each type of study design. For example, both cohort studies and case-control studies are susceptible to confounding; however, due to the typically retrospective nature of the collection of exposure data, case-control studies tend to be more susceptible to bias. Pre-established quality assessment instruments, such as the Newcastle-Ottawa scale, have separate scales for the different study designs assessing quality based on pertinent design features for each type of observational study.

9.3.5   Method of meta-analysis of observational studies

The stages in conducting a meta-analysis of observational studies are also much the same as for trials, with the main differences again relating to the methodological limitations of observational studies. The key issues are described in Table 9.3.3.

The most important additional issues for a meta-analysis of observational studies relates to the consideration of possible sources of heterogeneity between observational study results, particularly where it is planned to use a random-effects model. Sensitivity analyses must be conducted to

Table 9.3.3 Stages of a systematic review: intervention studies versus observational studies

Review stage	Section described for intervention studies	Issues to consider when considering review for observational studies
1. Check for funnel plot asymmetry as an indicator of publication bias.	Section 9.2.2	Same process.
2. Carry out and interpret a test for heterogeneity (Q-statistic and I^2 statistic).	Section 9.2.3	Same process. Heterogeneity is especially important for observational studies for reasons given in Section 9.3.3.
3. Calculate a pooled effect estimate using fixed-effect or random-effects meta-analysis.	Section 9.2.4	Same process, but paying particular attention to explaining heterogeneity if using a random-effects meta-analysis.
4. Present results (individual studies and pooled estimate) in a forest plot.	Section 9.2.5	Same process. The forest plot should present results separately for the different study designs included in the meta-analysis. Interpretation of the overall pooled result should be treated with caution.
5. Carry out a sensitivity analysis to investigate the influence of study attributes on effect estimate.	Section 9.2.6	Sensitivity analyses based on aspects of methodological quality is especially important for a meta-analysis of observational studies.

investigate the influence that aspects of methodological quality, especially in relation to bias and confounding, have on the effect estimate derived from the meta-analysis.

A good example of the importance of carrying out such a sensitivity analysis is given by Egger *et al.* (2003). They looked at how differential recall of past exposures could introduce bias in case-control studies included in a meta-analysis. A meta-analysis conducted by Nelemans *et al.* (1995) investigated the relationship between intermittent exposure to sunlight and risk of melanoma. The authors collected information on whether or not researchers had blinded the study participants of case-control studies included in the meta-analysis by hiding the study hypothesis from them. A sensitivity analysis based on whether or not the study participants had been blinded revealed a significant difference between the two groups of studies in terms of the pooled effect estimate ($p < 0.001$). For studies that had not blinded study participants, the pooled effect estimate indicated a significant increase in risk of melanoma from intermittent exposure to sunlight of 84 per cent (OR = 1.84, 95% CI = 1.52–2.25). However for studies that had incorporated some blinding of the study hypothesis, the increase in melanoma risk was more modest (OR = 1.17, 95% CI = 0.98–1.39, with the lack of statistical significance being in part due to the small number of studies that used blinding ($n=7$)). The overall pooled OR for the increased risk of melanoma from intermittent exposure to sunlight was calculated as 1.57 (95% CI = 1.29–1.91).

Summary: systematic reviews and meta-analysis of observational studies

- Systematic reviews of observational studies are important as these provide a means of synthesising information about aetiological hypotheses, and interventions that cannot be tested by a trial design for ethical and/or practical reasons.

- A meta-analysis based on a systematic review of observational studies provides a useful summary of the evidence from the review as a pooled effect estimate.

- Caution should be exercised in both the conduct and interpretation of meta-analyses as observational studies are generally more susceptible than intervention studies to bias and in particular to residual confounding.

- The methods of a systematic review of observational studies require additional information to be collected about methodological quality in terms of bias and confounding.

- The methods of a meta-analysis of observational studies require additional attention to explaining heterogeneity where this exists and to sensitivity analysis to investigate the impact of methodological differences between studies. Sensitivity analysis should pay particular attention to possible effects of bias, confounding and type of study design.

9.4 The Cochrane Collaboration

9.4.1 Introduction

In 1979 Archie Cochrane, a British epidemiologist, wrote:

It is surely a great criticism of our profession that we have not organised a critical summary, by specialty or subspecialty, adapted periodically, of all relevant randomised controlled trials. (Cochrane, 1979)

He recognised that people who wanted to make more informed decisions about health care did not have ready access to reliable reviews of the available evidence. He had already suggested the establishment of a central international register of clinical trials in an earlier book, *Effectiveness and Efficiency*, published in 1972, which caused little reaction at the time. Unfortunately he never lived to see his vision realised. Neither did he see the creation of the central register he had proposed become a reality in the form of the ***Cochrane Controlled Trials Register***, which was set up some years later (see below).

Shortly before his death in 1988, Cochrane referred to a systematic review of RCTs of care during pregnancy and childbirth as 'a real milestone in the history of randomised trials and in the evaluation of care', and suggested that other specialities copy the methods used. The NHS Research and Development Programme took this up and funds were provided to establish the ***UK Cochrane Centre*** which opened in Oxford in 1992. From the outset it was hoped that an international response might be established and a year later at a meeting in Oxford in 1993, 77 people from nine countries co-founded the *Cochrane Collaboration*. At the time of writing there were 15 Cochrane Centres around the world.

9.4.2 Cochrane Collaboration logo

The adopted logo of the Collaboration is the forest plot of the results of systematic review referred to by Cochrane in 1988 of care during pregnancy and childbirth. Only two trials showed statistically significant effects, but the pooled data from all seven studies strongly indicated that corticosteroids reduced the risk of babies dying from the complications of immaturity. The treatment was shown to reduce the odds of the babies dying by 30–50 per cent. No systematic review of these trials was published until 1989 and so most clinicians had not realised that the treatment was so effective.

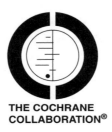

THE COCHRANE
COLLABORATION®

9.4.3 Collaborative Review Groups

The Cochrane Collaboration is an international organisation, consisting of a network of individuals and institutions, which aims to help people make well-informed decisions about health care and policy by preparing, maintaining and ensuring the accessibility of systematic reviews of the effects of health interventions.

It is organised around *collaborative review groups*, each of which focuses on a particular health problem. Each group uses methods designed to minimise bias, to identify relevant trials, and to prepare and maintain reviews that are then published on the *Cochrane Database of Systematic Reviews*. At the time of writing there were over 40 review groups, which covered most of the important areas of health. Each group has a coordinating editor and a supporting editorial team.

The many achievements of the Collaboration in such a short space of time reflect the goodwill and efforts of the individuals who contribute their time and effort, often without specific funding to do so. The organisations that do provide support tend to be public institutions such as government agencies and universities.

9.4.4 Cochrane Library

The Cochrane library consists of several databases together with a handbook on the science of reviewing research, a glossary of methodological terms and Cochrane terminology and contact details for review groups and other groupings in the Collaboration. The databases are listed below.

Cochrane Database of Systematic Reviews

Reviewers contribute their completed reviews and protocols to this database. Each review consists of a cover sheet giving details of the title, authors etc.; an abstract; a structured report of the review; discussion of the results; implications for research and practice; and a citation list and summary table of the studies included in the review, together with details of any eligible studies which were excluded, and tables of results.

Cochrane Controlled Trials Register (CCTR)

This was introduced in Section 9.2 and is a bibliographic database of all controlled trials identified by contributors to the Collaboration as part of the international effort to search systematically the world's health-care journals and other sources of information to create an unbiased data source for systematic reviews.

Database of Abstracts of Reviews of Effectiveness (DARE)

DARE includes structured abstracts of systematic reviews which have been critically appraised by reviewers at the NHS Centre for Reviews and Dissemination in York (UK) and by others, such as members of the American College of Physicians' Journal Club and the journal *Evidence-Based Medicine*.

Cochrane Methodology Register (CMR)

This is a bibliography of articles on the science of research synthesis.

NHS Economic Evaluation Database (EED)

This is a bibliography of published economic evaluations of health-care interventions.

The entire Cochrane library is available on CD-ROM. It can also be found on the National Electronic Libraries for Health (NELH) website (www.nelh.nhs.uk/).

The Collaboration has also developed software to assist in preparing and maintaining reviews, called *Review Manager* (**RevMan**). This allows entry of the review protocol, text commentary, characteristics of studies, comparison table, and study data. It can then be used to carry out all stages of the review, including meta-analysis and to present the results graphically as forest plots. RevMan is developed through a continuing process of consultation with its users. The software can be obtained (free of charge) at the Cochrane Collaboration's Information Management System (IMS) site: www.cc-ims.net.

9.5 Answers to self-assessment exercises

Section 9.1

Exercise 9.1.1

1. The objectives of the study are not clearly described, although the authors do state that the paper presents a systematic review of all published studies and a meta-analysis (where appropriate) looking at interventions in water quality, water supply, hygiene and sanitation in less developed countries. The meta-analyses were designed to identify the relative evidence of the effectiveness of these interventions in relation to diarrhoeal disease.

2. Yes, we are given a clear account of the populations to be studied, the interventions and the outcome to be investigated. The study population is described as incorporating 'less developed countries'. This is further defined as 'any country not within a class A region under the WHO comparative risk assessment' identified as not having very low mortality rates in both adults and children. The interventions are identified as those involving water quality, water supply, hygiene and sanitation, planned or occurring as natural experiments. The outcome is 'diarrhoeal disease occurring in non-outbreak conditions'.

3. The authors mention that they will consider 'all published studies' involving interventions, including meta-analyses if available, for inclusion in their review. This, as we shall see when we consider the implications of publication bias, might not have been the most appropriate choice for sourcing all relevant data.

Exercise 9.1.2

There were two selection criteria. First, the studies were required to have described a specific water, sanitation or hygiene intervention (or combination of these interventions). Second, studies had to report diarrhoea morbidity as a health outcome, measured under endemic (non-outbreak) conditions. Also, as mentioned previously, the authors required the studies to have been published 'to maintain quality (via peer review) and transparency'. We will return to this when we consider publication bias in Section 9.1.5. The authors state that 'no studies were excluded from the review on the basis of quality criteria alone'. They therefore included studies of recognised 'poor' quality. This, as we shall see, has potentially important implications for the results of a meta-analysis.

Exercise 9.1.3

1. The authors state that only published studies were included in the review because this ensured quality via peer review and transparency.

2. There is no guarantee that studies published in peer-reviewed journals are of good quality; as we saw above, published studies identified as 'poor quality' were still included in this systematic review. On the other hand, many studies of sufficient or 'good' methodological quality are not published in peer-reviewed journals. For example studies with non-significant or contradictory findings might be rejected for publication or not even put forward for publication.

Exercise 9.1.4

1. The authors searched the main English language databases (including Medline and EMBASE and the Cochrane Central Register of Controlled Trials). In addition they utilised foreign

language journal databases (LILACS and Pascal Biomed). Hand searching the extracted journal articles for further references is also described.

2. The search is fairly comprehensive and should identify most relevant published articles. However, there is no indication that the authors searched the grey literature to identify unpublished studies and ongoing relevant research. Although 'author-based' searches were carried out to identify subsequent work by the primary investigators, we are not told whether they were contacted directly to obtain more information.

Exercise 9.1.5

1. Previously established criteria were used to examine the quality of studies in the review (Blum and Feachem). However, details of these criteria and the procedure used to describe the quality of the studies, including the number of reviewers, are not given in the paper, but it is referenced so you can look it up. Poor quality studies were identified as having any of the following design flaws: inadequately defined control groups, no clear measurement or control of confounding factors, no specific definition of diarrhoea or the particular diarrhoeal health outcome being used, and a health indicator recall period of more than 2 weeks.

2. While an attempt was made by the authors to assess the methodological quality of studies selected for the review, they stated that 'no study was excluded from the review or meta-analysis on the basis of quality criteria alone'. They indicated that, where possible, they would examine issues of study quality as 'a source of possible heterogeneity between results (variation between studies)'. We will discuss the assessment of heterogeneity and sensitivity analysis, when we look at meta-analysis, so we will return to the question of how the authors dealt with poor-quality studies in Section 9.2.

Exercise 9.1.6

1. Two types of hygiene intervention were identified, those relating to hygiene / health education, (6 studies) and those relating to hand washing, usually in combination with hygiene education, (5 studies). This education varied between studies. Education on hygiene was aimed at the mothers, although the health outcome was measured in the children.

2. The information for each study was tabulated by intervention, country, study quality, health outcome, age group, effect estimate used and 95 per cent CI. It is relatively straightforward to compare descriptors of the individual findings for each study from such a summary table.

Section 9.2

Exercise 9.2.1

1. Publication bias was explored through the use of Begg's test, and a result with a p-value less than 0.2 was defined, a priori, to indicate the possible presence of bias.

2. Begg's test has a rather low sensitivity for meta-analyses based on fewer than 20 trials so typically a more conservative p-value of < 0.1 is used as opposed to the < 0.05 level commonly used for most statistical tests. In this study the authors chose a p-value of < 0.2: it is likely that they were erring on the side of caution in choosing this conservative cut-off for statistical significance, as they could be fairly certain that publication bias had not occurred if $p > 0.2$.

3. The subanalysis on hygiene interventions did indicate the presence of publication bias, since the Begg's test p-value was 0.19 (< 0.2). However, interpretation of this result is not straightforward, as we need to consider (i) the generally low sensitivity of the test, (ii) the fact that this subanalysis was based on 13 studies (relatively few), and (iii) that the p-value is very close to the very conservative cut-off for statistical significance the authors used ($p < 0.2$). A cautious interpretation would be to suspect that some publication bias does exist.

Exercise 9.2.2

1. They carried out a test for heterogeneity (although the Cochran's Q statistic has not been specified), setting the p-value for statistical significance to $p<0.2$, again a conservative estimate to allow for the low power of the test. The authors did not attempt to quantify the statistical heterogeneity between studies (using the I^2 statistic).

2. Yes: the subanalyses for hygiene interventions recorded a p-value of < 0.01.

Exercise 9.2.3

1. While the authors present results from both fixed-effect and random-effects models at the bottom of Table 9.1.3 (Table 1 from paper A), the pooled relative risk for the random-effects model is more appropriate; from the footnote on Table 9.1.3 we can see there was evidence of significant heterogeneity between the studies ($p < 0.01$).

2. The pooled estimate of the relative risk by the random-effects model was 0.63 (95% CI 0.52 to 0.77), indicating a significant reduction in risk of diarrhoea by hygiene interventions (the intervention group were 37 per cent less likely to experience diarrhoea, with a 95 per cent CI of 23 to 48 per cent lower risk of diarrhoea). However, any conclusions should be treated with caution, because of the tentative evidence of publication bias (Begg's test, $p < 0.20$), discussed in Exercise 9.2.1. The implication might be that unpublished studies finding no effect or an opposite effect were not found and hence not included in the analysis. The authors also state that they carried out a 'reanalysis of the data after exclusion of studies thought to be of poor quality'. This is sensitivity analysis and is discussed in more detail in Section 9.2.6.

Exercise 9.2.4

1. While the authors do not actually state that they carried out a sensitivity analysis based on the methodological quality of the studies included in their systematic review, they do attempt to see how excluding studies of poor quality affects pooled estimates of the relative risk for the separate interventions.

2. For hygiene interventions, removal of the poor-quality studies led to a 13 per cent increase in the observed treatment effect, with the relative risk reduced to 0.55, compared with the 0.63 observed when all studies were included. Inclusion of poor-quality studies in the meta-analysis appears to dilute the effect of the hygiene interventions on reducing diarrhoea risk.

Exercise 9.2.5

The funnel plot shows the desired symmetric shape and this is consistent with no or minimal publication bias.

Exercise 9.2.6

1. All of the 95 per cent CIs overlap suggesting no heterogeneity.

2. As the p-values are all > 0.1 we can conclude that there is minimal heterogeneity particularly for the overall test since, given the relatively large number of studies, the test will have good sensitivity at this level of significance ($p=0.1$). This conclusion is consistent with our observation from the 95% CIs in question 1.

3. The value of the I^2 statistic is -50.13, which (see Section 9.2.3) is set to zero. This value of the statistic is interpreted as showing no heterogeneity.

4. Given the results so far it is reasonable to use a fixed-effect model.

5. For hypovolaemia the pooled $RR = 1.46$ (95% CI: 0.97, 2.22) indicating a 46 per cent increase in risk, the increased risk is not quite statistically significant with a lower 95% CI just under 1.0. For burns, the pooled $RR = 2.40$ (95% CI: 1.11, 5.19), indicating almost a $2\frac{1}{2}$ fold increase in risk and, despite the wide 95% CI, this increase in risk is statistically significant. Overall, the total pooled $RR = 1.68$ (95% CI: 1.26, 2.23), indicating a 68 per cent increase in risk, a result that is clearly significant.

10

Prevention strategies and evaluation of screening

Introduction and learning objectives

Introduction

In this chapter we will look at the application of some important epidemiological concepts to prevention strategies, including screening programmes. We begin by exploring concepts of risk and the implications of these for strategies of prevention. We then look at how screening programmes are evaluated, the commonly used measures of validity of screening tests and the particular types of bias that arise in epidemiological studies of the effectiveness of screening. Finally, we examine how variations in patterns of mortality rates according to when people are born, or when they die, so-called cohort and period effects, can provide important information on disease causation. Although we will introduce some new ideas and terminology, this material mainly builds on ideas discussed in previous chapters.

Learning objectives

By the end of this chapter you should be able to:

- Define and compare, with examples, relative risk (RR) and attributable risk (AR).

- Calculate attributable risk (you are already familiar with calculation of RR).

- Describe what is meant by population attributable risk (PAR).

- Describe, with examples, the epidemiological background to high-risk and population approaches to prevention.

- Describe the advantages and disadvantages of high-risk and population approaches to prevention.

(Continued)

Quantitative Methods for Health Research   Nigel Bruce, Daniel Pope and Debbi Stanistreet
© 2008 John Wiley & Sons, Ltd

- Explain why the evaluation of screening programmes is important and list, with examples, the criteria commonly used for this purpose (Wilson–Jünger criteria).

- Define and calculate commonly used validation criteria (sensitivity, specificity, predictive values, likelihood ratio, accuracy) and interpret information provided by the receiver-operator characteristic (ROC) curve.

- Describe the most common types of bias that arise in epidemiological studies of the effectiveness of screening programmes.

- Describe what is meant by cohort and period effects, with examples; describe the graphical methods used to identify these effects and explain how they can contribute to identifying disease causation and the effect of preventive measures.

Resource papers

There are two resource papers for this chapter:

Paper A

Rose, G. (1981). Strategy of prevention: lessons from cardiovascular disease. *Br Med J* **282**, 1847–1851 (no abstract available).

Paper B

Gunnell, D., Middleton, E., Whitley, E. *et al.* (2003). *Br J Psychiatry* **182**, 164–170.

10.1 Concepts of risk

10.1.1 Concepts of relative and attributable risk

We will begin by comparing and contrasting two measures of risk, ***relative risk (RR)*** and ***attributable risk (AR)***. We discussed RR in Chapter 5 and this was defined as incidence in the exposed group/incidence in the unexposed group.

We can see that RR is a ratio. For example, the RR for smoking and lung cancer in a study might be reported as 10, meaning that the risk of lung cancer among smokers is 10 times that in non-smokers. As a measure of risk, RR gives us a good idea of the increased risk that an individual faces as a result of being exposed to the factor of interest. AR tells us something equally important, but rather different. We will explore this alternative perspective on risk through the following exercise.

 Self-Assessment Exercise 10.1.1

In the following table three activities are listed, together with injury and disease outcomes that can result from these activities. Two blank columns are provided for you to complete. In the first column (risk to individual), make some notes on the level of risk that engagement in each of the activities poses for the individual, that is, the RR. Make this assessment in everyday language such as very low, low, high, etc., do not try to guess actual values of the RR. For the second column (burden to society), think about the burden that each activity poses for society as a whole (the country, for example).

Activity	Outcome	Risk to individual	Burden to society
Base jumping (from buildings, bridges, etc., with a parachute)	Death from injury due to failure of parachute or hitting buildings		
Driving a car, or being a passenger	Death or serious injury in crash		
Smoking tobacco	Death from lung cancer or cardiovascular disease		

Answers in Section 10.5

In this exercise we have identified that:

- Some activities (e.g. base jumping) are dangerous for the people who engage in them, but lead to a very small burden of ill health for society because they are pursued by a tiny minority of people.

- Others, such as car occupancy, can result in a very substantial burden to health services and society, even though the risk to individuals on any given journey (or even over a year) is relatively low. The reason for this is that very large numbers of people travel in cars and very many journeys are made.

- Cardiovascular disease (CVD) is very common so that if smoking increases risk by two–threefold the impact on society, in terms of the numbers of cases of and deaths from CVD (burden of disease), will be very great.

The key elements here are (a) the risk to the individual associated with exposure, (b) the prevalence of the exposure in the population and (c) how common the disease or outcome is in the population. As we have said, the risk to the individual is measured by the RR. Another measure, AR, takes account of how common the disease outcome is and represents the incidence that can be attributed to the exposure. AR therefore gives us a better idea of the public health impact (or 'burden') of the exposure.

10.1.2 Calculation of AR

The calculation of AR is quite simple: it is the difference between the incidence for exposed people and the incidence for those who are unexposed (often referred to as the *risk difference*). It is defined as follows:

$$\text{Attributable risk (AR)} = \text{incidence in exposed group} - \text{incidence in unexposed group}$$
$$= I_{(\text{exposed})} - I_{(\text{unexposed})}$$

Note that, whereas RR is a ratio of incidence rates and therefore expressed as a number, AR is the difference between rates and is therefore expressed as a rate. You will have an opportunity to calculate and compare these two measures of risk in the next exercise.

If the association between a risk factor and a disease is causal, the AR indicates the number of cases among the exposed that can be attributed to the risk factor (cause). This is also the number that could (theoretically) be prevented if the exposure was eliminated. This notion is of course rather simplistic, since it assumes that any causes other than the risk factor being investigated have equal effects on the exposed and unexposed groups, but this is nevertheless a useful way to start thinking about what AR tells us. One can think of some examples where this is fairly clear. For example, the difference in incidence rates of liver cirrhosis among (a) heavy drinkers and (b) non-drinkers would, in a European country, indicate the rate of cirrhosis due to heavy alcohol consumption as this is by far the most important cause. We could apply a similar argument to smoking and lung cancer.

 Self-Assessment Exercise 10.1.2

The following table shows incidence rates for people exposed and unexposed over a lifetime to factor A, which increases the risk of a rare cancer, and factor B, which increases the risk of ischaemic heart disease (IHD), a disease that is far more common.

Risk factor	Disease risk	Rate/10 000 per year		Relative risk	Attributable risk
		Exposed	**Unexposed**		
Factor A	Cancer	1.2	0.4		
Factor B	IHD	660	220		

1. Calculate the RR and the AR for the rare cancer (factor A).

2. Calculate the RR and the AR for IHD (factor B).

3. Comment on what you find.

Answers in Section 10.5

Some of the other ways of expressing the concept of AR are summarised below. Perhaps the most important is ***population AR (PAR)***, which describes the disease burden attributable to a risk factor in a specified population.

Population attributable risk (PAR)

This is the excess rate of disease in the total study population (exposed and unexposed) that is attributable to the exposure. This is a useful measure as it translates the information we obtain from AR into the situation for the population of interest, such as the country. It is defined as:

$$PAR = I_{(whole\ population)} - I_{(unexposed)}$$

$$(or)\ PAR = AR \times (proportion\ of\ population\ exposed)$$

So, if the exposure is common and there is (at least) a small or moderately increased RR associated with exposure, then the PAR may be substantial. A good example of the application of this in practice can be seen with the respiratory and cardiovascular consequences of urban air pollution. If the ambient air of a city is polluted, it is very difficult for anyone to avoid exposure (a very high proportion of the population is exposed). In this situation, even a modest RR can translate into a substantial public health burden where common disease outcomes (such as chronic obstructive pulmonary disease, asthma, cardiovascular disease, etc.) are involved.

Population attributable risk percentage (PAR%)

This is the proportion of disease in the population that is attributable to the exposure and thus could be eliminated if the exposure was eliminated; it is defined as follows:

$$PAR\% = \frac{PAR}{I_{(whole\ population)}} \times 100$$

Preventive fraction

If the exposure is preventive, and the incidence in the exposed group is less than in the unexposed group, then the AR $(I_{(exposed)} - I_{(unexposed)})$ would be negative. This is rather meaningless (a negative rate), and in this situation an analogous measure is used, the ***preventive fraction (PF)***. This is defined as follows:

$$PF = \frac{I_{(unexposed)} - I_{(exposed)}}{I_{(unexposed)}}$$

 ### Self-Assessment Exercise 10.1.3

In a European country the prevalence of smoking among men is 30 per cent and coronary heart disease (CHD) mortality for all men is 200 per 100 000 per year. From various studies, estimates of the mortality rates among non-smokers is 150 per 100 000/year and among smokers is 317 per 100 000/year.

1. Calculate the RR and the AR.

2. Calculate and interpret the PAR.

3. Calculate and interpret the PAR%.

4. If the adult male population of the country is 20 million, how many deaths could theoretically be prevented if the smoking prevalence among men was reduced to 15 per cent? (you will need to recalculate the PAR).

Answers in Section 10.5

Summary: measures of risk

- RR: the ratio of the incidence rate of exposed and the incidence rate of unexposed groups (or more and less exposed respectively if we are dealing with degrees of exposure). The RR is a ratio and provides a measure of risk to the exposed individual.

- AR: the difference between the incidence rate among people who are exposed (or more exposed) and the incidence rate among those who are not (or less) exposed. AR is a rate and is a measure of the burden of disease attributable to a risk factor.

- PAR: takes into account the frequency of exposure in a population (e.g. the country) providing a measure of the burden of disease arising from that exposure in the defined population.

10.2 Strategies of prevention

10.2.1 The distribution of risk in populations

We will now look at why these concepts of risk, and in particular the way that risk is distributed in the population, have important implications for strategies of prevention. Much of this discussion is based on paper A: although published in 1981, this paper is worth studying as it illustrates very clearly how conclusions about prevention strategies can be derived from epidemiological principles and research findings. Exercise 10.2.1 and the subsequent discussion will help your understanding of these concepts. Please now read the excerpt from Rose (1981) (paper A) headed 'Absolute and Relative Risk', review Figure 2, and complete Exercise 10.2.1.

Absolute and Relative Risk

Life insurance experts concerned with charging the right premiums taught us that "high risk" meant "high relative risk," and in this until recently they have been abetted by the epidemiologists. Figure 2(a), taken from life insurance data,[1] shows for each of four age groups the relation of blood pressure to the relative risk of death, taking the risk for the whole of each age group as 100. The relative risk is seen to increase with increasing pressure, but the gradient gets a little less steep as age advances. That is perhaps not surprising, because a systolic pressure of 160 mm Hg is common in older men, and we would not expect it to be so unpleasant as at younger ages, when it is rare.

In figure 2(b) the same data are shown but with a scale of absolute instead of relative risk. The pattern now appears quite different. In particular, the absolute excess risk associated

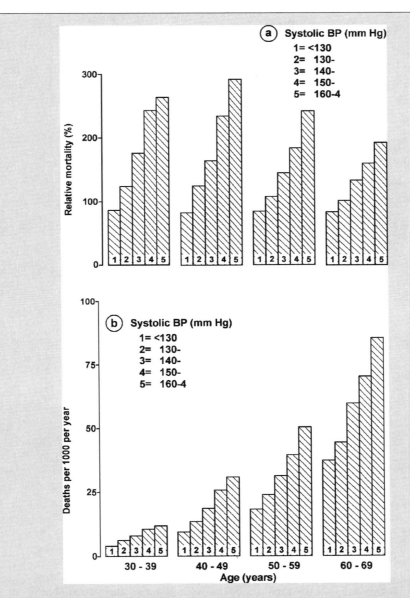

Fig 2 – Age-specific mortality in men according to blood pressure and age, from life insurance data: (a) relative risk, and (b) absolute risk

with raised pressure is far greater in the older men. A systolic pressure of 160 mm Hg may be common at these ages, but common does not mean good. To identify risk in relative units rather than absolute units may be misleading.

Self-Assessment Exercise 10.2.1

1. From Figure 2(b), the lower chart, estimate (as the actual values of the mortality are not given) the attributable risk of group 5 (systolic blood pressure 160–164) versus group 1 (systolic blood pressure <130), for age 30–39 years (you will need to estimate the difference between mortality rates).

2. Also from Figure 2(b) estimate the AR for group 5 versus group 1 at age 60–69 years.

3. Comment on what you find.

Answers in Section 10.5

We will now look at the implications of these findings for prevention strategies. Figure 3 from paper A is central to this discussion.

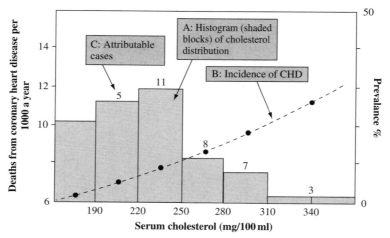

FIG 3—Prevalence distribution of serum cholesterol concentration related to coronary heart disease mortality (- - - -) in men aged 55–64. Number above each bar represents estimate of attributable deaths per 1000 population per 10 years. (Based on Framingham Study.[4])

*Conversion: SI to traditional units—*Cholesterol: 1 mmol/1≈38.6 mg/100 ml.

Figure 10.2.1   Distribution of cholesterol levels, risk and attributable cases. Reproduced from Figure 3 of paper A

Information in the diagram

Figure 3 presents three distinct pieces of information, each of which is highlighted by a box and arrow in Figure 10.2.1, and discussed further here. First (A), there is a histogram (shaded columns) illustrating the distribution of serum cholesterol levels in the Framingham study: the scale (prevalence per cent) is on the right-hand y-axis, and you will see that the distribution is slightly positively skewed. Second (B), the dashed line rising across the histogram is the incidence (mortality) rate, with the scale on the left-hand y-axis. The rate for the highest category of cholesterol is about twice that of the lowest. Hence the RR for the highest category versus the lowest is about 2.0. Third

(C), numbers are shown on top of the histogram: these are the estimates of the numbers of cases that can be attributed to the respective cholesterol levels, and we will discuss these further below.

Distribution of risk

From the histogram we can see that there are very few people with cholesterol levels that are associated with the highest RR. However the majority of the population, although not experiencing a RR as high as 2, does nevertheless have an elevated RR compared to the lowest cholesterol group, and this RR for 'the majority' is 1.2–1.5 times that in the lowest cholesterol group.

Attributable risk

When we look at the cases attributable to raised cholesterol (the numbers on top of the histogram) there is an important, and perhaps surprising, finding. These numbers have been obtained by applying the excess (attributable) mortality rates (deaths per 1000 population per 10 years) at each level of cholesterol to the numbers of people with those levels. We find that $5+11+8 = 24$ out of the total of 34 (70 per cent), that is, the majority of all the cases arise from the many people with 'typical' levels of cholesterol and moderately raised RR and not from the relatively few people with the high levels of cholesterol and high RR. This is a very important finding. In this population, 'typical' levels of cholesterol were not healthy. The implications of these observations for prevention strategies are now becoming apparent, and are discussed further in the next section.

10.2.2 High-risk and population approaches to prevention

In paper A, Geoffrey Rose discusses two approaches to prevention, termed ***high risk*** and ***population*** (or mass). The following sections and diagrams help to explain what is involved, for both approaches, in terms of the distribution of risk factors and associated RRs.

The high-risk approach

The high-risk approach is illustrated in Figure 10.2.2. The diagram is a schematic summary based on Figure 3 in paper A, and it shows:

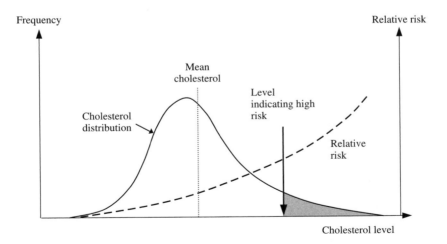

Figure 10.2.2 The high-risk approach to prevention

- The distribution of cholesterol levels as a skewed curve, including the mean (dotted line).

- The RR as a rising dashed line.

- A nominal cut-off level of cholesterol above which an individual is considered 'high-risk' (solid arrow with shaded portion of curve for values above the cut-off).

In the ***high-risk approach***, individuals with cholesterol levels above a value associated with high risk ('level indicating high risk' in Figure 10.2.2) would be identified through screening and then managed with advice on exercise and diet and, if necessary, cholesterol-lowering drugs. These people are represented by the shaded area under the distribution to the right of the cut-off arrow.

While this strategy is appropriate for those individuals with a high RR, you can see that it will have no impact on the majority of people with moderately raised RR. We will now consider the implications of this.

The population (or mass) approach

The population approach is illustrated in Figure 10.2.3. The diagram is also based on Figure 3 in paper A, as well as Figure 10.2.2 above, and shows:

- The original distribution of cholesterol levels as a skewed curve (A), including the mean (dotted line).

- As a new feature, a downward (left) shifted distribution of cholesterol levels as a skewed curve (B), including the mean cholesterol after the shift.

- The RR, as before, as a rising dashed line. Note that this does not change position or slope as the relationship between cholesterol level and RR has not changed.

- The same cut-off level of cholesterol above which an individual is considered to be at 'high risk'.

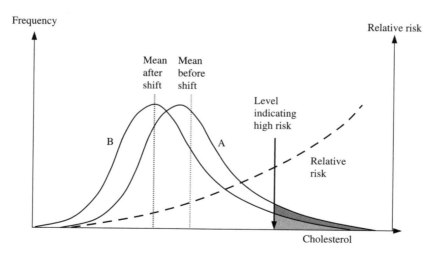

Figure 10.2.3 The population (mass) approach to prevention

With a population approach, measures (which we will consider shortly) are taken to move the whole distribution downwards (to the left). This has two effects:

- The RR of the majority of the population is reduced, since the central part of the distribution of cholesterol is now located over a lower portion of the RR curve. From our earlier discussion in which we found that most cases arise from the majority of the population towards the centre the distribution, this should have a substantial impact on the overall burden of disease.

- The proportion of the population that is now above the 'high-risk' cut-off has also been reduced, as shown by the reduced shaded area under the shifted distribution curve (B). Although this proportion is likely to be reduced somewhat with the population approach, it will not be eliminated.

Both strategies are required

From this examination of the distribution of risk we can see that neither strategy is sufficient on its own. The high-risk approach will not address the underlying problem of moderately raised risk among the majority of the population, whilst the population approach will leave a tail of individuals at high risk who, although fewer in number, still need to be identified and cared for.

The following exercise will help you to think about how these two approaches would be applied in practice to prevent heart disease by action on cholesterol levels. It also provides an opportunity to start thinking about some of the practical, political and social issues involved in implementing these strategies.

Self-Assessment Exercise 10.2.2

Make a list of the ways in which society might attempt to reduce the risk of IHD arising from elevated blood cholesterol through (a) a high-risk and (b) a population strategy.

Answers in Section 10.5

This exercise perhaps raised more questions than it answered, such as:

- What measures are likely to be most (cost)-effective?

- Which professional groups, institutions, etc., are best placed to implement these measures, and how?

- Are the many people with only moderately raised RR likely to take the advice being offered?

- What are the political and social implications of debate about individual freedom of choice?

Some of these issues are discussed in paper A. For a more detailed discussion, including the relevance to other health and social issues, see Rose (1992). For an example of the application of the concepts of high-risk and population prevention to a range of international public health issues, see the *World Health Report 2002* (WHO, 2002).

Safety and the population strategy

We have seen that the population strategy involves applying measures to large numbers of people, which may be the whole population or an important subgroup of the population. Please now read the excerpt 'Safety is paramount' from paper A, on the consequences of applying one of the early cholesterol-lowering drugs (clofibrate) to large numbers of people, and complete Exercise 10.2.3.

Safety is Paramount

The recent World Health Organisation controlled trial of clofibrate produced disturbing results.[8] In the treated group non-fatal myocardial infarction was reduced by 26% (about the effect predicted from the fall in cholesterol concentrations). Mortality from non-cardiac causes, however, increased by one-third, an effect rather unlikely to be due to chance. This finding is important to the strategy of prevention. Clofibrate has been in use for many years and has been given to enormous numbers of patients. Until the results of this trial appeared there was no suspicion that it might kill. Indeed, by clinical standards it can still be called a relatively safe drug, since the estimate of excess mortality works out at only about one death per 1000 patient-years. In patients with severe hyperlipoproteinaemia we would be prepared to take such a risk if it was thought that the drug might reduce their very high death rate.

Intervention for prevention where the risk is low is totally different. I suggested earlier that a large number of people exposed to a small risk might yield more cases in the community than a small number exposed to a big risk. There is a counterpart to that in regard to intervention. If a preventive measure exposes many people to a small risk, then the harm it does may readily—as in the case of clofibrate—outweigh the benefits, since these are received by relatively few. Unfortunately we cannot have many trials as large as the clofibrate study, nor are we able to keep such trials going for longer than a few years, usually five at the most. We may thus be unable to identify that small level of harm to individuals from long-term intervention that would be sufficient to make that line of prevention unprofitable or even harmful. Consequently we cannot accept long-term mass preventive medication.

 Self-Assessment Exercise 10.2.3

1. One strength of the population approach is that small reductions in risk achieved by many people can have a substantial impact on disease burden. How can this line of argument be applied to the safety of population prevention measures?

2. Why might it be difficult to identify the risks of a population prevention measure?

Answers in Section 10.5

The final exercise in this section will help to consolidate ideas about prevention strategies. Questions 1 and 3 require reading all of paper A, and reference to Rose (1992) is recommended if you are interested in more in-depth discussion.

Self-Assessment Exercise 10.2.4

1. In paper A, Geoffrey Rose refers to the 'prevention paradox'. What does this mean?

2. To which prevention strategy (high-risk or population) do the following statements best apply?

   a) shifting the mean of the distribution of a risk factor;

   b) screening for people with levels of a risk factor at or above a given point, and treating as necessary;

   c) screening for people with average levels of a risk factor, and treating as necessary;

   d) increasing tax on alcoholic drinks;

   e) water fluoridation (fluoride at around 1 ppm prevents tooth decay).

3. Prepare a summary list of the advantages and disadvantages of (a) the high-risk approach, and (b) the population approach.

Answers in Section 10.5

Summary: high-risk and population approaches to prevention

- The distribution of risk in a population has very important implications for planning prevention. For common diseases, where risk factors are widely distributed in the population, most of the cases may arise from the majority of people with only moderately raised RR, rather than the few with very high RR.

- The high-risk approach involves identifying and managing individuals with high RR, the tail of the distribution. This approach would typically be delivered through the health system.

- The population approach involves measures that can shift the whole exposure distribution, thereby reducing the RR for the majority. This approach will typically require social, economic and political action.

- It is very important that preventive measures applied to a population are safe – even a small risk can have disastrous results when applied to a very large number of people.

- Both high-risk and population approaches have advantages and disadvantages.

- A comprehensive prevention strategy requires both high-risk and population approaches to achieve the combined benefits of radical action to reduce population risk, and the identification and management of smaller numbers at high individual risk.

10.3 Evaluation of screening programmes

Cancer smear test errors killed 14 women
Staff and agencies, Thursday May 3, 2001

Fourteen women have died of cervical cancer despite being given the all-clear after smear tests, an audit into cervical screening services in Leicestershire revealed today.

The study of 403 women diagnosed with cervical cancer in a seven-year period showed that smear tests produced inaccurate results in nearly a third of cases.

Sixty-four more women eventually had to undergo radical treatment, including hysterectomies, after wrongly being given the all-clear at a time when their condition could have been treated with a simple operation, the Department of Health said.

The audit of women diagnosed with the disease between January 1993 and August 2000 found 122 discrepancies, of which 84 patients had a 'false negative' smear. Of those, 14 died and 64 underwent more radical treatment than they might otherwise have needed. The remaining women were not believed to have suffered any adverse consequences.

Speaking at a press conference at the Department of Health in central London, the government's cancer 'tsar', Mike Richards, said it was tragic that women had died and offered his condolences to bereaved relatives but stressed that Leicestershire was not failing.

He admitted the NHS had made mistakes but denied it had been negligent.

He said: 'That is why the audit was undertaken in the first place, to learn and then improve the service.'

Mr Richards said that the relatives of the 14 women who died would be told about the exact circumstances by Leicestershire health officials later today. He admitted that some could take legal action.

> 'No screening test can ever be 100% accurate, it is not an exact science.'

Women who have been diagnosed with cervical cancer in Leicestershire will be offered an appointment with their gynaecologist and counselling.

Mr Richards stressed that the cervical cancer screening programme in Leicestershire had to be understood in context.

'Leicester is not failing, it performs well on all qualitative assurance measures and death rates from cervical cancer are falling in line with national trends,' he said.

'We recognise this may and will cause distress to some of the patients. The NHS say sorry when they get things wrong. We want to put the audit into the public domain so that learning is not just in Leicestershire but all around the country.'

Government health figures show that the NHS Cervical Screening Programme saves around 1,300 lives a year. It is directly responsible for a 42 per cent drop in incidents of cervical cancer between 1988 and 1997. It is estimated that the programme has saved more than 8,000 lives in that time.

Mr Richards said it was unlikely that the problem of wrongly interpreted smears was restricted to Leicestershire. 'We can assume that around the rest of the country there will be other cases where diagnosis of cervical cancer or abnormality on the smear were not picked up.'

Philip Sturman, chief officer of Leicestershire Community Health Council, which represents patients, urged the public not to panic.

'It is important not to scare people with these results – screening saves lives,' he said.

The NHS cervical screening programme was set up in 1988 and is based in Sheffield. It has screened almost four million women in England each year with around 3,450 new cases of cervical cancer – the most common form of cancer in women aged under 35 – diagnosed.

Figures show that 83.7 per cent of women of screening age have had a smear in the last five years with 3.3m women aged 25 to 64 screened.

The smear test spots abnormal cells, but does not test for cancer itself.

From the *Guardian*, 3 May 2001

10.3.1 Purpose of screening

A screening programme is designed to assess people in the population who are at risk of a disease, and classify them as having either a high or low chance of actually having the disease, at an early stage. Those people with a high chance of having the disease can then be referred for a definitive assessment (for example, a biopsy) and treatment as necessary, while those with a low chance can be reassured.

In order to achieve this, a programme is required to carry out repeated examinations of large numbers of well people (who do not have, or are unaware of, symptoms), using a test that combines accuracy with simplicity, low cost, safety and acceptability. This is a substantial and demanding task. As the newspaper article illustrates, screening programmes are complex operations that have limitations. It emphasises that screening tests are not perfect and that evaluation is very important.

10.3.2 Criteria for programme evaluation

A number of criteria are commonly used in the evaluation of screening programmes, known as the Wilson–Jünger criteria. These are summarised in Table 10.3.1

Table 10.3.1 Criteria for the evaluation of screening programmes

Criterion	Discussion
Importance of condition.	There may be little value in developing a screening programme if the condition is not important, either in terms of severity, or incidence/prevalence, or both.
Natural history of condition is known.	It is important to know about the natural development of a disease that is being considered for screening; that is, how it develops without any human interference or treatment. This is called the ***natural history***. For example, does it always progress to a more serious stage requiring treatment? If not, in what proportion of people does it progress, from what stage, and what factors determine this progression?
Preclinical phase allowing early detection.	This relates to the natural history, but also to opportunities for treatment. For screening to have any chance of being effective, there must be a phase during which the disease can be detected, but before it has become too advanced to treat successfully.
Acceptability and safety of the screening test.	The test must be acceptable (not unduly painful or anxiety provoking) and safe. For example, it has been necessary to show that the radiation dose used in mammography (screening for breast cancer by radiography) is safe, and will not of itself cause breast cancer when used repeatedly during a woman's life.
Validity of the screening test.	A number of measures are used to assess how valid the screening test is compared to a definitive diagnostic test (the 'gold standard'). These measures are sensitivity, specificity, predictive value, accuracy and likelihood ratio. The discrimination of the test can also be analysed and displayed with a receiver-operator characteristic (ROC) curve. These are all explained in Section 10.3.3.

Table 10.3.1   (Continued)

Criterion	Discussion
Good coverage of at-risk population obtainable.	Unless good coverage can be achieved, the screening programme can have only a limited impact on the overall disease incidence. An example relevant to cervical screening programmes is the difficulty of contacting younger women living in some urban areas due to the inaccuracies of GP registers.
Effective management of confirmed cases is available, and resources exist to pay for treatment.	It would unacceptable to screen a population, detect a possibly serious disease, and then not be able to treat that disease effectively, or not be able to afford to treat everyone confirmed as having the disease.
Human and financial resources are available to operate the system for screening, definitive diagnosis, recall, quality control, etc.	Screening on a large scale, such as for breast and cervical cancer, is a major operation. Carrying out mammography requires expensive equipment, well-trained radiographers (to take X-rays), and radiologists (to read X-rays), and a good system for contacting and recalling women who require treatment or routine re-examination.
Cost-benefit ratio is acceptable.	The costs of preventing a case (incidence and/or mortality) should be calculated, and assessed in comparison with other procedures competing for resources.
Advice and counselling available.	Advice and support are necessary for people in various stages and categories of the screening process: • people who may be afraid of attending for screening; • people with a positive screening test, who turn out not to have the disease (false positive); • people with a positive screening test, who turn out to have the disease (true positive); • people with a negative screening test, who turn out to have the disease (false negative).

10.3.3   Assessing validity of a screening test

In Chapter 4 we looked at validity in relation to questionnaire design and measurement in surveys. Validity is a measure of accuracy and can be defined as the capacity of a test or question to give the true result. These concepts apply equally to screening tests, which, after all, are measurement tools used to establish whether or not an individual is likely or not to have a disease. We will now introduce an example that will help to illustrate these various measures of validity.

Example

Blood cholesterol testing is increasingly common, and many self-test machines are available. This is a form of screening (albeit mainly for a self-selected population), and it is of interest to assess how *valid* the results are. In the following (hypothetical) example, results on 100 people from a self-test machine have been compared (using the same blood sample) with a well-calibrated laboratory analyser, which can be treated as a *gold standard*. The results for each machine have been expressed in terms of the number (per cent) of people tested who had moderately or very high cholesterol (termed 'raised'), which, for the purpose of this example, is taken to be above ($\geq$) 6.5 mmol/l.

		Laboratory test		Total
		$\geq$ 6.5 mmol/l ('Raised')	< 6.5 mmol/l	
Self-test machine	$\geq$ 6.5 mmol/l ('Raised')	24	10	**34**
	< 6.5 mmol/l	3	63	**66**
	Total	**27**	**73**	**100**

Measures of validity

The following are commonly used measures of test validity and we will examine each in turn by reference to the above example.

Sensitivity: ability of the test to recognise people with disease

We will consider first how well the self-test machine recognises people who really have an elevated cholesterol, that is the 27 people testing high ($\geq$6.5 mmol/l) on the laboratory analyser, which is as close as we are going to get to the truth. Of these 27 people, the self-test recognised 24. Expressed as a percentage, this is 88.9 per cent, which we might judge to be good. This measure of test performance is called *sensitivity* and is defined as:

> The *sensitivity* of a test describes its ability to correctly identify people who have the characteristic that is being measured.

Sensitivity should be presented with the 95 per cent confidence interval (CI): it is a proportion, so the formula for the standard error (SE) and 95 per cent CI are as for a proportion (see Chapter 4). In this case, the SE is 6.05 (%) as shown below and the 95 per cent CI is $88.9 \pm (1.96 \times 6.05) =$ 77.1–100%.

$$SE(sensitivity) = \sqrt{\frac{p(1-p)}{n}} = \sqrt{\frac{88.9(100-88.9)}{27}} = 6.05$$

Specificity: ability of the test to recognise people without disease

There were 73 people whose test result on the laboratory analyser was < 6.5 mmol/l, and who therefore were not cases of 'raised' cholesterol. How well did the self-test do? Of these 73 people, the self-test reported 63 as having a cholesterol level of < 6.5 mol/l, which is 86.3 per cent, and is also quite good. This measure of test performance is called *specificity*, and is defined as follows:

> The *specificity* of a test describes its ability to identify correctly people who do not have the characteristic that is being measured.

Specificity should also be presented with the 95 per cent CI, which is 78.4–94.2 per cent. This is narrower than the 95 per cent CI for sensitivity as there are more cases ($n = 73$ versus 27) from which to derive the specificity estimate.

Predictive value: how trustworthy is the result predicted by the test?

By this we mean, if the test predicts that the person is (or is not) a case, how likely is it that the test is correct? We can examine this aspect of performance for a positive (case) and a negative (not a case) result.

- **Positive result:** Of the 34 people with a high result on the self-test machine, only 24 really had a high level according to the laboratory test, which is not so good. This is 70.6 per cent and is termed the *positive predictive value*. A good way to think about the implications of this is to imagine that you were one of the 34, thinking from the self-test that you had a raised cholesterol, only to discover later that it was not true. In practice, this would cause people a lot of anxiety (which might be a lot worse if you were dealing with a test for cancer), and in research would lead to serious bias in, for example, a *prevalence* estimate.

- **Negative result:** Of the 66 people testing negative on the self-test, 63 really were negative. This is 95.4 per cent, which is good. If anything, the problems caused by a poor *negative predictive value* would be worse than for a poor positive predictive value: we saw the effects of this in cervical cancer screening in the newspaper article.

Accuracy: how likely is it than any result is correct?

This measure considers all tests and asks what is the probability that any test, whether positive or negative, has provided the correct result. This is 24 (correct positive results) + 63 (correct negative results) divided by the total (100): this is 87 per cent, which is fairly good.

Likelihood ratio

As with predictive value, this can be determined for both a positive and a negative test.

- **Likelihood ratio for positive test:** this looks at how much more likely it is that a positive screening test result will be found in a person with the condition, as opposed to a person without the condition. This is calculated (with sensitivity and specificity as proportions rather than percentages) as:

$$Likelihood\,ratio\,(positive\,test) = \frac{Sensitivity}{1 - Specificity}$$

In this case, it is 6.49. We can interpret this as meaning that it is 6.5 times more likely that a positive test will be found in someone with the condition than someone without it.

- **Likelihood ratio for negative test:** this looks at how much more likely it is that a negative screening test result will be found in a person with the condition, as opposed to a person without the condition.

$$Likelihood\,ratio\,(negative\,test) = \frac{1 - Sensitivity}{Specificity}$$

In this case, it is 0.13.

Summary

A good way to help understand what these measures of test performance show, and to calculate them, is to present the situation as a general 2×2 table:

		True situation		Total
		Positive	**Negative**	
Test	Positive	**a** (true test positives)	**b** (false test positives)	**a+b**
	Negative	**c** (false test negatives)	**d** (true test negatives)	**c+d**
	Total	**a+c** (true positives)	**b+d** (true negatives)	**a+b+c+d**

This table can now be used to help in calculating the test measures:

Measure	Summary (performance of test)	Calculation
Sensitivity	Percentage of true positives detected	a/(a+c)
Specificity	Percentage of true negatives detected	d/(b+d)
Positive predictive value	Percentage of test positives that are correct	a/(a+b)
Negative predictive value	Percentage of test negatives that are correct	d/(c+d)
Accuracy	Percentage of test results that are correct	(a+d)/(a+b+c+d)

 ## Self-Assessment Exercise 10.3.1

In this exercise, the screening test is for a cancer that is much less common than the prevalence of raised cholesterol (27 per cent) in our earlier example. Comparison with the gold standard of biopsy provided the following results:

		Gold standard (biopsy)		Total
		Have disease	**Disease free**	
Screening test	**+ve on test**	325	450	**775**
	−ve on test	25	4800	**4825**
	Total	**350**	**5250**	**5600**

1. What is the prevalence of cancer in this example?

2. Calculate (with 95 per cent CI) and interpret the sensitivity of the test.

3. Calculate and interpret the specificity.

4. Calculate and comment on the positive and negative predictive values.

5. Calculate and comment on the accuracy of the test.

6. Calculate and interpret the likelihood ratios for (a) a positive test and (b) a negative test.

Answers in Section 10.5

The receiver-operator characteristic (ROC) curve

We have seen that a screening test is designed to classify individuals as having a high or a low risk of a disease. For most tests, a decision has to be made about the value (which may be a questionnaire score, a physiological measurement, or physical findings such as cells or an X-ray) that, if exceeded, will be taken as indicating high risk of having the disease. For any given test, if a higher value (or more definite finding) is used, it will be more certain that the person is at high risk; that is, the test will give a better specificity. The other side of this coin, however, is that there will also be an increased probability that people with the disease will be missed; that is, there is lower sensitivity. Conversely, if a lower (less definite) 'cut-off' level is taken, sensitivity will be increased at the expense of specificity.

These characteristics of a test, including the trade-off between sensitivity and specificity, can be described by the *receiver-operator characteristic* (ROC) curve. This also allows identification of the cut-off value giving the best discrimination optimising sensitivity and specificity. ROCs are so-called from their use with radar during the 1939-45 war. In that situation, ROC curves were used to identify settings that would best assist (radar) receiver operators in distinguishing between reflected signals from an object of interest (ship, aircraft) and other background objects or conditions that were not a threat. If the equipment was set too sensitive, there would be many false positives; for example, fighter planes being sent to intercept flocks of birds. If it was set too specific, there would be more risk that some incoming enemy aircraft would not be detected.

Example

In Chapter 4 we discussed validity in respect of designing a back pain disability questionnaire. Using this example, let's assume we have now scored the questionnaire responses on a scale of 0–30 obtained from 235 subjects in an occupational setting. We wish to determine the value of the disability score that best discriminates between the presence or absence of persistent back pain. The presence of back pain has been assessed by self-reports of the nature and duration of symptoms. Table 10.3.2 and Figures 10.3.1a and b provide some information on the distributions of the scores among those with and without back pain.

Table 10.3.2 Distributions of disability scores among cases and non-cases of back pain (output from SPSS)

Persistent back pain	Mean	N	SD	Median	Inter-quartile range	Minimum	Maximum	Range
No	5.66	116	3.580	5.00	3.0 – 7.0	0	19	19
Yes	10.23	119	4.938	9.00	7.0 – 13.0	1	30	29
Total	7.97	235	4.883	7.00	5.0 – 10.0	0	30	30

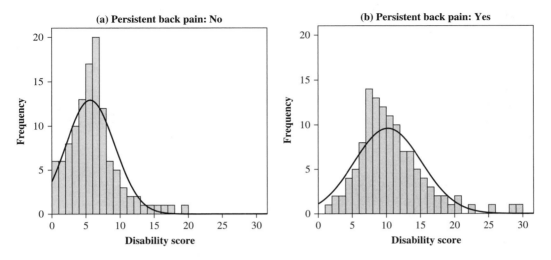

Figure 10.3.1 Distributions of disability score for (a) subjects without persistent back pain and (b) subjects with persistent back pain

 Self-Assessment Exercise 10.3.2

Using the information in Table 10.3.2 and Figures 10.3.1a and b:

1. Describe the distributions for those (a) with and (b) without back pain, including how the distributions differ.

2. What cut-off score would be needed to ensure that test positive results included only people with back pain? Approximately what proportion of people with back pain would be wrongly classified as a result?

3. What cut-off score would be needed to ensure that test negative results included only people without back pain; that is, all people with back pain had a test positive? Approximately what proportion of people without back pain would be wrongly classified as a result?

4. Hazard a guess at the score you think will discriminate best between those with and without back pain.

Answers in Section 10.5

Table 10.3.3 shows the sensitivity and 1 – specificity associated with values of the questionnaire disability score. These are shown over the full range of possible scores (0–30) with two extremes representing perfect sensitivity and worst specificity (−1) and perfect specificity with worst sensitivity (31). Figure 10.3.2 shows the ROC curve based on the data from the 235 respondents (SPSS output). We will now discuss the interpretation of these results.

Table 10.3.3   Sensitivity and 1 – specificity values associated with scores from the disability questionnaire

Positive if greater than or equal to	Sensitivity*	1 – Specificity*
−1.00	1.000	1.000
0.50	1.000	.948
1.50	.992	.897
2.50	.975	.828
3.50	.958	.741
4.50	.924	.629
5.50	.882	.483
6.50	**.815**	**.310**
7.50	.697	.207
8.50	.588	.155
9.50	.487	.112
10.50	.395	.086
11.50	.311	.069
12.50	.252	.052
13.50	.193	.043
14.50	.151	.034
15.50	.118	.026
16.50	.092	.017
17.50	.076	.009
18.50	.059	.009
19.50	.050	.000
21.00	.034	.000
23.50	.025	.000
26.50	.017	.000
29.00	.008	.000
31.00	.000	.000

*expressed as a proportion

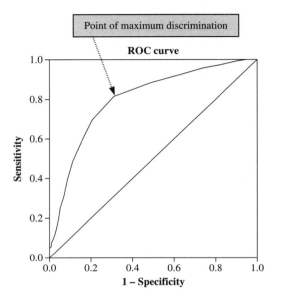

Figure 10.3.2   Receiver operator characteristic (ROC) curve for back pain score

The important results from ROC analysis are as follows:

1. The *area under the curve*, which quantifies the overall capacity of the test to discriminate between those who have the disease (back pain) and those who do not. This analysis yielded an estimate of the area at 0.802, with a standard error of 0.029 and 95 per cent CI 0.745–0.859, $p < 0.0001$ (SPSS output). A test with no power whatever to discriminate will have an area of 0.5 and is illustrated by the diagonal line in Figure 10.3.2, so the better the test, the larger the area to the left of the diagonal line. Our test is very much better than the zero discrimination line, and the 95 per cent CI shows that we have a fairly precise estimate of how much better. We interpret this result as follows: for a test where higher values are associated with greater likelihood of disease (as in this case), the area represents the probability that a randomly selected

person with the disease will have a higher test result than a randomly selected person who does not have the disease. In this case the probability is just over 80 per cent, or 8 out of 10.

2. The *point of maximal discrimination* (marked on Figure 10.3.2), which is the point furthest from the diagonal line of no effect. This also indicates the sensitivity and 1 − specificity at the points of maximal discrimination, which are approximately 80 per cent and 30 per cent, respectively (and therefore the specificity is 70 per cent).

3. The *sensitivity* and *specificity* associated with the full range of scores, including the point of maximal discrimination, are shown in Table 10.3.3. In this table it is very clear how sensitivity falls as specificity rises and vice versa (remember that column 3 is 1 − specificity). The values of sensitivity and specificity identified from the curve are associated with a score of just over 6.5 (bold, larger typeface in table), so an integer score of 7 would be taken as the cut-off: this is the answer to question 4 in Exercise 10.3.2. You can also see the results for the questions about cut-offs (2 and 3) in Exercise 10.3.2. Question 2 requires a specificity of 100 per cent (true negatives must be correctly identified), which is achieved at a score of 20 (only integer scores are possible). Question 3 requires a sensitivity of 100 per cent (all cases are to be included), which is achieved at a score of 1.

Which measures of validity are most useful?

All of these measures are useful, but there are some pointers to which are most informative in any given set of circumstances.

Sensitivity and specificity are particularly useful in assessing the overall performance of a test, as for a screening programme or in epidemiological studies. If we are trying to identify cases in a survey or cohort study, for example (or of course in screening), it is very valuable to know how good the test is at finding genuine cases. A test with a low sensitivity but very high specificity would, for example, not find all the cases, but it would be unlikely to identify people as cases if they did not have the disease. Conversely (and not infrequently in epidemiological studies), it may be useful to use an initial test with a high sensitivity and low specificity to identify cases and possible cases (thus missing very few real cases), and then apply a more rigorous test for the final case definition.

Predictive values, positive and negative, are particularly relevant to the health-care setting, where the results of an individual test will need to be discussed with a patient. These measures help with answering questions such as 'I have a negative test result − does that mean I definitely don't have cancer?' If the negative predictive value were 95 per cent, the response would be, 'It is unlikely, but there is still a small chance, about 1 in 20, that you could have the disease.'

10.3.4 Methodological issues in studies of screening programme effectiveness

Of the various epidemiological study designs available, RCTs and case-control studies are used most commonly to study the effectiveness of screening programmes. The design of these studies raises some quite complex issues, in particular the avoidance and/or interpretation of potential sources of bias that arise because it is a screening programme that is being studied. The three most important types of bias in epidemiological studies of screening programmes are summarised here.

Selection (volunteer) bias

People taking part in screening programmes may differ from those who do not. If this difference is associated in some way with their general health, severity of disease (for which they are being screened) and likely compliance with advice and treatment, then these are all ways in which the screened group may be biased towards a better outcome. This source of bias is more likely to arise with observational studies (e.g. case-control) than with RCTs, since randomisation should balance the characteristics of people screened and not screened.

Length-based sampling (prognostic) bias

This second source of bias results from the observation that screening may detect people with less rapidly progressing (less severe or aggressive) disease than the usual route of presenting to a doctor with symptoms or other problems. This occurs because the less rapidly advancing cases have a longer preclinical phase than the more severe cases. Thus, when screening is carried out, people with the less severe form are more likely to be picked up; there are in effect more person-years of preclinical 'less severe' disease around in the population than person-years of 'more severe' disease. If this bias occurs, the screened group will, on average, tend to have less severe disease and may consequently be observed to have better outcomes.

Lead-time bias

This third type of bias occurs because screening can pick up cases earlier in the natural history than when they present through the usual route; that is, to a doctor when symptoms arise. Of course, an effective screening and treatment programme might actually achieve a better outcome (longer survival, or cure) as a result of earlier detection, but that is **_effectiveness_**, not **_bias_**. What we are talking about here is the perception that survival is longer, simply because the diagnosis has been made through screening, say, 6 months or a year earlier than it would otherwise have been if the person had been diagnosed when symptoms arose and he or she visited a doctor. This is summarised in Figure 10.3.3.

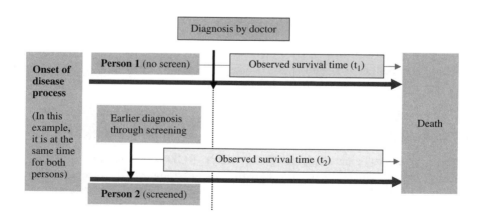

Figure 10.3.3 Illustration of lead-time bias

In this example, two people develop a disease that in fact runs exactly the same course from onset to death. Person 1, who is not screened, becomes ill, visits the doctor, and is diagnosed and after a period of time (t_1) dies. Person 2, on the other hand, is screened, and as a result, the diagnosis is made some time earlier for him than for person 1: this person subsequently dies after a period of time (t_2) that is longer than t_1. This gives the impression that person 2 survived longer, but in fact treatment following detection of the disease at screening is no more effective than treatment of disease diagnosed when the person became clinically ill. This situation could lead to a mistaken conclusion that screening and early treatment resulted in longer survival.

Summary: evaluation of screening programmes

- Although the validity of the screening test is very important, evaluation must include all aspects of the programme.

- The criteria and characteristics discussed in Sections 10.3.2 and 10.3.3 summarise the attributes that must be considered when planning a screening programme, or evaluating an existing one.

- Epidemiological studies designed to assess the effectiveness of screening programmes are subject to particular forms of bias.

10.4 Cohort and period effects

10.4.1 Analysis of change in risk over time

In Chapter 2 we considered how routine data collected on populations could be used to generate hypotheses about possible associations between risk factors (exposures) and a disease or outcome of interest. Detailed analysis of how risk (e.g. mortality) changes over time in groups of people of different ages or born at different times can be very informative. The two most important influences on risk that can be identified in this way are known as *cohort* and *period effects*, and these are now described.

Cohort effect

A group of people born at a particular time or over a relatively short period of years (known as a *birth cohort*) will experience a unique set of social and environmental conditions over the course of their lifetimes. These conditions will at times present exposures that carry some increased (or decreased) risk of disease. Such exposures might occur while their mothers were pregnant, at or around birth, or at a particular age in their lives such as teenage or young adult years. The increased risk of disease relating to one or more of these exposures will be identifiable among people born at a particular time in history. This is known as a *cohort effect* and is related in some way to the time these people were born, even though the exposure may occur at some later stage in their lives.

Cohort effects may be apparent in the incidence over time of diseases with a long interval between the cause and the onset of the disease. For example, increasing mortality rates among women from lung cancer have been attributed to smoking trends among different (birth) cohorts of women. In the UK, women in their late teens and early twenties at the time of the Second World War and during the years immediately afterwards became part of a growing trend of smoking among women. This trend was related to smoking being perceived as more acceptable and fashionable and also because the war years had resulted in many more women working in industry and offices. As a result it can be observed that women born in the 1920s and 1930s, who were therefore at a 'vulnerable' age (around 16-25 years old) during a period when smoking was being rapidly taken up by young women, have higher rates of lung cancer mortality than women born before the 1920s.

Period effect

A contrasting situation occurs when people (of all ages or any age) in a given population experience a change in exposure at a particular time (or period) in history. This is known as a **period effect**. This is often seen for health outcomes with more immediate causes, or those with a short latency period that affect all age groups (or at least a wide age range) at the same time. An example of this was the introduction in the UK of the law enforcing the wearing of front seat belts in cars, which resulted in a rapid and sustained reduction in mortality from road traffic accidents. When front seat belt wearing was made compulsory in the UK, compliance with the law was very good and the rate of wearing belts increased rapidly from less than half to around 90 per cent of all front-seat passengers. The effect was a dramatic reduction in deaths and serious injuries from road accidents (among car occupants, not pedestrians!). This is a **period** effect, and was not restricted to any one age group.

It can be appreciated that the identification of cohort and period effects can be very useful in relating observed rates of mortality and morbidity to the patterns of events and circumstances that have occurred over time in order to understand the aetiology of disease and the impact of prevention measures. Thus, specific studies can be designed to investigate these effects, incorporating **cohort** or **period analyses**, to help investigate possible causal associations. In the following example based on analysis of suicide trends in the UK, we will see how information about social trends can be related to observed cohort and period effects and how valuable this is in thinking about prevention and public health policy.

10.4.2   Example: suicide trends in UK men and women

In Chapter 2, we investigated some of the changing trends in suicide rates over the last 50 years by age and sex. We are now going to look at these trends in more detail. The following examples are taken from paper B (Gunnell *et al.*, 2003). In this study, trends in suicide were examined to see whether changes in the UK over time could be explained by cohort or period effects. We will begin by looking at trends in age-specific suicide rates.

Trends in age-specific suicide rates

Mortality rates for virtually all causes of death increase with age. Plotting death rates by age group over time is probably the most common way of illustrating trends in mortality and it is a method we have used previously. Figure 10.4.1, taken from paper B, illustrates trends in suicide since the 1950s for defined age groups.

Three-year moving averages

The presentation of data in Figure 10.4.1 involves the use of 3-year moving averages. This technique is used to smooth year-on-year fluctuations which are mainly random. The most common method of calculation is as follows. For year X, the smoothed rate $= [(0.25 \times$ rate for year X $- 1) + (0.5 \times$ rate for year X$) + (0.25 \times$ rate for year X $+ 1)]$.

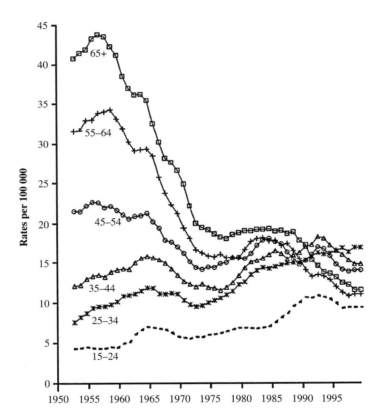

Figure 10.4.1 Age-standardised suicide rates: 1950-1999 England and Wales (3-year moving averages) in males
Figure 1(a) in paper B[1]

---

[1] Note that the y-axis on this and some of the following graphs has been altered to 100 000 as this was incorrectly labelled as 100 00 in the published paper.

Self-Assessment Exercise 10.4.1

1. From Figure 10.4.1 what can you say about trends in suicide deaths among men in the age groups illustrated?

2. You will notice that suicide rates fell across all age groups during the late 1960s. What kind of effect describes this pattern of decline in death rates?

3. Can you think of any possible explanations for the decline in suicide rates identified in question 2?

Answers in Section 10.5

Analysis of period effects

In Figure 10.4.2, reproduced from paper B, suicide rates in six age groups are shown for five periods of death, for males and females. This method of graphical analysis is used to identify whether there is any evidence of a period effect, since each line illustrates the death rates (i) for all age groups and (ii) at a particular time. If a period effect is occurring, this should be reflected in the suicide rates for deaths of all (or a wide range of) age groups at a particular period in history. On the graph, where a period effect is evident, we would therefore expect to see one or more of the lines with higher rates, and a tendency for the lines to be separated in a parallel way. The following exercise explores whether there is evidence of period effects for suicide among men and women.

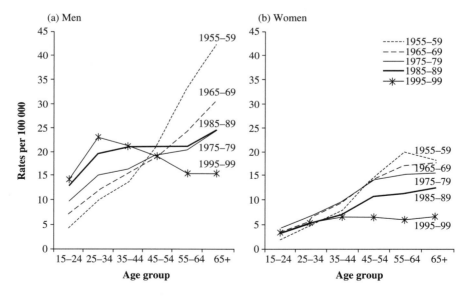

Figure 10.4.2 Suicide and undetermined death rates by time (of death) period and by age group in (a) men and (b) women in the UK (Figure 2 in paper B)

Self-Assessment Exercise 10.4.2

1) The x-axis of Figure 10.4.2 shows age groups: what are these ages?

2) What, approximately, is the suicide rate for men, dying at age 28 years, in 1977?

3) Does Figure 10.4.2 (a) provide evidence of a period effect among men?

4) Is there evidence in Figure 10.4.2 (b) of a period effect for women?

Answers in Section 10.5

Analysis of cohort effects

Graphical methods are also commonly used for analysis of cohort effects and this is illustrated in Figure 10.4.3, reproduced from paper A. The way in which this graph is plotted may seem unfamiliar at first, but if you work through the interpretation systematically, it is not difficult to understand.

To demonstrate cohort effects, we plot *age-specific (suicide) rates* (that is, age at death) for different birth cohorts. For example, the first group shown by the fine dotted line shows male suicide and undetermined death rates for those born between 1940 and 1945 and dying at different ages. The data range from the suicide rate among 15-19-year-olds (born 1940–44) on the far left, through to the suicide rate among 55-59-year-olds (born 1940–44) on the far right end of the dotted line.

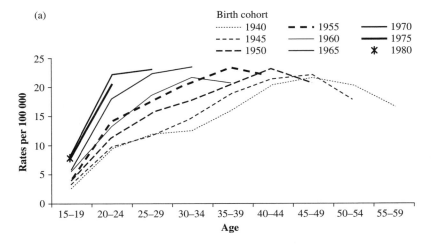

Figure 10.4.3 Rates of male suicide and undetermined death in successive 5-year birth cohorts by age group. The x-axis (age groups) shows age at death (Figure 3a in paper A)

This graph shows that for each successive birth cohort, suicide rates in young men (that is, up to the age of 30–34 years) have increased across all age groups. This indicates that, since 1940, we can identify an effect such that the more recently males are born, the greater is the risk of suicide up to age 34 years. This indicates a probable birth cohort effect. The question then is, what might be progressively increasing the risk of young male suicide in this way?

A second question arises from the observation (from data in Figure 10.4.3) that, as we look across from 'earlier born' cohorts (e.g. 1940–, 1945–, etc.) to 'later born' cohorts (1970–, 1975–, etc.), the suicide rates appear to peak at progressively younger ages. Thus, the peak for the birth cohort 1945–49 is age 45–49, which must therefore have occurred in the period of death 1990– (calculated by adding the age at death to the birth year). Similarly, the peak for the 1950–54 birth cohort is age 40–44, and the period of death is also 1990–. In fact, the peaks in death rates occurred around 1990 for all birth cohorts, indicating a *period effect*.

The final exercise looks at the data for males from paper B in more detail, and helps us draw some conclusions about what might be going on.

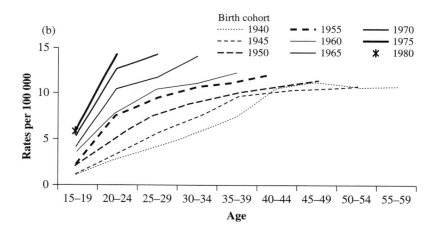

Figure 10.4.4 Rates of male suicide and undetermined death in successive 5-year birth cohorts by age group. The x-axis (age groups) shows age at death (Figure 3b in paper A)

 ## Self-Assessment Exercise 10.4.3

1. From Figure 10.4.4, what is the death rate (suicide and undetermined, excluding overdose and gassing) for men born in 1963 and dying at age 31 years?

2. How do the patterns of death rates for birth cohorts in Figure 10.4.4 differ from those in Figure 10.4.3, which was based on all methods of suicide.

3. What might be the explanation for the finding identified in question 2?

4. What can we conclude so far from the analyses of male suicides we have discussed in this section?

Answers in Section 10.5

Summary: cohort and period effects

- Cohort effects result from the experience of a group (cohort) born at a particular time and can be studied by examining death rates in relation to the year of birth.

- Period effects result from circumstances occurring at a particular time or period and can be studied by examining death rates in relation to the year of death.

- Cohort and period analysis can play a useful part in the study of disease causation and can help shed light on the associations between historical events; social, political and environmental trends and prevention measures; and patterns of disease incidence.

10.5 Answers to self-assessment exercises

Section 10.1

Exercise 10.1.1

Activity	Outcome	Risk to individual	Burden to society
Base jumping (from buildings, bridges, etc., with a parachute)	Death from injury due to failure of parachute or hitting buildings	High: this is a dangerous activity	Very low, because relatively few people do base jumping
Driving a car, or being a passenger	Death or serious injury in crash	Relatively low: the chances of an individual's being injured over a year or even a lifetime are not great*	Substantial, because even though individual risk is not high, it is a very common activity
Smoking tobacco	Death from lung cancer or cardiovascular disease (CVD)	High: it is estimated that one in three smokers will die of a condition related to smoking	Very high, because not only is the individual risk high, but at least one-third of the (UK) population smoke, or have smoked, and CVD is very common

* For some population subgroups, such as young males there are substantially higher risks to individuals.

Exercise 10.1.2

Risk factor	Disease risk	Rate/10 000 per year		Relative risk	Attributable risk
		Exposed	**Unexposed**		
Factor A	Cancer	1.2	0.4	3.0	0.8 per 10 000 per year
Factor B	IHD	660	220	3.0	440 per 10 000 per year

The RR is the same for both factors, but the AR is very different. Thus, although exposure to factor A carries a RR of 3.0, the exposure and cancer are relatively rare. As a result, there are only 0.8 cases per 10 000 population per year *attributable* to exposure to this factor. In contrast, although factor B has the same RR of 3.0 for IHD, 440 cases per 10 000 per year can be attributed to this exposure. This is because the exposure is very much more common, as is the disease. This emphasises two key points:

- Clearly the common exposure, factor B, has a far greater public health impact. This is very important in terms of reducing the burden of a common disease.

- For individuals exposed, both factors are of similar concern although the context can be expected to differ; for example, while factor B may be an exposure of concern to the general public, factor A might be restricted to a specific occupational setting.

In this exercise we found the attributable risk of IHD to be 440 per 10 000 per year: of every 10 000 people exposed, 440 per year will suffer IHD attributable to factor B. Thus, if exposure is eliminated for 10 000 people, 440 cases of IHD per year could be prevented (subject to related risk factors being unchanged).

Exercise 10.1.3

1. RR $= 2.11$; AR $= 167$ per 100 000 per year (which implies that 167 cases per 100 000 population per year can be attributed to smoking).

2. PAR $=$ AR $\times$ (proportion of population exposed) $= 167 \times 0.3 = 50$ per 100 000 per year (or if calculated by alternative formula 200 − 150 per 100 000 = 50 per 100 000 per year). Thus, in the specified country, 50 deaths from CHD per 100 000 total population can be attributed to smoking.

3. PAR% $= 50$ per 100 000/200 per 100 000 $= 25$%; that is smoking is responsible for 25 per cent of deaths from CHD in the country.

4. If smoking prevalence in men were reduced to 15 per cent, the PAR would be $167 \times 0.15 = 25$ per 100 000 per year, equivalent in this population to prevention of $20\,000\,000 \times 25/100\,000$ deaths from CHD $= 5000$ deaths each year. This assumes that effects of smoking in the past are nolonger a factor and that the influences of other risk factors are ignored.

Section 10.2

Exercise 10.2.1

1. At age 30-39, the AR is approximately 12/1000/year − 3/1000/year = 9/1000/year.

2. At age 60-69, the AR is approximately 87/1000/year − 37/1000/year = 50/1000/year.

We can see that, although the RR is larger in the younger age group, the AR is far larger in the older age group, since the absolute rates are much greater in the 60-69 year age group. As a result, raised blood pressure has a far greater public health impact at older ages than it does among young people.

Exercise 10.2.2

Strategies for reducing IHD risk associated with cholesterol

High-risk approach	Population approach
Screening based mainly in primary care, which would include:	• Dietary advice to the population (what is effective?).
• Detection of people with raised levels of cholesterol and of other related risk factors.	• Labelling of fat content and type on food.
	• Agricultural practices that reduce the fat content of meat, etc.
• Management by dietary advice, medical treatment (drugs), exercise, etc.	• Policies to address issues of accessibility and cost of healthier foods, especially for poorer people.
• Monitoring.	• Policy on exercise facilities and transport, etc., that can encourage greater physical activity.

Exercise 10.2.3

1. The argument about the benefits of the population strategy is essentially the same, but turned around, when considering safety. A small risk (associated with a prevention measure) applied to a large number of people may result in a disturbingly large number of adverse events (non-cardiac deaths in the case of clofibrate). For people at high risk of a disease, it may be reasonable to accept the small risk associated with the intervention. This would not be acceptable for the rest of the population made up of people with low individual risk.

2. It is rare for studies (ideally trials) of prevention measures to be carried out that are large enough to detect the small risks we are concerned with. Even a study with (for example) 20 000-30 000 subjects is small in comparison with the application of a prevention measure to a population of tens or hundreds of millions of people. In addition, such trials can rarely be continued for more than a few years, so problems emerging after 5–10 years may well be missed.

Exercise 10.2.4

1. 'The prevention paradox' is described as the situation in which a measure that brings large benefits to the community offers little to each participating individual. Thus, a preventive action that reduces the risk of the majority (and therefore substantially reduces the population burden of the disease) does little for the individual because the RR for most people is only moderately raised; as individuals, they are not very likely to suffer from the disease anyway. In contrast, a preventive measure targeted at individuals with high RR can bring a substantial benefit to them but may do little to reduce the population burden of disease.

2. The statements apply as follows:

   a) Population approach.

   b) High-risk approach.

   c) This statement does not really apply to either approach. Screening and treating individuals with average levels of the risk factor (around the mean) is not suitable for the population approach and is likely to be ineffective. It is very time-consuming, as there are so many people in this category and adopting an individual approach to reducing only moderately raised risk is difficult for both the professional(s) and the individual concerned.

   d) An example of government action that can reduce general alcohol consumption and that is consistent with a population approach.

   e) Another example of a population approach and also of the 'safety is paramount' issue which is seen with the controversy surrounding the safety of adding fluoride to drinking water for prevention of tooth decay. Let us consider, for the purposes of illustration, the consequences of adding to drinking water a substance with a small RR of serious disease (e.g. cancer). Since virtually everyone in the supplied area would use that water, the PAR would be substantial. The view that fluoridation may have serious adverse health effects is not accepted by those with responsibility for dental public health. However, widespread fear of such effects combined with freedom of choice arguments has effectively prevented the authorities in many parts of the country from proceeding with what is known to be a highly effective means of preventing tooth decay.

3. Summary of advantages and disadvantages of high-risk and population strategies

(a) High-risk strategy

Advantages	Disadvantages
Appropriate to the individual who is at high risk. Avoids interference with those who are not at special risk.	Prevention becomes medicalised. Success is only palliative and temporary. It does little to alter the situations that determine exposure, or the underlying causes of the health problem.
Readily accommodated within the ethos and organisation of medical care. Easy for doctors to see high-risk people as 'almost patients', and treat them accordingly.	The strategy is problematic because so much behaviour is determined by social norms and what peers do. The high-risk approach requires that individuals identified as at high risk should behave differently from most of the rest of society.
To be effective, interventions can be quite resource intensive. Focusing on those at highest risk offers more cost-effective use of resources.	Limited by the poor ability to predict the future outcome of individuals, even if in high-risk group.
Since interventions have costs (adverse consequences) as well as benefits, and assuming costs are similar for all, focusing on those at higher risk will improve the benefit-to-cost ratio.	Problems of feasibility and costs. Costs of screening, including human resources, and of treatment and monitoring may be high.
	The contribution to overall control of a disease may be disappointingly small.

(b) Population strategy

Advantages	Disadvantages
The strategy is radical, as it offers the chance to address the underlying causes.	May not be accepted easily, especially by the medical profession, although this is changing. Also it is difficult to see (and establish) the links between action and results, especially for individuals.
It is potentially powerful, as shifting the distribution of common risk factors can have substantial effects on the incidence of disease.	May not be feasible where political interests do not lie with the social, economic and environmental well-being of the population.
It is behaviourally more appropriate, as the social, cultural and economic determinants of behaviour are addressed. This means that individuals are not being asked to change their ways against the grain of society.	There may be substantial costs, with benefits being seen only in the long term, and they may be difficult to attribute to the investment.
	Safety is paramount and is a potential concern for population approaches. On p. 1850 of paper A, the potential hazards of applying an intervention to a substantial proportion of the population are discussed. The example discussed is of a drug, clofibrate, which was used to lower cholesterol. The conclusion was that if (as in this case) a drug has even a slightly elevated RR and is given to very large numbers of people, the resulting numbers of serious adverse effects are disturbingly large.

Section 10.3

Exercise 10.3.1

1. The prevalence of cancer is $350/5600 = 6.25\%$.

2. The sensitivity of the test $= 325/350 = 92.9\%$ (95% CI $= 90.2–95.6\%$). This sensitivity is high, and is estimated fairly precisely due to the numbers of people in the study with disease ($n = 350$).

3. The specificity $= 4800/5250 = 91.4\%$: this is also high. We have not calculated the 95 per cent CI, but this would be even more precise than for the sensitivity, as there are many more disease-free people in the sample.

4. The positive predictive value (PPV) $= 325/775 = 41.9\%$, which is very low. As a consequence, subjects with a positive test (only 42 per cent of whom will turn out to have the disease) would need to be managed carefully and considerately. This is a result of the low prevalence of the disease, despite high values for sensitivity and specificity. Note that sensitivity and specificity are fixed characteristics of a given test, but the predictive values depend on the prevalence of the disease or characteristics being screened for. The negative predictive value (NPV) $= 4800/4825 = 99.5$ per cent, so subjects with a negative test could be reassured with a high level of confidence.

5. The accuracy of the test $= (325 + 4800)/5600 = 91.5\%$, which is good for a screening test.

6. The likelihood ratios for (a) a positive test $= 92.9/(100 − 91.4) = 10.8$, so it is nearly 11 times more likely that a positive test will be found in a person with the disease than in a person who is disease free. For (b) a negative test $= (100 − 92.9)/91.4 = 0.08$, so there is only an 8 per cent chance that a negative test result will be found in a person with the disease compared to a person who does not have the disease.

Exercise 10.3.2

1. Both distributions are unimodal and positively skewed. The distribution for respondents without back pain has a mean of 5.7 (SD 3.6), a median of 5 (IQR 3.0–7.0) and a range of 0–19. The distribution for those with back pain has a mean of 10.2 (SD 4.9), a median of 9.0 (IQR 7.0–13.0) and a range of 1–30. Thus, the distribution for those with back pain has a larger range and spread, with higher measures of central tendency, but there is considerable overlap between the two distributions. (For hypothesis tests of no difference between the two distributions, $p < 0.0005$ for both t-test and Mann–Whitney test.)

2. The cut-off score needed to ensure that test positive results included only people with back pain is 20, as the people without back pain have scores up to, but not in excess of, 19. At this cut-off, the test would therefore have a specificity of 100 per cent. However, the great majority of cases of back pain would be wrongly classified as false negatives.

3. The cut-off score needed to ensure that test negative results include only people without back pain is 1, as only scores less than 1 (zero) include no people with back pain. At this cut-off, the sensitivity is 100 per cent, as all people with back pain are included in positive tests. The great majority of people without back pain are wrongly classified, as false positives.

4. We discuss the score with the best discrimination after introducing the receiver-operator characteristic (ROC) curve.

Section 10.4

Exercise 10.4.1

1. Suicide rates among older age groups have reduced markedly for men aged over 45 since the 1950s. However, for younger age groups there has been an increase. In fact, for men aged 15-44 rates doubled, although for males 15-24 and 35-44 rates have decreased since the early 1990s.

2. This shows a period effect. A decline was experienced by all age groups at a particular point in time (late 1960s), albeit more marked for older age groups.

3. The reason for the period effect in the late 1960s is probably related to the introduction of natural gas for domestic use. Studies examining suicides by cause of death during this time noted that the reduction was associated with a reduction in the rate of suicides by domestic gas asphyxiation.

Exercise 10.4.2

1. These age groups are for the age at death by suicide.

2. For men aged 28 years (age group 25-34) dying in 1977 (period of death 1975-9), the suicide rate is (approximately) 15 per 100 000.

3. For men, the lines do not show a consistent parallel separation. In fact, while the older age groups do show some evidence of progressive (and almost parallel) decrease across age at death periods, the youngest age groups show the opposite – an increase across age at death periods. Thus, we might conclude that there is no evidence of a consistent period effect across all age groups but one explanation could be different period effects affecting suicide in older and younger men in quite different ways. We did notice that the reduction in age-specific mortality seen in the 1960s, which we suggested in Exercise 10.4.1 may be evidence of a period effect resulting from gas detoxification, was much greater among older men. These findings from period effect analysis for men should also be considered in light of the cohort effect analyses, which are studied next.

4. For women in the age groups 35-44 and above there is consistent evidence of decreasing suicide rates across the time periods, with lines more or less parallel. This is indicative of a period effect. At younger ages, there has been very little change in the rates.

Exercise 10.4.3

1. The suicide rate is (approximately) 11 per 100 000.

2. In contrast to Figure 10.4.3, there is no evidence in Figure 10.4.4 that the suicide rates were peaking progressively earlier as we look from 'earlier-born' to 'later-born' cohorts.

3. Since all birth cohorts (with overdose and gassing excluded) now show similar patterns of rates without progressively earlier peaking, we can assume that the period effect identified in Figure 10.4.3 applies to suicide by overdose and/or gassing, but not to other methods. This fits the explanation we considered earlier, namely the detoxification of domestic gas. To this can be added the increasing use of catalysers in cars, which effectively remove carbon monoxide from the exhaust. To reiterate, these would result in period effects because (i) they are introduced

at a particular time in history, and (ii) they will tend to affect all (or at least a wide range of) age groups.

4. In conclusion, from the period and cohort analyses of male suicides, we can say that there does appear to be a period effect for suicide by overdose and gassing and we have some plausible explanations for this (domestic gas and catalysers). Figure 10.4.3 showed evidence of a birth cohort effect and the exclusion of overdose and gassing in Figure 4.4 illustrated this very clearly once the period effect was removed. A number of potential social, economic and method (of suicide) explanations for this progressive rise in suicide rates with later-born cohorts of males since 1940 are considered in the discussion of paper B.

11

Probability distributions, hypothesis testing and Bayesian methods

Introduction and learning objectives

You will by now be familiar with the concept of an hypothesis test, and have used a number of the most common ones, including the chi-squared and the two-sample t-test (and z-test). We have also introduced somewhat more specialised tests, such as McNemar's test, which is used for matched categorical data (for example, in matched case-control studies – Chapter 5).

We have also described and emphasised the assumptions for each test, and pointed out that these should be assessed prior to applying any given test. One such assumption concerns the distribution of the data and how this can be related to a theoretical probability distribution. For example, you will recall that the t-test requires that the distributions of the populations from which the samples are drawn should be (approximately) normal, and the standard deviations similar. We will begin this chapter by describing the main theoretical probability distributions to help your understanding of the theoretical basis of hypothesis testing. We will also introduce some important probability distributions not covered in previous chapters, such as the Poisson distribution, which can be used to make assumptions about count data for rare events, and the binomial distribution, which is useful in quantifying the accuracy of estimates of disease prevalence.

The rest of this chapter is aimed at extending your knowledge of hypothesis testing in a number of specific ways:

- We introduce you to other commonly used tests for particular situations, including the paired t-test, which is used for continuous paired (or matched) data; analysis of variance (ANOVA), which is used for continuous data with more than two groups; and the chi-squared test for trend, which is used for ordered categorical data to assess the significance of a trend in the relationship between an exposure and an outcome.

- We discuss the use of transformation to convert skewed data into normally distributed data, so that the assumptions of the hypothesis test can be met for continuous data.

Quantitative Methods for Health Research   Nigel Bruce, Daniel Pope and Debbi Stanistreet
© 2008 John Wiley & Sons, Ltd

- We discuss the use of non-parametric tests, which do not rely on the distribution of the data: these tests are a very useful alternative to transformation for use with continuous data, or with ordered categorical data.

- In the final section, we will discuss Bayesian methods, an interesting and very different approach to determining the probability of an outcome that is gaining increasing recognition and application.

Before introducing these new hypothesis tests, we will review the key ideas about probability and the nature of probability distributions, and see how these distributions apply to the common tests we have already used – such as the *t*-test and chi-squared test.

There is no resource paper for this chapter, although examples will be used to illustrate all of the new hypothesis tests.

Learning objectives

By the end of this chapter, you should be able to do the following:

- Describe the main theoretical probability distributions, and their uses.

- Describe when it is appropriate to use a paired test (as opposed to an independent sample test) and carry out and interpret this test.

- Describe what is meant by transformation of data and how to select the appropriate power of the transformation.

- Describe when it is appropriate to use ANOVA and interpret the results of this test.

- Describe the key features that distinguish between parametric and non-parametric hypothesis tests.

- Describe, carry out and interpret non-parametric hypothesis tests for continuous or ordered categorical data in different situations (comparing two or more groups and measuring associations).

- Describe what factors should be considered when choosing an appropriate hypothesis test.

- Select an appropriate hypothesis test for use with different types of data and analytic requirements (e.g. comparison, association).

- Determine whether a set of data complies with the assumptions of the selected test.

- Describe how the problem of multiple significance testing arises, and utilise a suitable correction method.

- Describe the main features of Bayesian methods.

11.1 Probability distributions

11.1.1 Probability – a brief review

We previously discussed the importance of using data from a sample to draw conclusions about the population from which it was selected. For example, let's say we have identified an improvement in survival from a new treatment compared to an old treatment, in a sample of patients taking part in a trial. What we really want to know is whether this improvement would be seen in the whole population of patients, or whether it could be due to chance (sampling error). We introduced probability theory in Chapter 4, Section 4.2 and considered how we could use it to relate samples to populations and hence to draw conclusions about populations.

Before discussing this application of probability distributions further, it is useful to review the main properties of probability.

- The probability of an event can be defined as the proportion of times that the event would occur if the experiment or observation were repeated a large number of times.

- Probability lies between 0 (the event never happens) and 1 (the event always happens).

- The probability of the complementary event (the event does not occur) is 1 minus the probability of the event occurring.

- If two events are mutually exclusive (that is, when one happens the other cannot happen), the probability that one *or* the other happens is the sum of their probabilities. For example, a die may show a five or a six, but not both. The probability that it shows a five *or* six $= 1/6 + 1/6 = 2/6$ (1/3).

- If two events are independent (that is, knowing when one has happened will not tell us anything about whether the other will happen), the probability that both will happen is the product of their probabilities. For example, if a coin is tossed twice, the probability of two heads occurring is $1/2 \times 1/2 = 1/4$. We will return to this example when we look at *probability distributions* in the following section.

11.1.2 Introduction to probability distributions

When collected together, data from a sample (observed data) form an *empirical* or *frequency distribution*. In introducing descriptive data, we graphically represented data from a continuous variable (particulate matter in air pollution, PM_{10}) in a histogram showing the frequency distribution of the data (Figure 11.1.1). We described this variable as having an approximately normal distribution.

Frequency distributions display the actual data for a variable taken from a sample. In contrast, a *probability distribution* is theoretical and shows how the total probability (which equals 1) is distributed among the different possible values of a variable. As with frequency distributions, probability distributions can be illustrated as a histogram. An important example of a probability distribution, the sampling distribution, was introduced in Chapter 4. You will recall that this was a theoretical distribution, showing the probability of different values of the mean of a variable assessed through repeated samples of a given size. The concept of a probability distribution can probably be most easily understood though a simple example: Figure 11.1.2 illustrates the probability distribution for obtaining heads after two tosses of a coin.

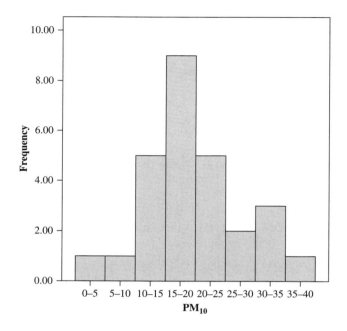

Figure 11.1.1 Frequency distribution of PM_{10} concentrations (same data as in Chapter 2)

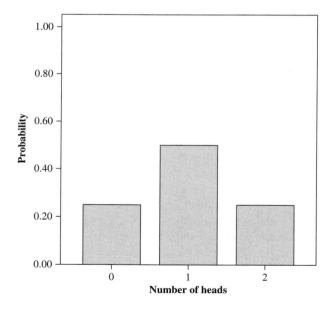

Figure 11.1.2 Probability distribution for obtaining heads after two tosses of a coin

The y-axis measures the probability for each value of the variable. We can see that the probability for obtaining zero (or two) heads is 1/4 (0.25), and it is the probability of obtaining a head after the first toss of the coin (1/2) multiplied by the probability of obtaining a head after the second toss of the coin (1/2). The probability distribution represents the probability of all possible events (no heads, one head and two heads), and therefore the total probability is 1.

This example only applies to discrete (categorical) variables (for example, tossing a coin can only result in two outcomes; a head or a tail). For continuous variables, the probability of any particular value is zero (as the number of possible values is infinite), so the ***probability density***, rather than the actual probability, is plotted on the y-axis. Figure 11.1.3 illustrates the probability distribution representing the probability density of the variable for the continuous PM_{10} data we studied in Chapter 2.

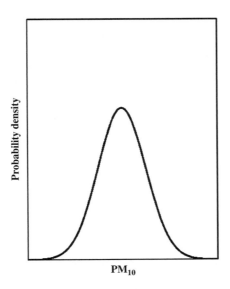

Figure 11.1.3 Probability distribution for PM_{10} data showing probability density

As with discrete variables, the probability distribution represents the probability of all possible values of continuous variables. Therefore, the total area under the probability density curve will be 1. The shapes of probability distributions are characterised by the same features as frequency distributions; for example, the number and position of modes (the values at which the probability (or probability density for continuous variables) reaches a maximum), the skewness of the distribution, etc.

When observed data form a frequency distribution which approximates a particular probability distribution, theoretical knowledge of that probability distribution can be used to answer questions about the data. The most common example is the normal distribution that was introduced in Chapter 4: we will now look at this in more detail, as well as other important probability distributions.

11.1.3   Types of probability distribution

We have already come across some of the more common probability distributions when we introduced hypothesis tests for continuous variables with a sample size of more than 30 (z-test) and a sample size of less than 30 (t-test, although applicable for all sample sizes) and for categorical variables (chi-squared test) (Table 11.1.1).

Table 11.1.1   Hypothesis tests and probability distributions described previously

Probability distribution	Hypothesis test	Where test described
Normal distribution	z-test	Chapter 5, Section 5.5.4
t-Distribution	t-test	Chapter 5, Section 5.5.4
Chi-squared distribution	Chi-squared test	Chapter 5, Section 5.5.3

There are a number of other probability distributions that are commonly used for data with various properties. Visual inspection of a set of observed data can often indicate which probability distribution is most suitable. Depending on whether the variable is continuous or discrete, the probability distribution can be continuous or discrete, examples of which are shown in Table 11.1.2.

Table 11.1.2   Example of continuous and discrete probability distributions

Continuous	Types of data
Normal (Gaussian) distribution	Continuous
Log-normal distribution	Continuous
t-Distribution	Continuous
Chi-squared distribution	Continuous
F-Distribution	Continuous
Binomial distribution	Categorical (dichotomous)
Poisson distribution	Discrete (counts)

Before we describe the practical application of probability distributions in making inferences from samples to populations, it is useful to summarise briefly each distribution and the **_parameters_** used to describe the distribution. Parameters are the mathematical properties that determine the shape and location of the distribution, allow the determination of the probability associated with specified sections of the distribution, etc. The mathematics involved in describing these probability distributions can be rather complex and is beyond the scope of this book. It is however, useful to be familiar with the different types of probability distribution, how these differ for different types of variable, and how each distribution is described by its parameters. This will help you understand the theory behind **_parametric_** hypothesis testing, and why we also sometimes need to use other procedures including **_transformation_** (Section 11.2) and **_non-parametric_** tests (Section 11.3).

1. Continuous probability distributions

Continuous probability distributions typically have no upper limit, and some have no lower limit. However, there are three other general points applicable to all continuous probability distributions, some of which have been touched on earlier. First, because a continuous variable has an infinite number of possible values, the probability of any particular value is zero. It is therefore only possible to calculate the probability that the variable will take a value within a specified range.

Second, as we saw in Figure 11.1.3, if all possible values of a continuous variable are plotted on a horizontal axis, we can draw a probability density curve. To do this, the equation of the probability distribution is used. The total area under this curve is 1 (equal to the total probability).

Third, to use a probability distribution, the area corresponding to a particular range of values is typically considered. We saw this when we introduced confidence intervals (CIs) in relation to the sampling distribution (Chapter 4). Because the sampling distribution has a **normal** probability distribution, we know that approximately 95 per cent of values lie between ± 1.96 times the standard deviation (σ) of the population mean (μ). Therefore we can say that there is a 95 per cent chance that we choose a sample whose mean lies in the interval $\mu +/- 1.96 \, \sigma/\sqrt{n}$.

(a) The normal distribution

The normal distribution is the most commonly used probability distribution. We described the normal distribution in detail in Chapter 4 (Section 4.4). A summary of what we already know about the normal distribution is given in the box below.

The normal distribution

- is described by two **parameters** (the **mean** (μ) and the **standard deviation** (σ))

- is **unimodal** and bell-shaped, symmetric about its mean

- usually has no upper or lower limits

- has a curve that is shifted to the right if the mean is increased and shifted to the left if the mean is decreased

- has a curve that is flattened if the standard deviation is increased and becomes more peaked if it is decreased

- is used to analyse continuous data from one or two large ($n > 30$) samples

- can be used to define **confidence intervals**.

As we shall see, other probability distributions (including discrete distributions) approximate the normal distribution under certain circumstances and therefore the normal distribution can often be substituted for these other distributions.

It is possible to test data statistically to determine whether they follow a normal distribution by either the Shapiro–Wilk W test or the Kolmogorov–Smirnov test. Details of these tests can be found in standard statistical reference books.

There are an infinite number of normal distributions depending on the parameters (mean (μ) and standard deviation (σ)) of the distribution. One frequently used normal distribution is the **standard normal distribution**. This distribution has a mean of 0 and a standard deviation of 1. The standard normal distribution is particularly useful because the probabilities relating to the distribution have been tabulated.

(b) The *t*-distribution

We used Student's *t*-distribution previously when carrying out an hypothesis test on samples with less than 30 subjects (the *t*-test) (Chapter 5, Section 5.5.4). The distribution has only one parameter, and this is the degrees of freedom, equal to the number in the sample minus 1 ($n - 1$). The *t*-distribution is similar in shape to the normal distribution but is more spread out with longer *tails* due to the typically small sample size. As the sample size increases, the shape of the *t*-distribution becomes increasingly like the normal distribution. This is one reason why the *t*-test is appropriate for both small and large samples.

The *t*-distribution is used for a number of hypothesis tests, including the two-sample (or independent sample) *t*-test and the **paired t-test** (introduced in Section 11.3 of this chapter). The distribution can also be used to calculate CIs for sample means.

(c) The chi-squared distribution

As we have seen, the chi-squared distribution is a particularly useful probability distribution for analysing categorical data (Chapter 5), although it is still a **continuous probability distribution**. This is because the critical value of the chi-squared test forms a chi-squared distribution. When we introduced this hypothesis test, we saw that the chi-squared probability distributions are characterised by their degrees of freedom. Typically, the chi-squared distribution is highly positively skewed; however, as the degrees of freedom increase, the shape of the distribution approaches normality.

In Chapter 5, we saw how the chi-squared distribution could be used in the chi-squared hypothesis test to compare two or more proportions. Later in this chapter, we shall look at other applications, as in comparing three or more groups of continuous or ordered categorical data when using the Kruskal–Wallis hypothesis test.

(d) The F-distribution

If two normally distributed populations have equal variances, the ratio of the variances of samples drawn from each should follow an F-distribution. The **F-test** is carried out using an **F probability distribution**, which is positively skewed. One important and common application is the use of the F-test prior to carrying out a *t*-test, in order to investigate whether the variances of the two groups to be compared are similar – one of the key assumptions that needs to be met for the *t*-test. Another common use is in comparing three or more means in one-way analysis of variance (ANOVA), which we will return to in Section 11.3.

2. Discrete probability distributions

As illustrated in Figure 11.1.2, for categorical variables it is possible to derive the probability of every possible value, and the sum of all these probabilities is 1. The two most common probability distributions for data with these properties are the binomial and Poisson distributions.

(a) Binomial distribution

If there are a number (n) of what are often termed 'trials' (a clear example being tosses of a coin) that are independent of each other, and in which the outcome is either 'success' (heads) or 'failure' (tails), the number of observed successes follows a **binomial distribution**. In our example in Figure 11.1.2, we had a variable describing the number of heads (successes) in two tosses of a coin, taking values of 0, 1 and 2. This was an example of the binomial distribution.

Let us now look at an example of the binomial distribution in a health context. If we carried out a survey investigating the prevalence of smoking in a population (π) and took a random sample, the probability of any subject chosen being a smoker is p. In effect, as we assess each person, we are carrying out a series of independent assessments (referred to as 'trials' above) where the person either does or does not smoke. In effect, we can think of this as having a series of independent trials, each with the probability of 'success' (being a smoker) of p.

If we were to repeat the study with a series of randomly selected samples, the number of successes (smokers) in these repeated samples will follow the binomial distribution. The properties of the binomial distribution enable us to say how accurate the estimate of prevalence obtained is. We can use the binomial distribution whenever we have a series of independent assessments (trials) with two possible outcomes. If we treat a group of patients, the number who recover has a binomial distribution. If we measure the blood pressure of a group of people, the number classified as hypertensive has a binomial distribution, and so on.

The binomial distribution has two **parameters**, the number of individuals in a sample (or repetitions of the individual assessments), n, and the true probability of success in each individual assessment, π. Because the number of different probabilities in a binomial distribution can be very large, we usually need to summarise these probabilities in some way. Just as a frequency distribution can be described by its mean and standard deviation (or variance, which is the square of the SD), so can a probability distribution and its associated variable. The mean (value for the variable we expect if we look at n individuals) is $n\pi$. The variance is $n\pi(1-\pi)$. When n is small, the distribution is skewed to the right if $\pi < 0.5$, and to the left if $\pi > 0.5$. As n increases, the distribution becomes more symmetric and approximates the normal distribution if both $n\pi$ and $n(1-\pi)$ exceed 5.

In studies of public health, the binomial distribution can be used if researchers are interested in whether or not a health event has occurred rather than the magnitude of the event. For example, when looking at a smoking cessation intervention we might be more interested in whether individuals successfully stop smoking rather than how much they have reduced their smoking in terms of numbers of cigarettes smoked. The binomial distribution is the most frequently used distribution to describe discrete data.

(b) Poisson distribution

Another important discrete probability distribution useful in health research is the **Poisson distribution**. This describes variation in the rate at which usually fairly uncommon events occur over time, or spatially, provided that these are:

- Independent of each other, meaning that the timing of an event (or its location) does not depend on another event that has already taken place;

- Occur randomly over time (or in space; for example, the pattern of cases across a Primary Care Trust area in the UK) (Figure 11.1.4).

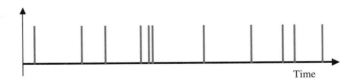

Figure 11.1.4 Events such as these that occur randomly in time and are not dependent on the timing of other events are described by the Poisson distribution

Examples of the Poisson distribution

A classic example of this distribution is radioactive emissions. You may be familiar with the Geiger counter that clicks as it is brought close to a radioactive source. These clicks speed up if either (a) the sensor is brought closer, or (b) there is a stronger source. Each click represents detection of an emission; that is, an event.

This is an example of a Poisson distribution because the timing of each detected emission (click) is independent of when others occur, and over time the pattern is random. Although a clear example, it is not particularly relevant to most health research. The same ideas can be applied to rates of disease (or death), where, for example, each new (incident) case is an event. Again, these must be independent and occur randomly in time or space. Some types of disease incidence, such as infectious disease, are not independent. Generally, however, so long as there is no strong evidence of 'clustering' of cases in time or space, it is acceptable to use the Poisson distribution.

Key features of the Poisson distribution

The shape of the Poisson distribution depends on just one parameter, the ***mean number of events*** occurring over periods of the same length (or over equal regions of space). This is called μ. Figure 11.1.5 shows the shapes of Poisson distribution for four different values of μ.

When events are very rare, there is a good chance of there being none or very few over the time period, and the distribution is therefore very positively skewed. However, as soon as we reach a mean of 10 or more, the distribution approximates closely to the normal distribution.

11.1.4   Probability distributions: summary

- A probability distribution shows the probabilities of all possible values of a variable.

- It is used to calculate the theoretical probability of different values occurring.

- All probability distributions are described by one or more parameters (e.g. the mean and standard deviation).

- The probability distribution will depend on the type of variable being analysed.

11.1.5   Probability distributions: implications for statistical methods

Many statistical methods are based on the assumption that observed data are a sample from a population and that the sample, if repeated, has a distribution with a known theoretical form. It is not possible to know whether this assumption is true, but only whether it is reasonable. If the assumption is reasonable, we can use methods making distributional assumptions (known as ***parametric methods***) that rely on probability distributions to calculate CIs and carry out hypothesis tests. We will look in more detail at the application of probability distributions to determining the standard error and precision of estimates and to comparison of groups using an hypothesis test later in the chapter.

If the assumption appears to be unreasonable, we need either to use statistical methods (e.g. hypothesis tests) that do not make such assumptions (***non-parametric methods***), or to ***transform*** our variable so that it does meet a distributional assumption. These techniques will be described in more detail in the following sections.

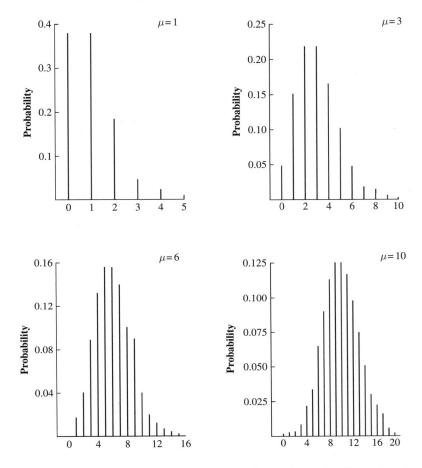

Figure 11.1.5 Poisson distribution for various values of μ Reproduced from Kirkwood B., *Essentials of Medical Statistics*. Wiley.

The following exercise will help to consolidate the ideas about probability and probability distributions we have covered in this section.

 Self-Assessment Exercise 11.1.1: Probability distributions

1. If the probability of a man aged 50 of having high blood pressure is 0.15 and the probability of his having a cold is 0.10, which of the following statements is correct?

   (a) The probability of his having both conditions is 0.015.

   (b) The probability of his having both conditions is 0.25.

   (c) If the man has high blood pressure, the probability of his also having a cold is 0.15.

2. Which of the following variables follow a binomial distribution?

   (a) The height of a sample of schoolchildren.

   (b) The proportion of adult men who smoke.

   (c) The number of admissions to hospital for a rare disease per month.

   (d) The number of people with back pain (assessed as yes or no) in a random sample of farmers.

3. Which of these statements is correct about the normal distribution?

   (a) It has a symmetric distribution about its mean.

   (b) It is followed by all continuous variables measured in humans.

   (c) It is the distribution towards which the binomial distribution will approximate as the number of trials (or the sample size) increases.

   (d) It is the distribution towards which the Poisson distribution will approximate as the number of events becomes rarer.

   (e) It is a common probability distribution followed by many variables.

Answers in Section 11.6

11.2 Data that do not 'fit' a probability distribution

As discussed in Section 11.1, there are often occasions when our data do not meet the assumptions required by statistical parametric methods using probability distributions. Parametric hypothesis tests are based on probability distributions and thus rely on more assumptions than do non-parametric tests. We must decide whether our data meet the requirements of a particular test by exploring the data (pictures and summaries) and using our own experience and knowledge of the situation. We may find, for example, that:

- the data are skewed, and do not appear to be from a normally distributed population; or

- the standard deviations of two samples are very different; or

- the relationship between two variables in a scatterplot looks curved, not linear.

When the evidence shows that the assumptions of a parametric test are not fulfilled, we may approach the analysis in one of three ways:

1. Rely on the *robustness* of the test we want to use (Section 11.2.1).

2. *Transform* the data into a new set of data that are consistent with the assumptions, and carry out the parametric test on the new data (Section 11.2.2).

3. Use a *non-parametric* hypothesis test (Section 11.2.3).

11.2.1   Robustness of an hypothesis test

We say that a test is **robust** to departures from the assumptions if we can still obtain valid results when the assumptions are not strictly met. For example, if we have large samples, the t-test can still be used even if the data are not from normally distributed populations: t-tests are robust to departures from the normal distribution for large samples. Also, as a rule of thumb, the two-sample t-test is fairly robust against unequal population standard deviations: if the ratio of the variances between the two groups is not more than 2, the t-test will generally remain valid at least when the sample sizes are similar. It is good practice, however, to carry out a test for equality of variance prior to conducting a t-test, and this is routinely done by software such as SPSS.

Since it may be difficult to decide just how far one can depart from the test assumptions, it is probably safer not to rely on robustness without seeking advice. If it is not safe to do so, we should consider either transforming the data or using a non-parametric test.

11.2.2   Transforming the data

The most common departure from parametric assumptions that we come across is skewed data. We know that survival-type data are generally positively (right) skewed, and so are many other measurements. Skewed data from human populations are almost always positively skewed, that is, with a long right tail, as in the example of survival data shown below in Figure 11.2.1, taken from Chapter 8.

We can sometimes overcome the problems of data that are skewed or not normally distributed by simply changing the scale of measurement; that is, by **transforming** the data. This means carrying out some calculation on the data. Examples of transformations include taking the logarithm of each data value (the most commonly used) and squaring each data value. If we can transform the data to a new set of values that meet the assumptions of a parametric test (e.g. that they have a normal distribution), we can carry out the appropriate hypothesis test on the transformed data.

The log transformation

The most widely used transformation for reducing positive skewness is the **log** (short for logarithmic) transformation, having the effect of stretching out the smaller values and squeezing together the larger values, and resulting in a more normally distributed set of data. This is known as the **log-normal probability distribution**. Figure 11.2.1 illustrates how log transformation results in a distribution that approximates the Normal distribution far more closely than the original skewed distribution.

We usually use the **natural logarithm** for this transformation. This is sometimes written ln instead of log, and the relevant key on most calculators is labelled **ln**. Note that it does not matter whether we use natural logs or logs to some other base (for example, the next most commonly used is base 10): the effect on the data is the same. However, we do need to know which base has been used when it comes to interpreting the results. We will now look at another example of skewed data and see how parametric assumptions can be applied.

Table 11.2.1 shows the vitamin D levels in the blood of 26 healthy men (Hickish, 1989). Plotting these data in a histogram shows them to be positively skewed, and that taking logs (natural) results in a distribution that approximates quite closely to the normal distribution (Figure 11.2.2).

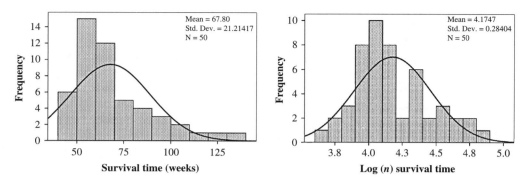

Figure 11.2.1   Log transformation of skewed survival data (from Chapter 8)

Table 11.2.1   Vitamin D levels in 26 healthy men (Hicklish *et al.*, 1989)

14	25	30	42	54
17	26	31	43	54
20	26	31	46	63
21	26	32	48	67
22	27	35	52	83
24				

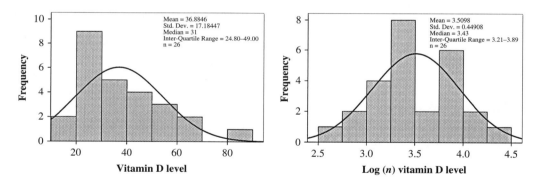

Figure 11.2.2   Skewed data on vitamin D levels (left) and log (natural) transformation (right)

The mean of the untransformed data is 36.88 (SD = 17.18) and the median is 31, consistent with quite marked positive skew. In view of this degree of skew, we would carry out analyses on the **transformed data**. For example, we can state that the mean of the log(n) vitamin D data is 3.51, and the 95 per cent CI for the population mean is 3.33–3.69. At present, these are still log(n) values of the vitamin D levels.

Interpreting the results

It is usually more meaningful to give results in the original scale. To do this, we have to do the opposite of taking logs, which is called **exponentiating**, or taking the **antilog**. We used this technique (exponentiation) to derive odds ratios from the regression coefficients in logistic regression, and hazard ratios in Cox regression. If x is an original data value, and $u = \log x$ is the transformed value, then $x = e^u$. This can also be written $x = \exp(u)$. When we exponentiate the mean of the logged data, we do not get back to the arithmetic mean of the original data. Instead, we obtain the ***geometric mean***.

The geometric mean is similar to the median of the original data and is always less than the arithmetic mean. It is not greatly influenced by very large values in a skewed distribution, so is a better representation of the average than the mean. Transforming our results back to the original scale, we have

$$e^{3.5098} = 33.44; \; e^{3.3284} = 27.89; \; e^{3.6912} = 40.09$$

So we can say that the estimate of the geometric mean is 33.44 with a 95 per cent CI (27.89–40.09). The geometric mean of 33.44 compares with 36.88 and 31.0 for the original mean and median, respectively, so it lies between the mean and median but slightly closer to the median. As an alternative, we could have summarised the untransformed vitamin D data by using the median (31) and interquartile range (IQR) (24.8–49.0). As we shall see when we look at non-parametric hypothesis tests in Section 11.3, the main advantage of using the mean and standard deviation derived from the transformed data is that we can still use ***parametric*** statistical methods, which not only produce CIs, but are also generally more powerful.

Other transformations of data

There are a number of other transformations that we can apply to positively skewed data, such as the square root ($\sqrt{x}$) or reciprocal ($1/x$) transformations, but these are less commonly used. The square root transformation is less dramatic than taking logs, but the reciprocal transformation is stronger and so can be useful for very skewed distributions.

Negatively skewed data can be made more normal with a power transformation, such as a square (x^2) or cube (x^3) transformation. There are many possible transformations: together, these are sometimes referred to as the ***ladder of powers***:

$$\ldots, x^{-2}, x^{-1}, x^{-1/2}, \log x, x^{1/2}, x^1, x^2, \ldots$$

The transformation x^1 leaves the value of x as it is. Provided $x > 1$, powers below 1 reduce the high values in a data set relative to the low values, and powers above 1 have the opposite effect of stretching out high values relative to low ones. The further up or down the ladder from x^1, the greater is the effect. Figure 11.2.3 illustrates the most common transformations for reducing skewness (x is the original data value).

Issues in interpretation of transformed data

The main problem in applying a transformation is how to interpret the results afterwards. The advantage of the log transformation is that the geometric mean and CI are directly related to the original data in an interpretable way. Unfortunately, no other transformation allows easy interpretation of the back-transformation in this way, and CIs in the transformed units are very difficult to interpret.

It is usually interpretability and the importance of a summary estimate and CI that determine whether the data should be transformed or not. It is quite common, for example, to see clinical laboratory measures which have a skewed distribution, such as serum bilirubin or lipoprotein, summarised by a geometric mean and CI (that is, a log transformation has been carried out). On the other hand, a clinical measure, such as time since diagnosis, might not be so easy to interpret after transformation, and so a non-parametric method could be adopted instead. However, this will be at the expense of difficulty in interpretation of CIs.

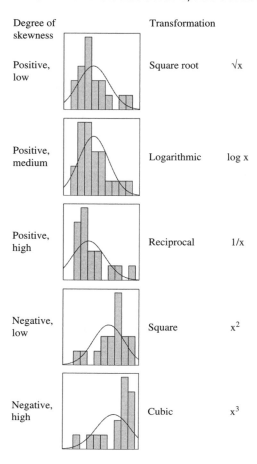

Figure 11.2.3 Common transformations for reducing the degree of skew in distributions

So, the decision about whether or not to transform the data will depend on a number of factors. Of course, there is also the option of using both transformation and non-parametric methods.

Summary: transformation of data

- Transformation is used to normalise data in order to apply parametric hypothesis tests.
- Data may be positively or negatively skewed: positively skewed data are much more common.
- There are a range of transformations that can be used, lying on a 'ladder' that defines the direction in which each alters the shape of the distribution, and the strength of that change.

- Log transformation, which may be to any base (natural, base 10, etc.), is most commonly used for positively skewed data. It is the transformation that allows the most meaningful interpretation of means and CIs.

- Analysis is carried out on the transformed data, and (for log transformations) values are exponentiated to obtain values for interpretation. The exponentiated mean derived from log transformation is known as the geometric mean.

- The decision about whether to use transformation or non-parametric methods for skewed data depends on a number of factors, including how interpretable geometric means will be, and the importance of being able to provide 95 per cent CIs.

- There is no reason why a combination of methods should not be used.

11.2.3 Principles of non-parametric hypothesis testing

We have seen that parametric methods for hypothesis testing require that assumptions pertaining to a probability distribution should be met. Where this is not the case, or it is not easy to check (as with a small data set), or it is decided that transformation would not be appropriate, **non-parametric** methods can be used. Such methods do not require the assumption of the normal distribution or any other probability distributions and are intended to overcome these problems.

Non-parametric hypothesis tests are sometimes called **distribution-free** tests, because the distribution of the outcome variable can take any shape and may be very skewed or non-normal. However, even though they do not have the strict assumptions of parametric tests with the appropriate probability distribution, this does not mean that the tests are assumption free. When we compare two independent groups of continuous observations, for example, the distribution of the values within each group is assumed to be similar in shape and have similar variance but the location of the distributions (e.g. medians) differs. Other assumptions will be outlined as we consider the more commonly used non-parametric hypothesis tests in more detail in Section 11.3.

Non-parametric methods can be used for continuous and ordered categorical data, such as scores. The most critical feature of these tests is that the **rank** ordering of the data is used, rather than the actual values themselves. The rank of a value shows its position in an ordered list of the data. For example, the ages 31, 57, 46, 65 and 49 have the following ranks:

Age	Rank
31	1
46	2
49	3
57	4
65	5

If two or more values are the same (tied), their rank is the average. In the following example where people are aged 49, ranks 2 and 3 are averaged, $(2+3)/2 = 2.5$.

Age	Rank
31	1
49	2.5
49	2.5
57	4
65	5

Using rank ignores the information in the actual numerical values. This is why these methods are also particularly suitable for data that are scores rather than measurements, whether the scores have many or few values.

Non-parametric tests are very useful when assumptions of the normal distribution are not met, but are less powerful than the corresponding parametric tests where assumptions for the latter are met. This means that if we use a non-parametric test we are less likely to reject the null hypothesis when it is false. So, if the assumptions are valid, it is better to use a parametric test.

The choice of statistical method will always depend upon several factors, such as the normality assumption, the importance of obtaining an estimate and CI, the ease of calculation and interpretation, and so on. We will frequently encounter non-parametric methods in the medical and health literature. In the next section we will look at non-parametric hypothesis tests alongside their parametric equivalents and discuss how and when each should be used.

11.3   Hypothesis testing

11.3.1   Introduction

In this section we will cover all the commonly used hypothesis tests. We have already introduced some of these in previous chapters, notably the chi-squared test and t-test, while others (including non-parametric tests) will be new. For those tests that have been previously described, we will revisit the circumstances in which they are used and refer to the relevant chapter and section of the book. Hypothesis tests that have not been covered elsewhere in the book will be described in detail with the use of worked examples. Section 11.4 provides a guide to help you choose an appropriate hypothesis test for any given comparison of data.

To start with we will review the key principles of hypothesis testing we have covered in previous chapters.

Review of hypothesis tests

We have seen that we use different tests for different data types and sample sizes (for example, categorical or continuous data, paired data, and small or large samples), and to answer different types of questions, such as (i) is there a difference between means? and (ii) are these two variables related? When we want to test an hypothesis, we must use a test that is appropriate to the data and to the question we want to answer. The following exercise will help you to recall some of the features of the two most commonly used hypothesis tests: the chi-squared test (Chapter 5, Section 5.5.3) and the t-test (Chapter 5, Section 5.5.4).

Self-Assessment Exercise 11.3.1

1. What assumptions should be met for the chi-squared test to be valid?

2. In respect of the two-sample t-test, (a) what assumptions do we make? and (b) how might you check that these assumptions are reasonable for your data?

Answers in Section 11.6

It is important always to check that the data meet the requirements of the proposed test – for example, by viewing a histogram to see whether we can reasonably assume that the data are from a normal distribution. If this is not so, the test may not be valid, and the results could be misleading.

Fundamentals of hypothesis testing

Let us also recall why we carry out hypothesis tests in the first place, and some general rules that all hypothesis tests follow. These points were described in detail in Chapter 5 (cohort studies) when we introduced the chi-squared test and t-test for looking at the results from the BRHS study.

Inference

We observed a number of interesting results in the BRHS; for example, that smoking was associated with an increased risk of IHD and that blood pressure differed between men with and without IHD. The fundamental question, however, was whether these results, observed in this sample of men, reflected the real situation in the population of middle-aged men in Britain from whom the sample was drawn. We noted that estimates from any possible sample vary from sample to sample (sampling error) and that hypothesis testing allows us to assess objectively whether the results observed in our sample are evidence of a real difference in the population or simply due to chance. Hypothesis testing, therefore, is an essential tool in the process of *inference*, relating findings from our sample to the population from which the sample was drawn.

The null hypothesis

Hypothesis testing essentially examines the probability that an estimate (e.g. the difference in mean systolic blood pressure) seen in the sample has occurred by chance and therefore does not reflect a true difference in the population. This premise means the starting point of hypothesis testing is to state the null hypothesis (H_0) (that there is no real association, difference in means, etc., in the population) and then the alternative hypothesis (H_1) (that there is a real association, etc.). If the null hypothesis is found to be unreasonable – that is, the data are not in agreement with such an assumption – we reject the null hypothesis in favour of the alternative hypothesis.

The test result – the p-value

We use an hypothesis test to determine the probability that the observed estimates from our sample occurred by chance, under the assumption that there is no true difference or association (H_0). We do this by using either probability distributions (parametric methods) or non-parametric methods.

The usual convention is that, if the probability of obtaining the observed difference (in this case), or one more extreme, is less than 0.05 (5 per cent, or 1 in 20) under the assumption of the null hypothesis (H_0), then it is sufficiently unlikely that we can reject the null hypothesis.

The acceptable level of probability for rejecting the null hypothesis is known as the significance level or p-value (alpha, α) and can be set at different levels depending on how certain we wish to be. However, while we might conclude that it is unlikely that estimates from our sample have arisen by chance under the assumption of H_0, we cannot say this establishes beyond all doubt that our sample estimates show there is a real difference in the population, but only that it is very likely. For example, with a significance level of 0.05, there remains a 1 in 20 chance that the observed difference could have arisen by chance; that is, it is a false positive, or Type I error.

Stages of hypothesis testing

Another important aspect we covered was the steps that should be taken in carrying out an hypothesis test.

1. Summarise data from the sample (e.g. difference in means, or in proportions with contingency table, etc.).

2. State the null hypothesis (H_0) and the alternative hypothesis (H_1) in relation to the sample estimate.

3. Carry out an hypothesis test appropriate to the type of data, having first checked that the relevant assumptions are met.

4. Obtain the test statistic (most commonly done by computer, which will also produce the result for step 5).

5. Assess the probability (p-value) of obtaining the observed test result (or one more extreme) by probability distribution-based (parametric) or non-parametric methods.

6. If the p-value is small (e.g. less than 0.05), reject the null hypothesis.

7. Where parametric methods have been used, state the estimate of difference or association, with the 95 per cent (or other level, as appropriate) CI.

We are now ready to look at specific tests in more detail, and will start with the type of data, comparison and test with which you are probably most familiar, a comparison of means from two groups, using the independent samples t-test.

11.3.2 Comparing two independent groups

We often want to compare two groups for a particular attribute measured on a continuous scale; for example, is the mean blood pressure of male smokers higher than non-smokers? These are independent samples because the groups are mutually exclusive; individuals cannot be in both groups. If the data conform to a particular probability distribution, we can use parametric hypothesis tests (the z-test or t-test) as long as the assumptions of the tests are met. If the data do not meet these assumptions, we will need to use a non-parametric, or distribution-free, method (e.g. the Mann–Whitney U test). Table 11.3.1 describes the main characteristics of hypothesis tests for comparing continuous data for two independent groups.

Table 11.3.1 Hypothesis tests used for comparing continuous data for two independent groups

Test	Parametric hypothesis tests Data/assumptions	Test	Non-parametric hypothesis tests Data/assumptions
z-test:	• Continuous data (sample size > 29) • Data have approximately normal distribution • Probability distribution (standard normal)	Mann–Whitney U test	• Continuous or ordered categorical data • No distribution assumption • Ranked data
	Reference: described in Chapter 5, Section 5.5.4		Reference: described in following section (11.3.2)
t-test:	• Continuous data (any sample size) • Groups have similar standard deviations • Data has approximately normal distributions • Probability distribution (t-distribution)	Wilcoxon signed rank test	• Continuous or ordered categorical data • No distribution assumption • Ranked data
	Reference: described in Chapter 5, Section 5.5.4		Reference: not described in this text. Produces identical results to the Mann–Whitney U test

The z-test and t-test were described in Chapter 5, Section 5.5.4. We will now look in detail at the non-parametric hypothesis test for continuous data (or ordered categorical data) for two independent groups – the Mann–Whitney U test. An alternative (Wilcoxon signed rank test) provides identical results to the Mann–Whitney U test and will therefore not be considered further.

The Mann–Whitney U test

As with all non-parametric hypothesis tests, the Mann–Whitney U test uses ranking of the data, rather than comparing the actual distributions. The following example describes how the test statistic is calculated and the result interpreted.

Calculation of the Mann–Whitney U statistic

Suppose that we have two groups of individuals with n_1 in the first group and n_2 in the second group. To carry out the test,

1. Rank **all** the measurements in ascending order

2. Sum the ranks of group 1 to give R_1

3. Calculate $U_1 = n_1 n_2 + \frac{1}{2} n_1 (n_1 + 1) - R_1$, and $U_2 = n_1 n_2 - U_1$

4. Set U to be the smaller of U_1 and U_2

Tables of critical values of the Mann–Whitney U statistic are available to determine the probability of obtaining the observed data under (H_0). These are tabulated for n_1 and n_2 less than 20. For larger values of n, the U statistic approximates the standard normal distribution.

Example

A study was set up to measure synthesis of alkaline phosphatase in two groups of patients: normal healthy subjects $(n = 6)$ and non-responsive patients with coeliac disease $(n = 7)$. The data for each group (including a histogram) are presented and displayed in Figure 11.3.1.

We can see that the data for both groups are not normally distributed, and therefore we should not compare the means of the two groups by the two-sample t-test. Instead we could compare the medians of the two groups and use a non-parametric test. The median and interquartile range (IQR) of alkaline phosphatase level for the two groups of patients are shown below.

Group	Median	IQR
Healthy subjects	0.485	0.450–0.613
Patients with coeliac disease	1.100	0.770–1.600

There does appear to be a substantial difference between the medians of the groups, but a non-parametric test is required to test whether this difference is statistically significant. We will now calculate the Mann–Whitney U statistic for $(n_1 = 6$ and $n_2 = 7)$ to check for significance, as follows:

1) Assign ranks to all the data (from both groups).

Healthy subjects	Rank	Patients with coeliac disease	Rank
0.42	1	0.75	6
0.56	5	1.60	12.5
0.46	2.5	1.10	10
0.51	4	1.60	12.5
0.46	2.5	0.77	7.5
0.77	7.5	0.80	9
		1.32	11
Total	$22.5 = R_1$		

2) Calculate the value of the U statistic, in this case,

$$U_1 = 6 \times 7 + \frac{1}{2} \times 6 \times (6+1) - 22.5 = 40.5$$

and

$$U_2 = 6 \times 7 - 40.5 = 1.5$$

Therefore, $U = 1.5$.

Note that either R_1 or R_2 can be used to find U_1 and U_2 (it does not matter which group is labelled as group 1), and that the ranks of equal (tied) values are averaged.

Healthy subjects
0.42
0.56
0.46
0.51
0.46
0.77

Patients with coeliac disease
0.75
1.60
1.10
1.60
0.77
0.80
1.32

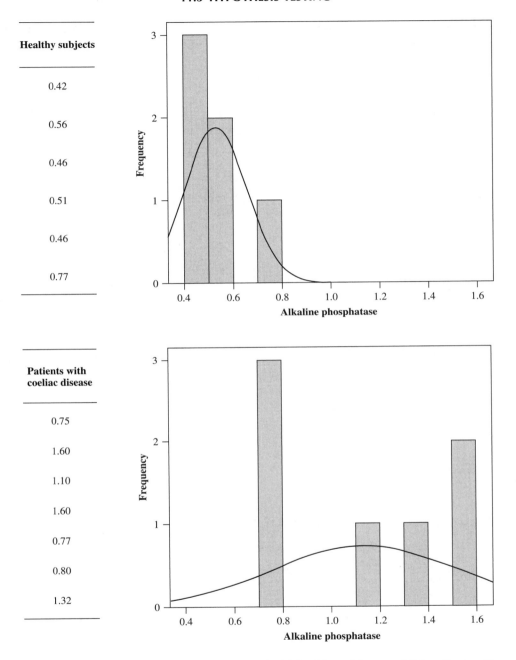

Figure 11.3.1 Alkaline phosphatase levels in (a) healthy subjects and (b) patients with coeliac disease

3) Compare the value of the U statistic to tabulated values of U. Below is an extract of the table of critical values for the U statistic (the values relevant to our example are shaded).

Table 11.3.2   Selected critical values of the Mann–Whitney U statistic

n_2	p-value	n_1					
		3	4	5	6	7	8
3	0.05	–	0	0	1	1	2
	0.01	–	0	0	0	0	0
4	0.05	–	0	1	2	3	4
	0.01	–	–	0	0	0	1
5	0.05	0	1	2	3	5	6
	0.01	–	–	0	1	1	2
6	0.05	1	2	3	5	6	8
	0.01	–	0	1	2	3	4
7	0.05	1	3	5	6	8	10
	0.01	–	0	1	3	4	6
8	0.05	2	4	6	8	10	13
	0.01	–	1	2	4	6	7

Using a significance level of 0.01 with sample sizes of $n_1=6$ and $n_2=7$, the critical value in the table is 3. The calculated value of U is 1.5, which is lower than the tabulated value. Note that, with this test, a value lower than the critical value denotes that the corresponding probability is achieved. Thus, the null hypothesis (there is no difference between the medians) is rejected ($p < 0.01$), and we can accept the alternative hypothesis (that there is a difference between medians). The box below summarises the main attributes of the Mann–Whitney U test.

Summary: the Mann–Whitney U test

Key features

- It is used to test the null hypothesis that the medians of two populations are equal.

- It is a non-parametric (distribution-free) hypothesis test.

- The data must be continuous or ranked (e.g. scores).

- The samples must be random.

- The samples must be independent (that is, a person cannot be in both samples).

Procedure
1. State the hypotheses

$$H_0: med_1 = med_2$$

$$H_1: med_1 \neq med_2$$

defining med_1 and med_2 as the population medians.

2. Decide on the significance level. Call this α (typically $\alpha = 0.05$).

3. Calculate the U statistic.

4. Compare the value of U with tabulated critical values of the U statistic, which is tabulated according to the sample size of the two groups (n_1 and n_2) to obtain the p-value.

5. If $p < \alpha$, reject the null hypothesis. Otherwise do not reject H_0.

6. State the conclusion and interpret the result.

11.3.3 Comparing two paired (or matched) groups

When we described intervention studies in Chapter 7, we introduced the idea of *paired* continuous data, with the example of before and after assessments of a sample of people with asthma. In this situation, we were interested in differences between the two assessments of a knowledge score in the same people. When our data are paired, we require a method to test the null hypothesis of no difference between the paired measurements. The parametric hypothesis test is the *paired t-test*, and the non-parametric equivalent is the *Wilcoxon signed rank test*. Table 11.3.3 describes the main characteristics of hypothesis tests for comparing continuous data for two paired groups.

Table 11.3.3 Hypothesis tests comparing continuous data for two matched/paired groups

Test	Parametric hypothesis tests Data/assumptions	Test	Non-parametric hypothesis tests Data/assumptions
paired t-test:	• Continuous paired data • Sample differences have normal distribution • Probability distribution (*t*-distribution)	Wilcoxon signed rank test	• Continuous or other ranked (e.g. scores) paired data • No distribution assumption • Ranked data
Reference: described in following section (11.3.3)		Reference: described in following section (11.3.3)	

The paired *t*-test and the Wilcoxon signed rank test are now described with examples in the following sections.

The paired *t*-test

For this hypothesis test, we will return to the before and after assessments in the sample of people with asthma. In this example, the two test scores for each patient are paired continuous data, and are shown in Table 11.3.4.

We saw that this gives us a series of differences $(A - B)$ for each person. The mean of these differences is 3.85, which is the difference between the mean of the 'after' scores (A) and the mean of the 'before' scores (B). As the data are paired, we need to use a paired hypothesis test. In this example we have continuous data (the scores), so we use a *paired t-test* rather than

Table 11.3.4   Test scores of asthma patients before and after attending a series of talks about asthma and its treatment.

Subject	Test scores		Difference (A − B)
	Before talks (B)	After talks (A)	
1	51	55	4
2	43	49	6
3	48	52	4
4	19	32	13
5	57	62	5
6	39	44	5
7	37	40	3
8	46	46	0
9	43	39	−4
10	43	52	9
11	53	50	−3
12	58	61	3
13	49	54	5
Mean	45.08	48.92	3.85

the independent-samples t-test. The calculation of this test is now described, using the data in Table 11.3.4 as an example.

Calculation of the paired t-test

As this is a paired test, we do not require the assumption of independence, nor do we need the assumption that each set of observations are drawn from populations that are normally distributed. We do need to be able to assume, however, that the differences between the paired observations (right-hand column in Table 11.3.4) are normally distributed.

In the example of subject 1 in Table 11.3.4 the difference between scores (After talks (A) minus Before talks (B)) is $55 - 51 = 4$. After calculating the differences between scores for each of the 13 subjects we have one sample of differences d_i with mean $\overline{d}$. To meet the assumptions of the paired t-test, we should check the distribution of the differences, and this is shown in Figure 11.3.2. Allowing for the small numbers, this can be accepted as normal. Generally, the distribution of differences tends to be normal, even if the original samples are skewed.

The next step is to test whether the mean difference is zero (that is, whether there is, on average, no difference between the measurements on each person). The paired t-test statistic is given by:

$$t = \frac{\overline{d}}{SE(\overline{d})},$$

where $SE(\overline{d}) = \dfrac{s}{\sqrt{n}}$ is the standard error of $\overline{d}$. The term s is the sample standard deviation of the differences and n the sample size – that is, the number of differences. Under the null hypothesis, this value comes from the same Student's t-distribution we used previously, on $n - 1$ degrees of freedom: note this is the number of pairs minus 1 (and of course is also the number

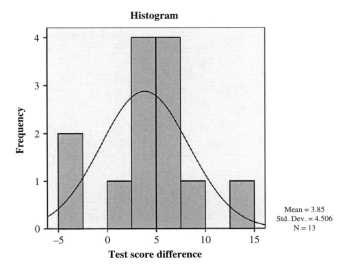

Figure 11.3.2 Distribution of the differences in the asthma test scores

of differences, -1). Therefore, we would reject the null hypothesis if our test statistic (ignoring whether it is negative or positive) were larger than the tabulated value at the required level of significance. Returning to our asthma example, we want to test whether the difference between the test scores for each individual is, on average, zero; that is, the talks have no effect on the patients' knowledge of asthma. More precisely, we test the null hypothesis:

$$H_0 : \mu_d = 0$$

where μ_d is the mean difference in test scores for the population of asthma patients. From Table 11.3.4, the mean of the sample of differences is as follows (note that four decimal places have been used to minimise rounding errors):

$$\overline{d} = \frac{50}{13} = 3.8462$$

and the standard deviation is $s = 4.506405697$.

The standard error of the mean difference is therefore

$$SE(\overline{d}) = \frac{s}{\sqrt{n}} = \frac{4.5064}{\sqrt{13}} = 1.2497$$

and the value of the t-statistic is

$$t = \frac{\overline{d}}{SE(\overline{d})} = \frac{3.8462}{1.2497} = 3.0777 = 3.08$$

We can then look up the value of t from tabulated critical values of the **t-*distribution*** (Table 11.3.5).

Table 11.3.5   Critical values of the t-distribution

Degrees of freedom	Two-tailed p-value			
	0.10	**0.05**	**0.01**	**0.001**
10	1.812	2.228	3.169	4.587
11	1.796	2.201	3.106	4.437
12	1.782	2.179	3.055	4.318
13	1.771	2.160	3.012	4.221
14	1.761	2.145	2.977	4.140

From the tabulated t-distribution on 12 degrees of freedom, we obtain $0.001 < p < 0.01$. There is strong evidence that the test scores differ, on average, in the population of asthma patients: the score obtained after attending the talks is higher than the score obtained before (positive mean difference). A 95 per cent CI for the population mean difference in test scores is given by:

$$\overline{d} \pm t_{n-1} SE(\overline{d})$$

where t_{n-1} is the two-sided 0.05 value of the t-distribution on $n-1$ degrees of freedom. The following exercise will help consolidate what you have learned about the comparison we are making and the hypothesis test.

 Self-Assessment Exercise 11.3.2

1. Calculate a 95 per cent CI for the population mean difference in scores (after - before) for the asthma example: you will need to use the critical value of Table 11.3.5 to do this.

2. Do you think the two-sided test was appropriate?

Answers in Section 11.6

Summary: the paired t-test

Key features

- It is used to test the null hypothesis that the population mean of the differences between matched pairs is zero.

- It is based on the t-probability distribution (will depend on its degrees of freedom $(n-1)$, where n is the number of pairs.

- The data must be continuous.

- The samples must be random.

- The samples must be paired (each subject appears in both samples or has a (well) matched partner in the other sample).

- The sample differences must be from a population with a normal distribution.

Procedure

1. State the hypotheses

$$H_0 : \mu_d = 0$$
$$H_1 : \mu_d \neq 0$$

defining μ_d, the population mean difference.

2. Decide on the significance level. Call this α. (Typically $\alpha = 0.05$).

3. Calculate the t-statistic.

4. Compare the value of t with the t-distribution on $n-1$ degrees of freedom and determine the p-value.

5. If $p < \alpha$, reject the null hypothesis. Otherwise do not reject H_0.

6. State the conclusion and interpret the result.

The Wilcoxon signed rank test

The non-parametric equivalent to the paired t-test is the ***Wilcoxon signed rank test***. This test is used with paired data when the distribution of differences in a continuous variable is not normal, or the variable is ordered categorical (e.g. scores).

Calculation of the Wilcoxon signed rank test

For n pairs of observations the procedure is as follows:

1. Calculate the signed differences between the pairs of observations (that is, observe whether the differences are negative or positive).

2. Rank the differences, ignoring the signs.

3. Sum the ranks of the negative differences to give $T-$ and the positive differences to give $T+$.

4. Set T to be the smaller of $T-$ and $T+$.

Tables of critical values of T for the Wilcoxon signed rank test are available to ascertain the probability that the observed data would arise under the assumption of the null hypothesis (H_0). These are tabulated for $n < 50$. For larger values of n, the T statistic will approximate the standard normal distribution.

Example

Eight pairs of identical twins were assessed for the effect of nursery school attendance on children's social perceptiveness scores. One twin was chosen at random to attend nursery school. After one term, the following results were obtained:

Pair	Score of 'nursery' twin	Score of 'home' twin	Difference	Rank +	Rank −
a	82	63	19	7	
b	69	42	27	8	
c	73	74	−1		1
d	42	37	5	3	
e	58	51	7	4	
f	56	43	13	5	
g	76	80	−4		2
h	82	65	17	6	

The median scores for nursery and home groups are 72.5 and 55, respectively, quite a substantial difference. The Wilcoxon signed rank test is used here to test for significance because (i) the data are paired by virtue of these being identical twins (so although two separate groups of individuals are being compared, they are very closely matched and can be treated as paired), and (ii) the distribution of the differences is not normal. In fact, the very small sample size makes it difficult to determine whether the distribution is normal, but it is assumed to be non-normal in this case.

Here $T- = 3$ and $T+ = 33$, and so $T = 3$. We can then look up this value in a table of critical values of T (Table 11.3.6).

Table 11.3.6 Critical values of T (for Wilcoxon signed rank test distribution)

n	Two-tailed p-value			
	0.10	**0.05**	**0.01**	**0.001**
5	0	–	–	–
6	2	0	–	–
7	3	2	0	–
8	5	3	1	0
9	8	5	3	1

From the tables, we can see that this result is just outside statistical significance at $p = 0.05$. Therefore, there is not quite sufficient evidence to reject the null hypothesis that nursery school experience does not affect the social perceptiveness of children. This could be regarded as an overcautious interpretation, as the p-value is right on the cut-off for statistical significance.

It should be noted that zero differences are discounted, n is decreased accordingly, and (as with the Mann–Whitney U test), tied values are assigned the average of the ranks covered. In an alternative approach, rather than rank the differences, sometimes the number of positive differences is used to calculate a test statistic that is then compared with a binomial distribution (or normal distribution for large samples). This is called the **sign test** and will not be considered further here.

Summary: the Wilcoxon signed rank test

Key features

- It is used to test the null hypothesis that the population median of the differences between matched pairs is zero.

- It is a non-parametric (distribution-free) hypothesis test.

- The data must be continuous or ranked (e.g. scores).

- The samples must be random.

- The samples must be paired (each subject appears in both samples or has a (well) matched partner in the other sample).

Procedure

1. State the hypotheses

$$H_0 : med_{\mathrm{d}} = 0$$

$$H_1 : med_{\mathrm{d}} \neq 0$$

   defining med_{d} as the population median difference.

2. Decide on the significance level. Call this α (typically $\alpha = 0.05$).

3. Calculate the T statistic.

4. Compare the value of T with tabulated critical values of the T statistic (tabulated according to the sample size of the number of pairs (n)).

5. If $p < \alpha$, reject the null hypothesis. Otherwise do not reject H_0.

6. State the conclusion and interpret the result.

11.3.4 Testing for association between two groups

We described how to summarise the relationship between two continuous variables when we introduced the principles of correlation in Chapter 2, Section 2.4. We found that if two continuous variables have an approximately linear relationship (as illustrated by a scatterplot), a correlation coefficient can be calculated to indicate the strength and direction of the relationship. The hypothesis test for assessing the probability of the null hypothesis being true is based on the value of the correlation coefficient (r). The method used for calculating r and its related p-value is the **Pearson** *(product moment) correlation*. This is the parametric hypothesis test for calculating a correlation coefficient. The non-parametric alternative is *Spearman's rank correlation* (Table 11.3.7).

Table 11.3.7 Hypothesis tests to study strength and direction of association between two groups

Test	Parametric hypothesis tests Data/assumptions	Test	Non-parametric hypothesis tests Data/assumptions
Pearson (product moment) correlation	• Continuous data • Both groups have approximately normal distributions • Linear relationship • Probability distribution (t-distribution)	**Spearman's rank correlation**	• Continuous or ordered categorical data • No distribution assumption • No assumption of linearity • Ranked data
Reference: described in Chapter 2, Section 2.4.5		Reference: described in following section (11.3.4)	

Spearman's rank correlation

Like the Pearson correlation coefficient, *Spearman's rank correlation coefficient* (r_s) can take a value between -1 and $+1$, and the interpretation of the value of the coefficient is essentially the same (although note that an equivalent coefficient of determination cannot be derived by taking the square of Spearman's coefficient). We may prefer this measure of correlation if any of the following are true:

• The data are not normally distributed.

• One or both variables are ordinal (have ordered categories).

• We require a measure which is not dependent on linearity.

Calculation of Spearman's rank correlation coefficient

For n pairs of observations $(x_1, y_1), \ldots, (x_n, y_n)$, this coefficient is most efficiently calculated as follows:

> 1. Rank each variable in ascending order.
>
> 2. Calculate the difference, d_i, between the two ranks for each individual i.
>
> 3. Calculate the sum of the squared differences; i.e. $D = \sum d_i^2$.
>
> 4. Spearman's rank correlation coefficient is then $r_s = 1 - \dfrac{6D}{n(n^2 - 1)}$.

Example

A sample of 10 students training as clinical psychologists were evaluated by a tutor at the end of the course according to suitability for their career (measure X) and their knowledge of psychology (measure Y). The scores on both measures were found to be highly positively skewed, so Spearman's correlation was chosen to study the association. The first two steps, the ranks and their differences, are presented below:

Student	A	B	C	D	E	F	G	H	I	J
Rank on X	4	10	3	1	9	2	6	7	8	5
Rank on Y	5	8	6	2	10	3	9	4	7	1
d_i	−1	2	−3	−1	−1	−1	−3	3	1	4
d_i^2	1	4	9	1	1	1	9	9	1	16

Hence, $D = 52$ and

$$r_s = 1 - \frac{6 \times 52}{10(100 - 1)} = 0.68.$$

We can then use a table of critical values of Spearman's correlation coefficient (r_s) to determine whether or not r_s differs significantly from zero (Table 11.3.8).

Table 11.3.8 Critical values of r_s (for Spearman's rank correlation)

n	Two-tailed p-value		
	0.05	**0.01**	**0.001**
5	1.000		
6	0.886	1.000	
7	0.786	0.929	1.000
8	0.738	0.881	0.976
9	0.700	0.833	0.933
10	0.648	0.794	0.903

We can see that our value of r (0.68) lies between the critical values for 0.05 and 0.01 with $n = 10$, so it is statistically significant. This can be expressed as $0.01 < p < 0.05$, and we can reject the null hypothesis that the correlation between suitability for career (measure X) and knowledge of psychology (measure Y) is equal to zero.

In addition to Spearman's rank correlation, you may also come across Kendall's tau (τ), which is a similar non-parametric correlation coefficient. We will not discuss that test further here.

Summary: Spearman's rank correlation hypothesis test

Key features

- It is used to test the null hypothesis that the population correlation coefficient is equal to zero.

- It is a non-parametric (distribution-free) hypothesis test.

- The data must be continuous, or ordered categorical (e.g. scores).

- The samples must be random.

- There is no assumption of linearity between the two variables, as it is the ranks that are being correlated. The data should be pictured on a scatterplot to allow meaningful interpretation of the Spearman correlations coefficient.

Procedure

1. State the hypotheses

$$H_0 : r_p = 0$$

$$H_1 : r_p \neq 0$$

defining r_p as the population correlation coefficient.

2. Decide on the significance level. Call this α (typically $\alpha = 0.05$).

3. Calculate the r_s correlation coefficient, and obtain the p-value (using tabulated critical values, from computer output).

4. If $p < \alpha$, reject the null hypothesis. Otherwise do not reject H_0.

5. State the conclusion and interpret the result.

11.3.5 Comparing more than two groups

We have seen how to compare continuous data for two groups by using the independent-samples z-test or t-test for normally distributed data, or alternatively by using the non-parametric Mann–Whitney U test for data when the assumptions for the parametric tests are not met. We might also wish to compare continuous data between more than two groups. The parametric method for comparing more than two means is ***analysis of variance (ANOVA)***, and its non-parametric equivalent for continuous or ordered categorical data is the ***Kruskal–Wallis test*** (Table 11.3.9).

Analysis of variance (ANOVA)

We will study this test with an example of data on systolic blood pressure (SBP) obtained from samples of four occupational groups in an industrial setting. The distributions for each group are almost normal and the variances similar (Figure 11.3.3), so we could use the t-test for comparing the mean SBP values for any two groups.

If we wish to compare mean SBP values for all four groups, we need to use ***one-way ANOVA***. This is simple enough to carry out with software such as SPSS.

Table 11.3.9 Hypothesis tests to compare continuous data for more than two groups

Test	Parametric hypothesis tests Data/assumptions	Test	Non-parametric hypothesis tests Data/assumptions
Analysis of variance (ANOVA)	• Continuous data • Three or more independent groups with normal distributions • Groups should have similar standard deviations • Probability distribution (F-distribution)	**Kruskal–Wallis**	• Continuous data • Three or more groups • No distribution assumption • Ranked data
Reference: described in following section (11.3.5)		Reference: described in following section (11.3.5)	

ANOVA separates the total variability in the data into that which can be attributed to differences between the individuals from the different groups (the **between-group variation**), and to the random variation between the individuals within each group (the **within-group variation**).

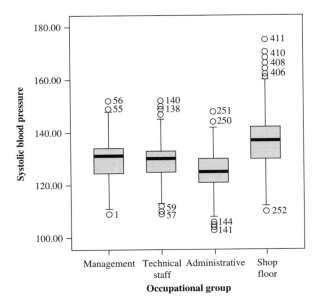

Figure 11.3.3 Box and whisker plot described below showing systolic blood pressure for four occupational groups

A box and whisker plot illustrates the distribution of continuous data. The box shows the median (thick black horizontal line) and the 25th and 75th centiles (bottom and top of the box, respectively) – hence the inter-quartile range (IQR). The whiskers, extending above and below the box show the range of values within 1.5 IQR below the 25th centile and 1.5 IQR above the 75th centile. Values outside this range are denoted as outliers and are indicated by subject id so these can easily be checked.

These components of variation are measured by variances (hence ANOVA). Under the null hypothesis, the group means are the same. If, however, there are important differences between the groups, the between-group variance will be larger relative to the within-group variance. The hypothesis test for one-way ANOVA is based on the ratio of these two variances and follows the **F-distribution**. In fact, it is the mean square of the variances that are compared – as explained in the example below.

As with other parametric (distribution-based) tests, there are assumptions that should be met, namely: (i) the data should be (approximately) normally distributed in the population, and (ii) the variance for each group is (approximately) equivalent: we saw from Figure 11.3.3 that this was the case. The mathematics involved in carrying out one-way ANOVA is complex and will not be considered further here. Standard software packages, including SPSS, provide output in the form of descriptive information and an ANOVA table displaying the value of the **F-ratio** and the associated p-value, and this is shown for the current example in Table 11.3.10. The first table shows mean values, data on the distributions, and 95 per cent CIs for each mean. The second (ANOVA) table shows the results for the significance test of the difference 'between groups' ($p < 0.0005$).

Table 11.3.10   Results from one-way ANOVA comparing mean SBP for four occupational groups

Staff group	N	Mean	SD	SE	95% CI		Min	Max
					Lower bound	Upper bound		
Management	56	129.9	9.5	1.27	127.4	132.5	109.0	152.0
Technical staff	84	129.4	8.4	0.92	127.6	131.3	109.0	152.0
Administrative	111	125.2	8.3	0.78	123.6	126.8	103.0	148.0
Shop floor	160	137.0	11.8	0.93	135.2	138.9	110.0	175.0
Total	411	131.3	11.1	0.55	130.2	132.4	103.0	175.0

ANOVA table Systolic blood pressure

	Sum of Squares	Df	Mean Square	F	Sig.
Between groups	9796.420	3	3265.473	32.849	.000
Within groups	40458.825	407	99.407		
Total	50255.246	410			

A clearer understanding of this test can be gained from looking at the ANOVA table in more detail. This shows the sums of squares (variance), degrees of freedom, mean squares (sums of squares divided by the df), the F-ratio (the ratio of mean squares), and the p-value.

The degrees of freedom for between groups is calculated as the number of groups (k) minus 1, so in this case, $4 - 1 = 3$. The degrees of freedom for within groups is calculated as the total number of subjects (n) minus the number of groups being compared (k); that is, $411 - 4 = 407$. The F-ratio (3265.473/99.407) is compared to tables of the F-distribution with ($k - 1 = 3$) and ($n - k = 407$) degrees of freedom, as shown in Table 11.3.11.

Table 11.3.11 Critical values of the F-distribution

df of denominator	p-value	Degrees of freedom (df) of the numerator				
		1	2	3	4	5
10	0.05	4.96	4.10	3.71	3.48	3.33
50	0.05	4.03	3.18	2.79	2.56	2.40
100	0.05	3.94	3.09	2.70	2.46	2.31
407	0.05	3.86	3.02	2.63	2.39	2.24
	0.01	6.70	4.66	3.83	3.37	3.06
	0.001	10.99	7.03	5.53	4.71	4.19
1000	0.05	3.85	3.00	2.61	2.38	2.22

We can see that our value of the F-ratio is considerably greater than the value for $p < 0.001$ for the relevant degrees of freedom in the table and is sufficiently large to indicate that the H_0 of no difference between groups is very unlikely. This result is consistent with the SPSS output, which showed $p < 0.0005$. We can therefore reject the H_0, although we need to look to the data to see which mean varies from which other mean. Exercise 11.3.3 takes you through this.

 Self-Assessment Exercise 11.3.3

1. From Figure 11.3.3, which groups do you think might have significantly different mean SBP?

2. Using the 95 per cent CIs in Table 11.3.10, summarise the differences between groups that appear to be significant.

Answers in Section 11.6

Summary: one-way analysis of variance (ANOVA)

Key features

- Is used to test the null hypothesis that the means of three or more populations are equal.

- Is based on the F probability distribution (will depend on its degrees of freedom).

- The data must be continuous.

- The samples must be random.

- The samples must be independent (that is, a person cannot be in more than one group).

- The samples must be from populations with normal distributions.

- The populations must have similar standard deviations.

Procedure

1. State the hypotheses:

    H_0: all group means in the population are equal

    H_1: at least one group mean in the population differs from the others.

2. Decide on the significance level. Call this α (typically $\alpha = 0.05$).

3. Calculate the F-ratio.

4. Compare the value of the F-ratio with the ***F-distribution*** for $k-1$ and $n-1$ degrees of freedom and determine the p-value ($k =$ no. of groups; $n =$ no. of observations).

5. If $p < \alpha$, reject the null hypothesis. Otherwise do not reject H_0.

6. State the conclusion and interpret the result.

The Kruskal–Wallis test

Staying with our example of the four occupational groups from the previous section, one of the other variables available from this occupational data set is alcohol consumption, in units per week. Figure 11.3.4a shows the differences between the groups and Figure 11.3.4b the distribution for one of these groups (administrative workers). You will see that the distribution is positively skewed due to a large number of non-drinkers, in addition to a small number of very heavy drinkers. We

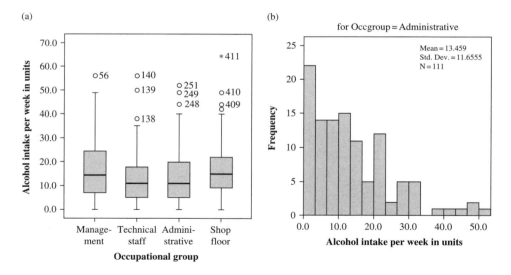

Figure 11.3.4 (a) Box and whisker plot showing alcohol intake (units per week) by four occupational groups and (b) distribution of alcohol intake (units per week) for administrative workers

could try log-transformation to normalise the distribution, but this is unlikely to help greatly due to the shape. A reciprocal transformation may be more effective, but will be difficult to interpret. In this situation it is more appropriate to use a non-parametric test to compare the average alcohol consumption between the four groups. The non-parametric equivalent to one-way ANOVA is the Kruskal–Wallis test.

Like other non-parametric hypothesis tests, the Kruskal–Wallis test uses ranking to compare groups and is an extension of the Wilcoxon signed rank test. Under the null hypothesis of no differences in the distributions between the groups, the sums of the ranks in each of the k groups should be comparable. After all the values in each of the groups have been ranked and the ranks summed, a test statistic can be calculated and compared to the chi-squared probability distribution for k (number of groups) minus one degrees of freedom.

For the alcohol consumption data, the chi-squared statistic is 15.84 (for three degrees of freedom). The p-value for obtaining a chi-squared statistic this large by chance (under the H_0) is p=0.001. Hence, we can reject the null hypothesis of no difference in alcohol consumption between groups.

This result does not tell us which group differs from which other group, and we have to go back to the data to assess this (Figure 11.3.4a and Table 11.3.12). Mann–Whitney U tests could be carried out to compare pairs of groups that appear to differ the most.

Table 11.3.12 Distributions for alcohol consumption by occupational group

Group	Median	IQR	Mean	SD	95% CI	Min	Max
Management	14.5	17.8	17.7	13.6	14.1 – 21.4	0	56.0
Technical	11.0	13.0	13.0	11.2	10.6 – 15.4	0	56.0
Administrative	11.0	15.0	13.5	11.6	11.3 – 15.6	0	52.0
Shop floor	15.0	13.0	16.9	10.8	15.2 – 18.6	0	64.0

Summary: Kruskal–Wallis test

Key features

- Is used to test the null hypothesis that each group has the same distribution of values in the population.

- Is a non-parametric (distribution-free) hypothesis test.

- The data must be continuous or ordered categorical.

- The samples must be random.

- The samples must be independent (that is, a person cannot be in more than one sample).

- The sample size should be sufficiently large for the analysis.

Procedure

1. State the hypotheses:

   H_0: each group has the same distribution of values in the population
   H_1: each group does not have the same distribution of values in the population.

2. Decide on the significance level. Call this α (typically $\alpha = 0.05$).

3. Calculate the test statistic.

4. Compare the test statistic with the chi-squared probability distribution for $k - 1$ degrees of freedom and determine the p-value (k = no. of groups).

5. If $p < \alpha$, reject the null hypothesis. Otherwise do not reject H_0.

6. State the conclusion and interpret the result.

11.3.6   Association between categorical variables

We have already come across the hypothesis tests for comparing whether there is a difference in proportions (or per cent) between independent groups (***chi-squared test***) or matched groups (***McNemar's test***) by a 2×2 contingency table. We used the chi-squared test to investigate whether there was a significant relationship between exercise and cancer in the chapter on cohort studies (Chapter 5, Section 5.5.3), and McNemar's test to investigate the null hypothesis that the population odds ratio was 1 for a matched case-control study (Chapter 6, Section 6.3). In this section we will see how a variation of the chi-squared test can be used to look for evidence of a ***dose-response*** relationship between an ordered categorical variable and an outcome of interest (***the chi-squared test for trend***). We will also introduce another hypothesis test that should be used if the assumptions of the chi-squared test are not met (***Fisher's exact test***). These tests are summarised in Table 11.3.13.

Table 11.3.13   Hypothesis tests to compare categorical data for two or more independent groups

Test	Data/assumptions
Chi-squared test	• Categorical data
	• Independent groups
	• >5 expected in 80% of cells
	• Probability distribution (chi-squared distribution)
Reference: described in Chapter 5, Section 5.5.3	
McNemar's test	• Categorical data
	• Matched/paired groups
	• Probability distribution (chi-squared distribution)
Reference: described in Chapter 6, Section 6.3.3	
Chi-squared test for trend	• Ordered categorical data
	• Independent groups
	• >5 expected in 80% of cells
	• Probability distribution (chi-squared distribution)
Reference: described in following section (11.3.6)	

| | Fisher's exact test | • Categorical data |

Fisher's exact test

- Categorical data
- Independent groups
- Typically used when < 5 expected in $>20\%$ of cells
- Probability distribution (F-distribution)

Reference: described in following section (11.3.6)

Chi-squared test for trend

For this test, we will use data from the occupational back pain data set (see Preface). Table 11.3.14 shows the proportion of women working in the manual occupational settings with back pain, stratified by age in three groups. We can see that there appears to be a greater proportion of women with back pain in the older ages.

Table 11.3.14 Proportion of female manual workers with low back pain by age group

| | Age group | | | | | | |
| | 18-29 | | 30-39 | | 40-49 | | |
	No	%	No	%	No	%	Total
Low back pain	30	22.1	49	24.6	64	36.6	143
No low back pain	106	77.9	150	75.4	111	63.4	367
Total	136	100	199	100	175	100	510

Using the chi-squared test detailed in Chapter 5, Section 5.5.3, we could test the null hypothesis that there is no relationship between self-reported back pain and age against the alternative hypothesis that there is a relationship. The chi-squared statistic is calculated as 9.88 for two degrees of freedom ($p < 0.01$); therefore, the null hypothesis can be rejected.

The chi-squared statistic would be the same no matter what the order of the rows and columns, and the test ignores the natural ordering of the columns. It can be seen that the percentage of women with back pain increases progressively with age. It is of interest to know whether there is evidence that the prevalence of back pain increases with increasing age; that is, there is evidence of a *trend*. You will recall that demonstrating an *dose–response relationship* is one of the features that Bradford Hill described as being indicative of causation. To test the null (H_0) hypothesis of no trend, we use the *chi-squared test for trend*, which has one degree of freedom.

Calculation of the chi-squared test for trend

Although the calculation of this test requires application of a detailed formula, the steps are not intuitively hard, and working through the procedure provides the most useful explanation of how the test identifies a trend within the data. This is explained in the following statistical reference section, using data from the back pain example (Table 11.3.14).

RS: Statistical reference section

The first step in calculating the test statistic is to derive the following information from the samples of individuals to be compared (Table 11.3.15).

Table 11.3.15 Observed frequencies and assigned scores for contingency table

Characteristic	Column 1	Column 2	Column 3	...	Total
Present (1)	x_{11}	x_{12}	x_{13}	...	R_1
Absent (0)	x_{01}	x_{02}	x_{03}	...	R_2
Total	C_1	C_2	C_3	...	n
Score	s_1	s_2	s_3	...	

The values required for the chi-squared statistic include the numbers of people with the characteristic (cells x_{11}, x_{12}, x_{13}...), the row total for those people with the characteristic (R_1), the column totals for each ordered category (C_1, C_2, C_3...), and a score assigned to each column of the ordered categorical variable (s_1, s_2, s_3...) – these scores are typically successive values, 1, 2, 3... Such equally spaced out values allow us to estimate whether there is a linear trend. Finally, we also need the total number in the sample (n).

The next step is to calculate the chi-squared statistic under the null (H_0) hypothesis of no trend by the formula:

$$\chi^2 = \frac{\left(\sum s_i x_{1_i} - R_1 \sum \frac{s_i C_i}{n}\right)^2}{\frac{R_1}{n}\left(1 - \frac{R_1}{n}\right)\left(\sum C_i s_i^2 - n \left(\sum \frac{s_i C_i}{n}\right)^2\right)}$$

While this formula seems quite daunting, all the values are easily obtained from the contingency table, and we shall look at an example using the data from Table 11.3.14.

Example

To investigate whether there is a significant trend of increasing back pain prevalence with increasing age, we:

(1) State the null and alternative hypotheses:

   H_0: there is no linear association between age and back pain in women in manual occupations.
   H_1: there is a linear association between age and back pain in women in manual occupations.

(2) Collect the information required to calculate the chi-squared test statistic from the contingency table.

   Taking the data from Table 11.3.14 and the template shown in Table 11.3.15, we get the following values:

Individuals with back pain in each category:	$x_{11} = 30, x_{12} = 49, x_{13} = 64$
Row total for individuals with back pain:	$R_1 = 143$
Column totals for each age category:	$C_1 = 136, C_2 = 199, C_3 = 175$
Scores for each column of age category:	$s_1 = 1, s_2 = 2, s_3 = 3$
Total in sample	$n = 510$

(3) Calculate the value of the chi-squared statistic specific to H_0:

$$\chi^2 = \frac{\left([(1 \times 30) + (2 \times 49) + (3 \times 64)] - 143 \times \left[\left(\frac{1 \times 136}{510}\right) + \left(\frac{2 \times 199}{510}\right) + \left(\frac{3 \times 175}{510}\right)\right]\right)^2}{\frac{143}{510} \times \left(1 - \frac{143}{510}\right) \times \left([(136 \times 1^2) + (199 \times 2^2) + (175 \times 3^2)] - 510 \times \left[\left(\frac{1 \times 136}{510}\right) + \left(\frac{2 \times 199}{510}\right) + \left(\frac{3 \times 175}{510}\right)\right]^2\right)}$$

$$= 8.54$$

(4) Compare the value of the chi-squared statistic to values from the chi-squared probability distribution with one degree of freedom, using a table of values for the chi-squared distribution, an extract of which is provided in Table 11.3.16.

Table 11.3.16 Critical values for the chi-squared distribution

Degrees of freedom	Two-tailed p-value			
	0.10	0.05	0.01	0.001
1	2.706	3.841	6.635	10.827
2	4.605	5.991	9.210	13.815
3	6.251	7.815	11.345	16.266
4	7.779	9.488	13.277	18.466
5	9.236	11.070	15.086	20.515

We can see that the value we obtained for the chi-squared statistic (8.54) is greater than the value for $p = 0.01$ but less than the value for $p = 0.001$ (one degree of freedom). Therefore, we can reject the null hypothesis that there is no linear association between age and back pain in this sample of women with $p < 0.01$.

 RS ends

Fisher's exact test

We saw that for 2×2 tables, the chi-squared test is not valid if any of the expected frequencies are less than 5. In this situation, we can use ***Fisher's exact test***. The test works by evaluating the probability associated with all possible 2×2 tables which have the same row and column totals (sometimes called marginal totals) as the observed data, under the assumption that the null hypothesis is true.

Calculating Fisher's exact test

We start with the 2×2 table, for which the row totals r_1 and r_2 and column totals c_1 and c_2 are fixed at those in our data:

	Yes	No	Total
Group A	a	b	r_1
Group B	c	d	r_2
	c_1	c_2	N

The probability of obtaining the cell frequencies a, b, c and d under the null hypothesis is given by:

$$\frac{r_1!r_2!c_1!c_2!}{N!a!b!c!d!}$$

where $x!$ is called 'x factorial' and means that we multiply together all integers from x down to 1; e.g. $4! = 4 \times 3 \times 2 \times 1 = 24$ (note $0!=1$). We use this formula to calculate the probability of observing each of the different tables into which the N individuals can be arranged, keeping the same fixed row and column totals. From this information, we can calculate the *exact probability* (p-value) of obtaining the observed set of frequencies, or a set that is more extreme, under the assumption of the null hypothesis.

Example

Data from a study of teenagers' eating behaviour (n = 16) were collected. Table 11.3.17 shows the number of males and females that were or were not dieting at the time of the study. We might hypothesise that the proportion of dieting teenagers is higher among women than men. Therefore the null hypothesis is that there is no difference between the proportion of male and female teenagers who are dieting.

Table 11.3.17 Numbers of male and female teenagers who are currently dieting.

	Males	Females	Total
Dieting	1	5	6
Not dieting	8	2	10
	9	7	16

Initially, we rearrange the 2×2 table so that the smallest value is in the top left-hand cell if this is not the case. The number of possible sets of frequencies which add up to the observed row and column totals (including the observed data) is shown in Table 11.3.18, together with the probabilities of observing such data if the null hypothesis were true, calculated by the above formula.

The observed data are shown in Table 11.3.18(ii) and the probability of observing such data if the null hypothesis were true is calculated as

$$\frac{6!10!9!7!}{16!1!5!8!2!} = \frac{6 \times 9 \times 7 \times 6 \times 5 \times 4 \times 3}{16 \times 15 \times 14 \times 13 \times 12 \times 11} = 0.02360$$

The other probabilities are calculated in a similar way. Notice how the factorials simplify by cancelling out sequences that appear on the top and bottom of the formula. If we do not simplify, the factorial multiplication might exceed the storage capacity of a calculator. We can check our calculations by adding up the probabilities for each table, which should sum to one.

Table 11.3.18 All possible 2×2 tables with fixed marginal based on data in Table 11.3.17, with exact probabilities

(i)	$\begin{array}{cc} 0 & 6 \\ 9 & 1 \end{array}$	$p = 0.00087$	(v)	$\begin{array}{cc} 4 & 2 \\ 5 & 5 \end{array}$	$p = 0.33042$
(ii)	$\begin{array}{cc} 1 & 5 \\ 8 & 2 \end{array}$	$p = 0.02360$	(vi)	$\begin{array}{cc} 5 & 1 \\ 4 & 6 \end{array}$	$p = 0.11014$
(iii)	$\begin{array}{cc} 2 & 4 \\ 7 & 3 \end{array}$	$p = 0.15734$	(vii)	$\begin{array}{cc} 6 & 0 \\ 3 & 7 \end{array}$	$p = 0.01049$
(iv)	$\begin{array}{cc} 3 & 3 \\ 6 & 4 \end{array}$	$p = 0.36713$			

The probability of obtaining a difference between the two groups as large as or larger than the observed difference is found by adding up the probabilities for the tables that correspond to the observed data and those that would give a more extreme difference between the two groups, which in this case is just Table 11.3.18(i) and (ii):

$$p = (0.00087 + 0.02360) \times 2 = 0.049.$$

The probability is doubled ($\times 2$) because we are using a ***two-sided*** test. This is the most common approach, and allows for the fact that the difference between groups could be in either direction; that is, more or less females are dieting than males. A ***one-sided*** test is less common and is used when the difference could only be in one direction. In our example, therefore, we can conclude that there is some evidence ($p < 0.05$, just) to suggest that the proportion of dieting teenagers is higher in females than in males.

An alternative way of deriving the p-value for a two-sided test, which is sometimes adopted, is to add together the probabilities of all the tables that have probabilities less than or equal to that for the observed data. In our example this would give

$$p = 0.00087 + 0.02360 + 0.01049 = 0.035.$$

This method always gives a p-value that is less than or equal to the first method, so it is less conservative (more likely to result in rejecting the null hypothesis).

11.4 Choosing an appropriate hypothesis test

11.4.1 Introduction

This section is designed to help in the process of selecting the appropriate hypothesis test (or tests – as often there may be more than one suitable method) for the commonly encountered types of data and analytic procedures. Table 11.4.1 serves as a guide for making these choices: we will shortly work through one example to illustrate how to use the table, and this is followed by some exercises for you to try.

We have emphasised on several occasions the importance of checking, summarising and displaying data before carrying out any hypothesis test, and the methods for doing this have been covered in previous chapters. Once we are satisfied that the data are 'clean', and we are familiar with how they are distributed and so on, it is time to select the right test. The following exercise provides some revision on the correct steps, before we look in detail at Table 11.4.1.

 Self-Assessment Exercise 11.4.1

List all of the issues that need to be considered when choosing an appropriate hypothesis test.

Answers in Section 11.6

11.4.2 Using a guide table for selecting a hypothesis test

Table 11.4.1 presents all of the basic hypothesis tests discussed in this chapter, together with the main features of each, and the situations for which they are most appropriate. The following example will illustrate how the table is organised.

Let's say we have two groups of primary school-age children living in poor areas of two cities (A and B) of a middle-income country where lead in paint is still common. Both groups have been sampled using random methods so that they represent the two cities. In one of the cities (B), a campaign has been running for the last few years to educate families about the danger of lead and to reduce the availability of paints with high lead content. The children's blood lead levels have been measured, and the distributions are found to be highly skewed, though more so in city A than city B, but are more or less normalised by log transformation. The variances for the two samples are not dissimilar, but that for city B is about 75 per cent of that in city A.

We wish to compare the blood lead levels obtained from the two cities to see whether the campaign has started to have any impact, given that a similar study carried out 5 years earlier found no difference between the cities. We have calculated means and SDs, and medians and IQRs, and it does appear that the levels in city B are lower than those in city A. Which test should we use to determine whether this difference is statistically significant?

So let's look at Table 11.4.1 and work through the steps. Blood lead levels are continuous data, and the children are in two independent groups; this takes us to the first two columns on the left of the table. We are making a comparison of means, so we look in the row labelled 'hypothesis test for comparison', which shows *t*-test, *z*-test and Mann–Whitney U test. Although the standard deviations are not too dissimilar for use of the independent sample *t*-test, we know the distributions are markedly skewed, and in fact more or less log normal, which raises doubts about using one of the parametric tests (t-test or *z*-test). So now we have two options, either to transform the data and use an independent sample *t*-test, or to use the non-parametric Mann–Whitney U test.

The final choice will depend on how we wish to present the data, and at this point you may wish to refer back to Section 11.2.2 on transformation. If we want to retain information about a mean difference and 95 per cent CI, we may opt for log transformation and the *t*-test, though this will provide a geometric mean and 95 per cent CI. If we want to retain the untransformed values, we can present medians and IQRs and use the Mann–Whitney U test. Alternatively, we can use both approaches.

Table 11.4.1 Table for selecting hypothesis tests according to main attributes: data, comparison groups, data type, distribution and purpose of test. In selecting an individual test, be sure that the assumptions for that test are met (these are not stated in full in this table)

Data	Continuous (and ordered categorical)					Categorical			
Comparison groups	Two groups		Three + groups		Rare count data	Two groups		Three + groups	
	Independent	Matched or paired	Independent			Independent	Matched or paired	No order	Ordered
Data type	Parametric / Non-parametric	Parametric / Non-parametric	Parametric / Non-parametric						
Distribution	Normal / Skewed	Normal / Skewed	Normal / Skewed		Skewed/ Poisson	Chi-square/ binomial	Chi-square/ binomial		
Hypothesis test for comparison	z-test (n ≥ 30) / t-test (n < 30) — Mann–Whitney U Test($)	Paired t-test / Wilcoxon signed rank test($)	Analysis of variance (ANOVA) / Kruskal–Wallis test($)	Poisson hypothesis test		Chi-squared test* (n ≥ 5 expected in 80% of cells); Fisher's Exact (n < 5 expected in ≥20% of cells)	McNemar's test	Chi-squared test* (n ≥ 5 expected in 80% of cells); Fisher's Exact (n < 5 expected in ≥20% of cells)	Chi-squared test for trend
Hypothesis test for association (~)	Pearson product moment correlation / Spearman's rank correlation		Pearson correlation matrix (#) / Spearman's correlation matrix (#)			Chi-squared test* (n ≥ 5 expected in 80% of cells); Fisher's Exact (n < 5 expected in ≥ 20% of cells)	McNemar's test	Chi-squared test* (n ≥ 5 expected in 80% of cells); Fisher's Exact (n < 5 expected in ≥ 20% of cells)	Chi-squared test for trend

If distributional assumptions not met (e.g. skewed), we can consider normalisation with transformation and then use the appropriate parametric hypothesis test. otherwise use a non-parametric hypothesis test.

~ Whilst correlation coefficients indicate the strength of an association for continuous (or ordered categorical) data, hypothesis tests for associations with categorical data do not.

* Note: With small numbers a Yates continuity correction is required.

$ Non-parametric tests can also be used if assumptions of parametric tests are not met (e.g. equality of variance for independent t-test).

Whilst correlation matrices have not been covered in this book they present the results of multiple simple correlations (depending on the number of groups being looked at).

Try using Table 11.4.1 in answering the questions in the next exercise. Detailed information about the nature of the data and whether assumptions are met is not given, so you will need to think about the options you have for different tests.

 Self-Assessment Exercise 11.4.2

Which statistical test would you use to analyse the following:

a) To compare the number of cigarette smokers among cancer cases and age/sex-matched healthy controls?

b) To look at the relationship between cigarette smoking and presence/absence of respiratory symptoms in a group of people with asthma?

c) To look at the relationship between cigarette smoking (yes/no) and sex (male/female) in a small pilot study of 40 undergraduate students in their first year?

d) To examine the change in respiratory symptom prevalence in a group of people with asthma from winter to summer?

e) To compare the serum thyroxine levels during pregnancy of the mothers of two groups of babies? The first group of seven mothers had babies who died and the second group of 13 mothers had babies who survived.

f) To compare the number of cigarette smokers among a group of cancer cases and a random sample of the general population?

g) To compare mean peak flow rate values (l/min) in a group of women as measured by two different instruments.

h) To compare knowledge scores about dangers of alcohol among groups of Year 10 children in four schools?

i) To investigate the association between (i) lead levels in a sample of children from one of the two cities in the example discussed above, and (ii) the same children's scores from a 15-point reading aptitude test?

Answers in Section 11.6

11.4.3   The problem of multiple significance testing

When we carry out multiple hypothesis tests on a number of different comparisons, there is an increased probability of finding a significant difference just by chance. Using a significance (alpha) level of 0.05, each test has a 5 per cent chance of a false-positive result when there is no real difference (type I error). So, if in a study we carry out, say, 22 comparisons with hypothesis tests, the probability of at least one false positive is greater than 5 per cent.

To deal with this problem there are a number of statistical methods aimed at controlling the overall type I error rate at no more than 5 per cent (or some other specified level). The disadvantage of all of these methods is that they are conservative and are likely to err on the side of safety (non-significance).

For example, we will consider a commonly used method of correction for multiple significance testing, the Bonferroni method (Altman, 1991, p. 211). This is the most conservative method of correction, and is carried out as follows: if we perform k comparisons, we should multiply the p value from each test by k; that is, we calculate p(corrected) $= k$p. So, if we have 10 tests, a p-value will have to be $< (0.05/10)$ or < 0.005 to be accepted as significant.

There are other, less conservative, methods of correction for multiple significance testing (for example, Duncan's multiple range test), and you will find that different statistical packages use different multiple comparison procedures. It is advisable to consult a statistician before using one of these statistical correction methods.

11.5 Bayesian methods

11.5.1 Introduction: a different approach to inference

In all the material we have covered so far, there has been a common theme of inference from sample to population, using hypothesis tests to determine the probability that we could obtain the observed data (e.g. a difference in means) under an assumption of the null hypothesis (H_o; no effect). If that probability is low (less than 5 per cent), we conventionally reject the null hypothesis and conclude that there is a real difference. This approach is sometimes referred to as *frequentist*, since it is based on frequency distributions of statistics (e.g. the mean) seen with all possible samples from a given population (see Chapter 4).

Bayesian methods, named after Thomas Bayes, who first published (posthumously) on these ideas in 1763, takes an alternative approach. In essence, the existing view about the probability of an event or effect (known as the *prior probability*) is first stated, and then modified by the current assessment (for example, a diagnostic test, or trial of a drug) to produce a new judgement about the probability of that effect or event (known as the *posterior probability*). The process is described by a formula, which is discussed in the following section, together with an exercise to work through.

Bayesian methods are considered controversial, not least for what is seen by 'frequentists' to be the potentially arbitrary and subjective way in which the prior probability is established. Supporters argue, however, that the flexibility of the method and the nature of its outcome (the posterior probability) have a number of advantages over traditional methods, and greater relevance to policy and practice. These issues are briefly discussed in Section 11.5.3.

11.5.2 Bayes' theorem and formula

A reasonably accessible way to understand the application of Bayes' theorem can be appreciated through the example of a screening test to establish the probability of a person having a disease. In this context, the theorem is described by the following formula:

Posterior odds of a disease $=$ prior odds $\times$ likelihood ratio of a positive test result.

You will recall that we introduced and calculated the likelihood ratio in Chapter 10 (validation of screening tests), and formulae for this and for the odds required to make the calculations are shown below:

$$[1] \text{ Prior odds} = \frac{\text{Prior probability}}{1 - \text{prior probability}}$$

$$[2] \text{ Likelihood ratio (for positive test)} = \frac{\text{Sensitivity}}{1 - \text{specificity}}$$

$$[3] \text{ Posterior probability} = \frac{\text{Posterior odds}}{1 + \text{posterior odds}}$$

We will now see how to apply Bayes' theorem through the following exercise.

 ### Self-Assessment Exercise 11.5.1

A woman aged 36 attends the GP for contraceptive advice. She smokes 20 cigarettes per day, has had more than five sexual partners in the last few years, and has tended to avoid barrier contraception. She also mentions that she may have noticed some vaginal bleeding. The GP sees from the records that the woman is due for a cervical smear test, and notes that she has several risk factors for cervical cancer (smoking, multiple partners and lack of barrier contraception), and possibly an important symptom (bleeding). The GP establishes a moderately high prior probability, which we will state as 40 per cent (0.40).

1. Calculate the prior odds.

2. The GP takes a smear test. Assuming the sensitivity of the test is 80 per cent and the specificity is 70 per cent, calculate the likelihood ratio for a positive test.

3. The smear test is positive. Calculate the posterior odds, and hence the posterior probability that the woman has cervical cancer.

4. Can you obtain the same result (approximately) by using Fagan's nomogram (Figure 11.5.1). This chart is used by running a line from the prior probability, through the likelihood ratio, to find the posterior (post-test) probability.

5. Interpret the result in the light of what we have discussed about Bayesian methods.

6. If the woman had a history indicating a very low risk (this is a routine smear, she is a non-smoker, unmarried and without a sexual partner for more than 5 years, and with no bleeding), the GP may assume a much lower prior probability; let's say 0.05 (5 per cent). This implies the GP thinks cervical cancer is unlikely, although it is still possible. This woman also has a positive smear test. Use the nomogram (Figure 11.5.1) to obtain the posterior probability that she has cervical cancer, and interpret the result.

Answers in Section 11.6

11.5.3 Application and relevance

Bayesian methods are used in many different disciplines, including 'engineering, image processing, expert systems, decision analysis, gene sequencing, financial predictions and increasingly in complex epidemiological models' (Spiegelhalter *et al.*, 1999). The method is thought to be intuitive

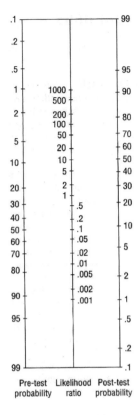

Figure 11.5.1 Fagan's nomogram

and conforms to practice: a common example (as we have seen with Exercise 11.5.1) being clinical practice in which a physician has some judgement (prior probability) about a patient having a particular disease, which is modified by current assessment (history, clinical examination and diagnostic tests) to help the doctor decide on the probability of the diagnosis (the posterior probability). In health research, Bayesian methods have been applied quite extensively with trials and meta-analyses, although the results do not yet have the same level of acceptance as traditional frequentist methods.

A number of advantages of Bayesian methods are described, however, including:

- Decisions about the prior probability (which, remember, must be stated) can make explicit assumptions and raise issues that often are not openly acknowledged in traditional approaches. Sources for the prior probability can include a wide range of information, including previous studies in the literature, meta-analyses, and expert opinion. The prior probability can be deliberately set as 'sceptical' if caution seems warranted, or alternatives can be used in sensitivity analysis to see how much influence variation across a range of prior probabilities might have.

- The conclusion, that is, the posterior probability, tells us how the latest piece of evidence should change what is currently believed and/or done. This has been argued to be of greater relevance to policy and practice than the output of traditional methods.

It is not possible in a brief introduction to do justice to the debates around the use and interpretation of Bayesian methods, and interested readers should look to more detailed publications on the topic (for example, Bolstad, 2004).

11.6 Answers to self-assessment exercises

Section 11.1

Exercise 11.1.1

1. (a) True. Events are independent, so the probabilities are multiplied.

   (b) False. The probability for both must be less than that for each one.

   (c) False. The events are independent. This means that the probability of having a cold will still be 0.10.

2. (a) No. This is a continuous variable and therefore will follow a continuous probability distribution.

   (b) No. It is the number of adult male smokers that will follow the binomial distribution, not the proportion. Proportions follow the chi-squared distribution.

   (c) No. As it is rare (count data), this variable should follow the Poisson distribution.

   (d) Yes. This variable will follow the binomial distribution, as there are only two possible events (back pain or no back pain).

3. (a) True.

   (b) False. Continuous random variables can also be positively or negatively skewed. We will consider this in more detail in section 11.2.

   (c) True.

   (d) False. The Poisson distribution becomes more normal as its mean increases.

   (e) True.

Section 11.3

Exercise 11.3.1

1. Data should be from independent groups, the comparison must be of categorical data and in the form of counts (numbers), and at least 80 per cent of cells must have an expected value of 5 or more.

2. (a) Data should be from independent groups and continuous. Data are from population(s) with (approximately) symmetric normal distribution(s). It is the appropriate test for small samples ($n < 30$), but can be (and usually is) used for larger sample sizes. The standard deviations of the two groups being compared should be similar.

   (b) It should be clear from the description of the data whether they are continuous, and the samples independent. Histograms could be used to assess whether the data appear to be from normal distributions, although this can be difficult to assess with very small samples. The sample variances should be checked to see whether they are similar: if the larger sample variance is more than twice the smaller variance, the samples may be from populations with unequal standard deviations. This can be tested by the F-test (and F-distribution), a check made routinely by statistical analysis software such as SPSS.

Exercise 11.3.2

1. The 95 per cent CI is calculated with the critical value of the t-distribution for the relevant degrees of freedom, and the level of certainty we require (5 per cent). The critical value for 12 df at 0.05 probability level is 2.179, so the 95 per cent CI is given by:

$$\overline{d} \pm 2.179 SE = 3.8462 \pm 2.179 \times 1.2497 = (1.1, 6.6)$$

This should be stated to one more decimal place than the data.

2. It could be argued in this example that attending the talks cannot decrease patients' knowledge, so if there is any change in test score it can only be an increase; that is, a one-sided test is appropriate. But is it possible that patients could become more confused by the talks, and do worse in the second test? As we have noted, one-sided tests are rarely appropriate in practice. If in doubt, use a two-sided test!

Exercise 11.3.3

1. Administrative and shop-floor staff are most likely to differ from each other, but each may also differ from management and technical staff. Management and technical staff have very similar means and distributions.

2. The 95 per cent CIs for administrative and shop-floor staff clearly do not overlap. The upper limit for administrative staff is also below the lower limits for both management and technical staff. The lower limit for shop-floor staff is also above the upper limits for both management and technical staff.

Section 11.4

Exercise 11.4.1

The following need to be considered:

- the number of groups for analysis
- whether the groups are independent of each other, such as boys and girls (the general rule is that an individual cannot be in more than one group), or whether each set of observations are paired (that is, made on the same individual) or closely matched (when individuals in one group are individually matched with a member of the other group
- the type of data, whether continuous, categorical or ordinal
- the distribution of the data
- the size of the sample
- the objective of the analysis.

Exercise 11.4.2

a) Matched/paired categorical data therefore McNemar's test.

b) Independent categorical data therefore chi-squared test (symptoms may be present/absent or on an ordinal scale, in which case adjust for trend).

c) Chi-squared test, but we may get < 5 expected in one cell; hence, we should consider Fisher's exact test.

d) Matched/paired categorical data therefore McNemar's test.

e) Independent continous data therefore two-sample t-test (or could consider using Mann–Whitney U test if the data did not meet assumptions of t-test).

f) Independent categorical data therefore chi-squared test.

g) Paired continous data therefore paired t-test (or could consider using Wilcoxon signed rank test if the data did not meet the assumptions of the paired t-test).

h) We could use ANOVA or Kruskal–Wallis, depending on distributions and variances and whether it is appropriate to treat the scores as continuous.

i) We know that the distribution of blood lead is markedly skewed, though we could transform this and use log lead levels with Pearson correlation so long as the reading test score distributions meet assumptions, but Spearman's rank correlation may be more suitable.

Section 11.5

Exercise 11.5.1

1. Calculation of prior odds $= \dfrac{0.4}{1-(0.4)} = 0.66$

2. Calculation of likelihood ratio (for positive test) $= \dfrac{0.8}{1-(0.7)} = 2.67$

3. Hence, the posterior odds $= 0.66 \times 2.67 = 1.76$, and posterior probability $= \dfrac{1.76}{1+1.76} = 0.64$

4. Fagan's nomogram produces a consistent result (it is difficult to read this precisely).

5. This example shows how the probability of the woman's having cancer (posterior probability) is determined by not only the result of the smear test but also the GP's view that, given the risk factor history and symptoms of bleeding, there is a moderately high chance of cancer.

6. In the case of the second woman, the history led the GP to a very low prior suspicion of cancer (prior probability = 5 per cent); using the nomogram, the posterior probability is only (approximately) 0.15 (15 per cent) despite the positive smear test. In other words, there is a high chance that the smear result is a false positive (though, of course, the smear result would need to be followed up carefully in the usual way).

References

Altman, D. (1991). *Practical Statistics for Medical Research*. Chapman & Hall: London.

Antman, E. M., Lau, J., Kupelnick, B. *et al.* (1992). A comparison of results of meta-analyses of randomized control trials and recommendations of clinical experts. Treatments for myocardial infarction. *JAMA* **268**, 240–248.

Begg, C. B. and Mazumdar, M. (1994). Operating characteristics of a rank correlation test for publication bias. *Biometrics* **50**, 1088–1101.

Bilton, T., Bonnett, K., Jones, P. *et al.* (2002). *Introductory Sociology* (4th edn). Macmillan: London.

Bolstad, W. M. (2004). *Introduction to Bayesian Statistics*. Wiley: New York.

Bowling, A. (1997). *Measuring Health: A Review of Quality of Life Measurement Scales* (2nd edn). Open University Press: Milton Keynes.

Bowling, A. and Ebrahim, S. (2005). Handbook of health research methods: Investigation, measurement and analysis. McGraw-Hill International. Open University Press.

Bradburn, N., Sudman, S. and Wansink, B. (2004). *Asking Questions: The Definitive Guide to Questionnaire Design for Market Research, Political Polls and Social and Health Questionnaires* (2nd edn). Jossey-Bass: San Francisco, CA.

Cochrane, A. L. (1979). 1931–1971: A critical review, with particular reference to the medical profession. In *Medicines for the Year 2000* (pp. 1–11). Office of Health Economics: London.

Cochrane Injuries Group Albumin Reviewers (1998). Human albumin administration in critically ill patients: systematic review of randomised controlled trials. *Br Med J* **517**: 235–240.

Davey, B. (1994). The nature of scientific research. In L. McConway (ed.), *Studying Health and Disease* (pp. 9–21). Milton Keynes: Open University Press.

DerSimonian, R. and Laird, N. (1986). Meta-analysis in clinical trials. *Control Clin Trials* **7**, 177–188.

Egger, M., Davey Smith, G. and Altman, D. G. (eds.) (2003). *Systematic Reviews in Health Care: Meta-Analysis in Context* (2nd edn). BMJ Publishing: London.

Egger, M., Davey Smith, G., Schneider, M. *et al.* (1997). Bias in meta-analysis detected by a simple, graphical test. *Br Med J* **315**, 629–634.

Gardner, M. J. and Altman, D. G. (eds) (2000). *Statistics with Confidence* (2nd ed). British Medical Journal Books: London.

Green, J. and Thorogood, N. (2004). *Qualitative Methods for Health Research*. Sage: London.

Griffiths, C. and Rooney, C. (1999). The effect of the introduction of ICD-10 on trends in mortality from injury and poisoning in England and Wales. *Health Stat Q* **19**, 10–21.

Hennekens, C. H. and Buring, J. E. (1987). *Epidemiology in Medicine*. Lippincott, Williams & Wilkins: Philadelphia, PA.

Hickish, T., Colston, K. W., Bland, J. M. and Maxwell, J. D. (1989). Vitamin D deficiency and muscle strength in male alcoholics. *Clin Sci* **77**, 171–176.

Jadad, A. R., Moore, R. A., Carroll, D. *et al.* (1996). Assessing the quality of reports of randomized controlled trials: is blinding necessary? *Control Clin Trials* **17**, 1–12.

Kirkwood, B. (2003). *Essential Medical Statistics* (2nd edn). Blackwell Science: Oxford.

Mathews, P. M. and Foreman, J. (1993). *Jervis on the Offices and Duties of Coroners (with Forms and Precedents)* (11th edn). Sweet & Maxwell: London.

Morris, J. N. (1957). *Uses of Epidemiology*. E & S Livingstone: London.

Nelemans, P. J., Rampen, F. H. J., Ruiter, D. J. *et al.* (1995). An addition to the controversy on sunlight exposure and melanoma risk: a meta-analytical approach. *J Clin Epidemiol* **48**, 1331–1342.

Office for National Statistics (2002). *Mortality Statistics: Childhood, Infant and Perinatal. Review of the Registrar General in England and Wales 2002* (ONS Series DH3 no. 35). Office for National Statistics: London.

Office of Population Census and Surveys (1981). *Third National Morbidity Study*. Morbidity statistics from General Practice 1981–1982. Office for National Statistics: London.

Pocock, S. (1984). *Clinical Trials*: a practical approach. Wiley: New York.

Popper, K. (1959). *The Logic of Scientific Discovery*. Hutchinson: London.

Prentice *et al.* (1988). In *Epidemiology*. L. Gordis (ed.).W.B. Saunders Company: London p. 169.

Rose, G. (1992). *The Strategy of Preventive Medicine*. Oxford University Press: Oxford.

Shulz, K. F., Chalmers, I., Hayes, R. J. *et al.* (1995). Empirical evidence of bias: dimensions of methodological quality associated with estimates of treatment effects in controlled trials. *JAMA* **273**, 408–412.

Spiegelhalter, D. J., Myles, J. P., Jones, D. R. *et al.* (1999). Methods in health service research: an introduction to bayesian methods in technology assessment. *Br Med J* **319**, 508–512.

Wadsworth, J., Field, J., Johnson, A. M. *et al.* (1993). Methodology of the National Survey of Sexual Attitudes and Lifestyles. *Journal of the Royal Statistical Society*. Series A **156** (3), 407–421.

Warrell, D. A., Weatherall, D. J., Cox, T. M. *et al.* (1987). *The Oxford Textbook of Medicine* (2nd edn). Oxford University Press: Oxford.

Wells, G. A., Shea, B., O'Connell, D. *et al.* (2000). The Newcastle-Ottawa Scale (NOS) for assessing the quality of non-randomised studies in meta-analyses. Paper presented at 3rd Symposium on Systematic Reviews: Beyond the Basics, Oxford.

World Health Organisation (2002). *The World Health Report 2002. Reducing risks, promoting healthy life.* World Health Organisation: Geneva.

World Health Organisation (2007). *World Health Organisation Mortality Database, Statistical Information System (WHOSIS)*. Online publication at: http://www.who.int/whosis/en/. Retrieved 15 June 2007.

Yusuf, S., Peto, R., Lewis, J. *et al.* (1985). Beta blockade during and after myocardial infarction: an overview of the randomized trials. *Prog Cardiovasc Dis* **27**, 335–371.

Index